Sexual and Reproductive Justice

Critical Perspectives on the Psychology of Sexuality, Gender, and Queer Studies

Series Editors: A.L. Jones (Alice Miller School), Damien Riggs (Flinders University), and Rebecca Stringer (University of Otago)

Mission Statement

The series seeks to publish scholarship that engages critically with the social and political uses of psychological knowledge, and with transformative paradigms that address obstacles to change. The series is open to a wide range of approaches that may be classified as "psychological," including manuscript proposals that focus on well-being, subjectivities, clinical practice, discourse, and their intersections.

Advisory Board Members

Meg John Barker, Virginia Braun, Chris Brickell, Heather Brook, Victoria Clarke, Charlotte Patterson, Elizabeth Peel, Esther Rothblum, and Gareth Treharne

Books in Series

Sexual and Reproductive Justice

From the Margins to the Centre

Edited by
Tracy Morison and
Jabulile Mary-Jane Jace Mavuso

LEXINGTON BOOKS
Lanham • Boulder • New York • London

Published by Lexington Books
An imprint of The Rowman & Littlefield Publishing Group, Inc.
4501 Forbes Boulevard, Suite 200, Lanham, Maryland 20706
www.rowman.com

86-90 Paul Street, London EC2A 4NE

British Library Cataloguing in Publication Information Available

Library of Congress Cataloging-in-Publication Data

Names: Morison, Tracy, editor. | Mavuso, Jabulile Mary-Jane Jace, editor.
Title: Sexual and reproductive justice : from the margins to the centre / edited by Tracy Morison and Jabulile Mary-Jane Jace Mavuso.
Description: Lanham : Lexington Books, [2022] | Series: Critical perspectives on psychology of sexuality, gender, and queer studies | Includes bibliographical references and index.
Identifiers: LCCN 2022002821 (print) | LCCN 2022002822 (ebook) | ISBN 9781793644206 (cloth) | ISBN 9781793644220 (paperback) | ISBN 9781793644213 (ebook)
Subjects: LCSH: Reproductive rights. | Sexual rights, | Feminist jurisprudence.
Classification: LCC HQ766 .S49 2022 (print) | LCC HQ766 (ebook) | DDC 363.9/6—dc23/eng/20220121
LC record available at https://lccn.loc.gov/2022002821
LC ebook record available at https://lccn.loc.gov/2022002822

Contents

List of Figures and Tables

FIGURES

TABLES

Introduction

Diversifying Reproductive Justice Scholarship: Marginalised Voices and Overlooked Issues

Tracy Morison and Jabulile Mary-Jane Jace Mavuso

Reproductive Justice has been acknowledged as among the most significant shifts in contemporary reproductive politics and feminist scholarship (Ross 2017). Since its inception over 30 years ago, this cross-disciplinary feminist framework has gained traction and is drawn on increasingly as an approach to activism and work in sexual and reproductive health and rights, and more recently as an analytic lens (Luna and Luker 2013). Despite the growing popularity of the Reproductive Justice framework among scholars studying sexual and reproductive issues, there remain overlooked areas, marginal topics, knowledges, and locations. We turn our attention to topics and perspectives hitherto un/under-addressed in Reproductive Justice scholarship (chapters 1–7) and showcase work offering original approaches and perspectives to more established topics (chapter 8 onward). Our aim is to make place for and amplify new voices and counter perspectives which expand ideas about whose sexual and reproductive lives, rights and freedoms matter.

In addition to expanding the scholarship in this way, as part of this Book Series on *Critical Perspectives on the Psychology of Sexuality, Gender, and Queer Studies* we wish to help address the limited engagement with the Reproductive Justice framework in psychology (Eaton and Stephens 2020; Morison 2021). To date, psychologists have drawn on Reproductive Justice to address a range of topics (e.g., breastfeeding, childbirth, human trafficking, intimate partner violence) (e.g., Chrisler 2012), but this work continues to be largely Euro-American in origin (cf. Eaton and Stephens 2020). There is still much work required within the various critically oriented branches of psychology that may offer new insights into sexual and reproductive oppressions.

Indeed, scholars and practitioners have called on the discipline to be involved in the project of understanding, documenting, providing support for, and eliminating sexual and reproductive injustices (Grzanka and Frantell 2017). Considering this call, the contributions in this volume, many authored by psychologists, have relevance for psychology, stimulating further consideration around how the discipline can engage with Reproductive Justice, participate in societal transformation, and help to achieve and expand Reproductive Justice goals.

THE HISTORY AND FOUNDATIONS OF (SEXUAL AND) REPRODUCTIVE JUSTICE

The Reproductive Justice movement is founded upon a long legacy of a commitment to struggling against racial, sexual, heterosexual, and class oppression. The movement was born in the 1990s in the United States as a product of several new ways of thinking about sexual and reproductive health (Ross and Solinger 2017). In 1994, the notion of reproductive rights as *human rights* was ushered into the global vernacular at the International Conference on Population and Development. This development signified a fundamental shift away from a focus on population control, largely through the regulation of women's fertility, to the acknowledgement of the importance of women's reproductive autonomy and human rights (Hartmann 2016). At the same time that this global shift towards human rights thinking was occurring, the notion of intersectionality was growing in popularity (Crenshaw 1989) and played an essential role in the development of Reproductive Justice as a framework for understanding and for sociopolitical intervention (Zavella 2016).

The reproductive justice movement emerged in response to the dominant 20th century, single-axis reproductive rights activism focussed on privileged, White, cisgender, and heterosexual women. Black feminists, like Collins (1991), Crenshaw (1989), and Lorde (1984), sought to show how racist and classist ideologies re/produce power inequalities between groups of women that limit the ability to make choices and support "stratified reproduction" in which reproduction is dis/encouraged on the basis of race and class (Luna and Luker 2013). Low-income, Indigenous, and Black women are discouraged or actively prevented from having "too many" children, through targeted contraceptive programming, forced sterilisation, and other means (Smith 2005). At the same time, government scrutiny regularly intrudes into the bodies and homes of marginalised women (e.g., removal of children from families, welfare surveillance, and penalties), limiting their parental freedoms (Ross and Solinger 2017). Women of Colour, Indigenous, and poor women are distinctly burdened by restrictions on their right to have and to raise children, unlike the White and/or middle-class women upon whose interests the mainstream Women's Movement was predicated.

Thus, Reproductive Justice was born out of an assertion that Black and of colour, Indigenous, and/or poor women's freedom and means to realise their reproductive preferences and desires are as important as the issues of bodily integrity and autonomy centred in the mainstream Women's Movement, focussed largely on contraceptive and abortion access and to some extent still does (SisterSong 2007). To this end, the founders of the Reproductive Justice movement sought to develop a comprehensive framework based on social justice thinking to consider the nuanced and contextual factors that differentially shape women's reproductive lives and experiences. One of the founders, Loretta Ross (2017) explains, "we spliced together the concept of reproductive rights and social justice to coin the neologism, 'reproductive justice.'" This new term encapsulates two foundational aspects of the framework (discussed in more detail further below), namely: (1) its human rights underpinnings and (2) a concomitant focus on social justice that brings sexual and reproductive politics into focus (Zavella 2016; Collins 2017).

Understandings of the intersectionality of gender were (and often still are) limited to addressing its race and class dimensions, with much of the Reproductive Justice scholarship and activism centring the experiences of cisgender and heterosexual women. In recent years, however, the Reproductive Justice movement has formed alliances and coalitions with Lesbian, Gay, Bisexual, Transgender, and Intersex (LGBTI) movements, working towards common causes (Nixon 2013; Price 2019). For example, Nixon (2013, 82) cites the rationale for expanding the scope of their work given by the *National Latina Institute for Reproductive Health*:

> The reproductive health and justice movements are about bodily autonomy for all, and particularly those whose gender is marginalized. Though this movement has traditionally been about women's control over their own bodies, we recognize now that this is not enough. As people whose genders have been marginalized, not just cisgender women, but transgender and gender non-conforming people too are consistently and systemically denied full bodily autonomy.

Such coalitions draw on intersectionality to address a range of *gendered* oppressions and privileges that are less visible in reproductive politics and scholarship, and so enlarge meanings of Reproductive Justice beyond the original cis-heterocentric focus, though there is more work to be done in this area. Some now refer to "*Sexual* and Reproductive Justice" to capture the conscious inclusion of sexuality and sexual justice issues (Price 2010). The frame is therefore expanded to include sexual health and rights, including but not limited to: access to relevant services and information, bodily integrity, sexual agency, and freedom from sexual violence (Armas 2007). As we highlight in this chapter and throughout the text, more recent scholarship has contributed to moving beyond the confines of cis-heteronormativity and the privileging of various identities and perspectives, evident in research on fat (e.g., Parker, Pausé, and Le Grice 2019; LaMarre et al. 2020; Ward and Mcphail 2019; Friedman, Rice, and Lind 2020), disability/crip (Jarman 2015; Hillard 2018), trans (Chace 2018; Riggs and Bartholomaeus 2019), and queer Reproductive Justice (Luna 2018; Smietana, Thompson, and Twine 2018; Silver 2020). This work continues to shed light on and challenge normative sexual and reproductive subjects in Reproductive Justice scholarship.

THE CORE TENETS OF SEXUAL
AND REPRODUCTIVE JUSTICE

Although it encompasses a raft of issues and topics of concern, Reproductive Justice is in essence a framework about power (Ross and Solinger 2017). The framework takes an expanded rights-based perspective that balances notions of rights and justice: "the human right to make personal decisions about one's life, *and* the obligation of government and society to ensure that the conditions are suitable for implementing one's decisions" (Ross and Solinger 2017). In line with the original impetus to go beyond pro-choice politics based upon liberal, individualised notions of rights, the Sexual and Reproductive Justice movement draws on human rights discourse to link the fulfilment of human rights with the achievement of social justice (Rebouché 2017). This expanded view allows a stronger claim to be made for injustices than recourse to national legal frameworks (Luna and Luker 2013). The core principles of the Reproductive Justice movement are based upon the human rights to have children or not, to have children under chosen conditions, and to raise them in supportive, safe, and healthy conditions (SisterSong 2007).

The notion of intersectionality explicitly connects these reproductive rights with social justice issues (e.g., economic disparities, education, immigration) by highlighting social factors that limit people's ability to exercise rights and make choices (viz., differential access to resources, socio-material conditions, and power relations within and among groups) and thus the need for socio-structural and systemic change (Rebouché 2017; Zavella 2016; Price 2010). The focus therefore goes beyond the individual to take account of a broad and interconnecting assemblage of reproductive and social issues and the systems of power shaping them (Oaks 2016).

Intersectionality theory draws attention to what Collins (1989) refers to as "the matrix of domination": the network of power relations that enables and restricts people's ability to exercise their sexual and reproductive rights. This matrix incorporates (i) structural and systemic dynamics, (ii) social relations shaped by gender, race, class, and other social categorisations, and (iii) socio-cultural discourses and practices (Chiweshe, Mavuso, and Macleod 2017). It shows that reproductive in/justice occurs along multiple and intersecting lines of privilege and oppression, including, age, gender, sexuality, class, race/ethnicity/indigeneity, immigration/citizenship status, carceral status, weight/size, and physical/mental dis/ability (SisterSong 2007). In this view, systems of oppression are seen as interlocking and interacting, a view that enables holistic analyses and practice (Smietana, Thompson, and Twine 2018).

(SEXUAL AND) REPRODUCTIVE JUSTICE SCHOLARSHIP

The Reproductive Justice framework gained traction somewhat more slowly in scholarship than in sexual and reproductive activism and programming (Luna and Luker 2013). A snapshot of the growing body of knowledge shows various engagements with this conceptualisation of reproductive (and, to a lesser extent, sexual) decision-making and experiences. There is geographical/regional and topical variation in the ways and extent to which Reproductive Justice has been engaged with as a conceptual framework. Much contemporary Sexual and Reproductive Justice scholarship is produced from and grounded in Global North contexts, largely due to the framework's emergence and development in the United States, as well as Global North-South power relations around knowledge production. This body of work has mostly focussed on the ways that social inequities limit reproductive options for variously marginalised, cisgender heterosexual women, including Women of Colour and low-income women who have historically been positioned as unfit reproducers/parents (Heinz and Roth 2019).

We provide an (admittedly partial) overview of Reproductive Justice scholarship highlighting the politics of location in this knowledge production in which work emerging in/from the Global North[1] (i.e., Western or Euro-American countries) forms the centre of scholarship, and work from regions typically marginalised in global patterns of knowledge production is at the periphery. There has been considerably less engagement with Reproductive Justice scholarship outside of Euro-American contexts and below we include research with marginalised communities beyond Euro-America as well as work conducted in Global South contexts. Our overview is partial and restricted to English-language scholarship.

The Right to Have Children

The Reproductive Justice movement in the Global North has drawn attention to historical and ongoing coercive contraception and sterilisation of minoritised women (Smietana, Thompson, and Twine 2018; Harris and Wolfe 2014). In this regard, Reproductive Justice scholars and advocates draw attention to the "contraceptive paradox": the notion that "contraception can be both a source of empowerment and agency for women who wish to control their fertility and a source of oppression for women deemed socially undesirable reproducers" (Gomez, Mann, and Torres 2018). Racism and eugenics have been highlighted as central to the determination of who is "fit" to reproduce and parent. Black women's reproductive capacities have long been entwined with paradoxical racist discourses portraying them as hyper-fecund yet devoid of the nurturing motherly qualities required to raise healthy, moral offspring. Such depictions continue to influence social policy and practices concerning Black women's reproductive abilities, desires, and needs (Jones 2013). This has been highlighted, for example, by several studies showing how Women of Colour and young women are frequently discouraged from having more children and are pressured to use Long-Acting Contraceptives (Brandi et al. 2018; Gomez and Wapman 2017; Senderowicz 2019).

This topic has also been researched in the Global South (Vasquez Del Aguila 2020; Mavuso 2020). For instance, Mavuso (2020) analyses news media coverage of an investigation by the South African Gender Commission into the forced sterilisation of pregnancy-capable women at public hospitals. The news coverage focussed solely on HIV-positive status, but Mavuso's findings show that reproduction is forcibly denied to a range of people considered "undesirable" reproducers along the cross-cutting lines of class, age, race, *and* HIV serostatus. Mavuso (2020) shows that the reproductive potential of young, Black, working-class, and/or HIV-positive women is cast as a "risk" or "burden" to the country and therefore as "needing" to be controlled.

Researchers have also considered pathways to parenthood other than biogenetic parenthood (often referred to as "natural" parenthood). Considering the issue of transnational adoption, Yook and Kim (2018) analyse Korean women's reflections on the decision to place their children for adoption. Their analysis identifies systemic and structural impediments to caring for children (e.g., denigration and lack of state support for sole parents/mothers) and illuminates these women's complex positioning and experiences as neither (silent) victims of poverty nor agents of self-mastery.

Others have attended to the complex issue of transnational commercial surrogacy. Using a Reproductive Justice lens, scholars have examined how this practice is constructed in public discourse. For example, routine descriptions of transnational commercial surrogacy as "humanitarian aid" for birth mothers in poor nations or the positioning of wealthy intended parents as benevolent obscures the structural conditions shaping decision-making and experiences. Such representations shift attention from power imbalances in surrogacy contracts or how those acting as surrogates are disadvantaged by surrogacy arrangements (e.g., receive a fraction of profits; risk injury, infertility, and death; poor reproductive healthcare) (Fixmer-Oraiz 2013; Mohapatra 2012).

Reproductive Justice scholars remind us that reproductive freedom is about more than access to technologies. It is also about *who* these technologies are serving and why (Boydell and Dow 2021). Taking up this idea, work from the Global South adds nuance and complexity to both the mainstream and Reproductive Justice scholarship. Much of this work addresses the lack of attention to the women/mothers providing reproductive labour in transnational adoption and surrogacy markets, most often poor Women of Colour. For example, Saravanan's (2016) research on surrogacy arrangements in India highlights class-based reproductive injustices against Indian women who act as surrogates for those from affluent contexts.

At the same time, some scholars show how transnational surrogacy can *challenge* hetero-patriarchal regulation of reproduction and family formation (Mohapatra 2012). Transnational surrogacy allows queer couples and others excluded from surrogacy by discriminatory domestic laws to realise their reproductive desires. In this vein, Ho (2019) shows how lesbians' use of assisted reproduction technologies in Taiwan subverts heteronormativity and repro-normativity. Nevertheless, despite the often taken-for-granted potential of these technologies to democratise access to biological parenthood, they remain largely the preserve of White economically privileged, cis-heterosexual couples (Luna 2018).

The Right to Supportive Conditions for Birthing and Parenting

The lack of supportive conditions for marginalised (cisgender) women's birthing and parenting was an important catalyst of the Reproductive Justice movement. This issue continues to be a focus among Northern scholars considering issues such as: health outcomes for mothers and infants (Davis 2019), reproductive health services and antenatal care (Julian et al. 2020), obstetric policies and practices (Kane 2020), obstetric violence (Davis 2018; Delay and Sundstrom 2019; Salter et al. 2021), and birth justice (Yam 2020).

A recent example is the work of US scholar Davis (2018, 2019, 2020), which spotlights the role of systematised racism in inferior, negligent, and abusive medical treatment received by pregnant and birthing Black women. She uses the frameworks of "obstetric racism" and "medical racism" to explore and understand compromised reproductive "care" during the pre- and postnatal period, maternal health outcomes, and birth outcomes among Black women (2018, 2019). Her participants report "various forms of racism during medical encounters while they were pregnant or during labor and delivery" (Davis 2020, 56) and she shows how such racism results in the increased likelihood of Black women experiencing premature births and dying from pregnancy-related complications.

Such reproductive oppression has also been addressed in Southern scholarship, although to a lesser extent, including, for example, domestic violence and maternal mortality (Madhok, Unnithan, and Heitmeyer 2014); the Israeli state's restrictions on Palestinian-Arab women's freedom, rights, and dignity during pregnancy, childbirth, and post-birth (Hamayel, Hammoudeh, and Welchman 2017); and obstetric violence (Majety and Bejugam 2016; Oluoch-Aridi, Jackline, Smith-Oka, Dailey, and Milan 2021).

In terms of the ability to parent children under supportive conditions, research in the United States highlights how the state has intervened to prevent marginalised people from parenting their children, including those who are poor, of colour, and/or Indigenous (Luna and Luker 2013; Solinger 2010). Welfare policies have been shown to disproportionately target and criminalise poor Women of Colour in the Global North. For instance, policies restricting the number of children eligible for welfare benefits target these women for "maternal neglect" (Solinger 2010). Women of Colour have also been targeted for drug use during pregnancy, and welfare programmes have applied "caps" on family size, requiring the use of long-acting reversible contraceptives or sterilisation as a condition for receiving further welfare assistance that the state *should* provide (Smith 2005).

Similarly, the over-representation of children of colour in the US child welfare system is in part due to the targeted removal of Native American children from their parents, families, and communities. The denigration of Native American parenting and communities often results in placement of children in the care of White communities and families, reinforcing White-supremacist and colonial discourses that privilege and valorise White parenting/parenthood and communities (Benson 2019; de Bourbon 2019).

State intervention and violence also constrains marginalised people's parenting in other ways. For instance, in the context of often-fatal routine violence of police brutality, African American parents raise children amid constant fear of violence being perpetrated against their children and themselves (Rogers 2015). Young mothers experience insidious structural and symbolic violence, with real material consequences; they struggle to access resources and support as they are positioned as inadequate parents within racist, classist, and adultist discourses (Hans and White 2019).

The Right Not to Have Children

Reproductive Justice has also been applied to understanding access to and experiences of the right to not have children. This work, largely focussed on heterosexual, cisgender women whom pro-natalist discourses have centred and responsibilised as reproductive subjects, includes scholarship on abortion and contraception. There is almost no research considering the issue of voluntary childlessness from a Reproductive Justice perspective (Morison et al. 2016; cf. Lynch et al. 2018).

Work that considers contraception in a nuanced light, as a source of both agency and domination, particularly for those who are positioned as falling short of the ideals of motherhood (Gomez, Mann, and Torres 2018), has contributed significantly to Reproductive Justice knowledge production. For instance, situating contraceptive programming within global reproductive politics, Smith (2014) locates the lack of contraceptive access in the Philippines within a (neo)colonial history of imposed neoliberal policies which require global South nations to take measures to reduce their population in exchange for international financial aid for economic development.

Research on long-acting reversible contraception has also interrogated contraceptive programming, viewing contraceptives as both a potential source of empowerment and oppression (Gomez, Mann, and Torres 2018) and exploring the possibility of coercive practices, especially against Women of Colour (Holt et al. 2018; Jones 2013; Carvajal and Zambrana 2020) and younger or poor women (Higgins, Kramer, and Ryder 2016; Grzanka and Schuch 2020). For instance, several studies in the Global North indicate that Women of Colour may experience direct and subtle coercion during contraceptive counselling (Brandi et al. 2018; Gomez, Mann, and Torres 2018; Gomez and Wapman 2017).

Teenagers' and young people's right to refrain from having children has been considered in relation to access to sexual information. For instance, Foulkes (2008) shows how abstinence-only sex education programs in US state-funded schools disproportionately impact teens who are queer, of colour, and/or come from low-income communities. Such programs act as a barrier to preventing unwanted pregnancy and impinge upon sexual and reproductive health and rights more broadly.

Abortion has continued to be a primary focus in what has perhaps become "mainstream" Reproductive Justice scholarship (Macleod, Beynon-Jones, and Toerien 2017). There is, however, work by Northern scholars on abortion access and politics which draws strength from and expands Reproductive Justice scholarship in novel ways. For instance, considering disability alongside Reproductive Justice, Smith (2005) and Jarman (2015) show how both anti-abortionists and pro-choice supporters mobilise ableist constructions of disability that are rooted in class- and race-based understandings of abortion.

Proposing an alternative to bifurcated political positions mobilised around "choice," Shaw (2013) argues for framing Canadian reproductive politics in terms of Reproductive Justice. This would allow access to abortion and entail broad support for the right not to have children, as well as enabling people to determine the conditions under which they choose to give birth (e.g., non-medicalised birthing), thereby upholding the right to have children in a supportive context.

In a similar vein, Southern scholars have added complexity to abortion research by drawing on Reproductive Justice. For example, scholarship on Zika virus infection during pregnancy (which can result in foetal microencephaly) highlights the tension between reproductive rights (i.e., to end pregnancy) and disability rights (i.e., preventing eugenic approaches and practices). Mohapatra (2019) illuminates the operation of ableism in efforts to contain the spread of the Zika virus and provide medical and reproductive healthcare to pregnant women who have contracted it. She argues along with Puerto Rican scholars Rabionet, Zorrilla, Rivera-Viñas, and Guerra-Sánchez (2018) that, in order to uphold reproductive autonomy, those who have contracted the Zika virus while pregnant need access to abortion *as well as* informational and economic support for parenting a disabled child.

Global South scholars have also explored abortion politics. Chiweshe and Macleod (2018), for example, analyse United Nations discussions about abortion. They highlight the deleterious consequences of constructions of abortion as "un-African" (which homogenises African cultures) and of assumptions that pregnant people have "choice" and autonomy in sexual and reproductive decision-making. Transnational studies of reproductive politics, which include comparisons between Global South countries as well as North-South comparisons, usefully illuminate equivalences across contexts and local specificities. These findings can help tailor the approaches taken to achieving sexual and reproductive justice to fit the context (Macleod, Beynon-Jones, and Toerien 2017; Macleod, Reynolds, and Macleod 2021). A good example of this transnational analysis is Chiweshe, Mavuso, and Macleod's (2017) narrative-discursive exploration of abortion decision-making in Zimbabwe and South Africa. Their analysis highlights similarities across the data in relation to the role of stigma and common rhetorical strategies used to justify pregnancy termination. They also show variations in ways of accounting for decision-making, which they connect to differences in the local conditions rendering pregnancy unsupportable (i.e., physiologically, emotionally, and cognitively unfeasible due to insufficient support at the individual and structural levels).

GAPS AND NEW DIRECTIONS IN
KNOWLEDGE PRODUCTION

Body Diversity: Extending Understandings
of Bodily Oppression

Sexual and Reproductive scholarship has interrogated how sexual and reproductive agency and the right to have children are circumscribed within systems that privilege certain bodies, denying this right to those whose bodies are deemed "abnormal" in various ways. Little work has attended to the reproductive privileging of normalised bodies. More research using a Sexual and Reproductive Justice lens to investigate bodily oppression and diversity is required to understand all the various ways that bodies are normatively privileged and oppressed in relation to sexuality and reproduction.

Disability has been neglected in *both* mainstream and Sexual and Reproductive Justice work on sexuality and reproduction (O'Connell 2016). Sexual and Reproductive Justice scholars have tended to focus on foetal disability and abortion access (see Jarman 2015). Accordingly, Bagenstos (2019) highlights the need to address the full range of reproductive issues that intersect with disabilities, like the right to parent, sexual autonomy, accessing sexual and reproductive services, sexual violence, and coercive sterilisation or contraceptive practices. Some noteworthy exceptions to the abortion focus include recent research on contraception for intellectually and developmentally disabled women (Hillard 2018; Wu et al. 2018), and weight stigma/fat oppression (LaMarre et al. 2020; Ward and Mcphail 2019; Friedman 2014; Friedman, Rice, and Lind 2020), including the ways that current Western discourses about pregnancy fatness are racialised and construct fat people as *non*-reproductive (Parker, Pausé, and Le Grice 2019).

Often marginalised in queer approaches to Reproductive Justice, engagement between trans* justice and Reproductive Justice scholarship and advocacy in the Global North highlights how transgender people, especially trans People of Colour, face obstacles to genetic parenthood through, for example, anti-trans legislation, contestation of parenting rights, removal of children, costs of fertility preservation and retrieval, and fatal anti-trans violence (Cárdenas 2016; Chace 2018; Nixon 2013; Honkasalo 2018).

In Australia, Riggs and Bartholomaeus (2019) investigated how cisnormativity regulates paths to parenthood for transgender and non-binary people. The researchers conducted a series of studies about fertility preservation with healthcare professionals, transgender and non-binary adults, and parents of transgender and non-binary children. Their findings highlight the need for access to fertility preservation as well as the challenging of wider social discourses and prohibitions that restrict trans and non-binary people's reproductive lives and freedom. More broadly, trans Reproductive Justice scholarship highlights how eradicating the wide range of cisnormative/anti-trans violence is crucial for trans, non-binary, and gender non-conforming people's reproductive dignity.

Similarly, there is little scholarship applying a Sexual and Reproductive Justice lens to the experiences of intersex people, whose bodies are frequently viewed as "aberrant" and "requiring" medical intervention. Despite long-standing advocacy by intersex rights movements, the issue of so-called normalising surgeries and procedures to "correct" gender non-normative bodies remains largely overlooked in the Sexual and Reproductive Justice literature. Few scholars investigate these practices as forms of bodily *and* symbolic violence that contribute to the sexual and reproductive injustices experienced by intersex people (George 2020; Rubin 2019).

Widening the lens to *Sexual* and Reproductive Justice

Reproductive issues seem to have gained primacy in research, even though the Reproductive Justice framework has always acknowledged the interdependence of sexual and reproductive autonomy (Ross and Solinger 2017). "Reproductive justice is not just about one's ability to reproduce. It's about autonomy, it's about respect, it's about shared principles based in the human right to health and a desire for real social change" (Perez 2007, 1). Thus, alongside the reproductive rights discussed above, the framework includes sexual rights to engage in sexual activity without state intervention and free from (the fear of) violence, disease, or unwanted pregnancy. To foreground this, some explicitly adopt the term *Sexual* and Reproductive Justice, but usage of this nomenclature is not consistent (Ross and Solinger 2017). More commonly, scholarship tends to discuss sexual oppressions under the rubric of sexual citizenship.

Despite the focus on reproduction and parenthood, there is some research that uses a Sexual and Reproductive Justice framework to show the linkages between sexual and reproductive oppressions. Such scholarship is varied, often focussing on specific marginalised groups. Cohen and Caxaj (2018), for example, focus on undocumented immigrant women working as farm workers in Canada, demonstrating how these "migrant women theoretically have the right to make free choices about their sexuality and reproduction" but "in reality . . . contend with multiple barriers when attempting to avail themselves of those rights" (p. 110). Rios and Hooton (2005) concentrate on Latinx communities in the United States showing how the sexual and reproductive oppressions they face are produced by the enactment of racist, anti-poor, and anti-immigrant welfare and immigration measures. Focussing on youth sexuality, Morison and Herbert's (2019) analysis of Aotearoa New Zealand's sexual and reproductive health policy shows how the dominant risk discourse in which policy is framed disadvantages young people and further marginalises Māori youth in particular.

A Note on Terminology

Sexual and Reproductive Justice Theory is intended to be anti-essentialist, recognising that "categories such as gender and race are socially contrived, [but that] they are also embodied sites of reproductive oppression" (Ross 2017a). Accordingly, attending to power must also mean recognising that language and discourse matter deeply in representational practices and knowledge production, including our scholarly writing. This is especially the responsibility of scholars who do not belong to the marginalised groups they are representing. We as editors and the contributors have therefore endeavoured to take language, discourse, and representation seriously: problematising essentialising and taken-for-granted social categories and the systems through which they are produced, using terms that are inclusive, and follow marginalised groups' self-naming practices. Language is ever-changing and shifting across time and place, and ought to move towards socially just practices, as must our practices.

CONCLUSION

In this chapter, we have provided an overview of extant research and the work that remains to be done in Reproductive Justice scholarship. Our aim in this collection is to contribute something new to discussions on Sexual and Reproductive Justice, in ways that increase our capacity to achieve just, systemic transformation that enables us all to live our lives with freedom and dignity. In this respect, the chapters in this collection articulate the various questions we have posed in this introduction, and sometimes suggest answers. It is only possible to do so much in one relatively short text, but we hope that in addition to contributing to the scholarship, this text will spark further critical questions, novel thinking, ongoing dialogue, and contribute to social change.

NOTE

1. We use this descriptor to invoke the politics of location and the dominant positioning of countries in historical and contemporary geopolitics, including those governing knowledge production, notably the United Kingdom and United States.

REFERENCES

Armas, Henry. 2007. "Whose Sexuality Counts? Poverty, Participation, and Sexual Rights." 294. Brighton, United Kingdom. https://opendocs.ids.ac.uk/opendocs/bitstream/handle/20.500.12413/4150/Wp294.pdf?sequence=1.

Bagenstos, Samuel R. 2019. "Disability and Reproductive Justice." *Harvard Law & Policy Review* 14 (2): 273–92. https://doi.org/10.2139/ssrn.3468736.

Benson, Krista L. 2019. "Indigenous Reproductive Justice after Adoptive Couple v. Baby Girl (2013)." In *Reproductive Justice and Sexual Rights: Transnational Perspectives*, edited by Tanya Saroj Bakhru, 84–104. New York: Routledge.

Bourbon, Soma de. 2019. "White Property Interests in Native Women's Reproductive Freedom: Slavery to Transracial Adoption." In *Reproductive Justice and Sexual Rights: Transnational Perspectives,* edited by Tanya Saroj Bakhru, 15–32. New York: Routledge.

Boydell, Victoria, and Katharine Dow. 2021. "Adjusting the Analytical Aperture: Propositions for an Integrated Approach to the Social Study of Reproductive Technologies." *BioSocieties*, no. 0123456789. https://doi.org/10.1057/s41292-021 -00240-w.

Brandi, Kristyn, Elisabeth Woodhams, Katharine O. White, and Pooja K. Mehta. 2018. "An Exploration of Perceived Contraceptive Coercion at the Time of Abortion." *Contraception* 97 (4): 329–34. https://doi.org/10.1016/j.contraception .2017.12.009.

Cárdenas, Micha. 2016. "Pregnancy: Reproductive futures in trans of color feminism." *TSQ: Transgender Studies Quarterly* 3 (1–2): 48–57.

Carvajal, Diana N., and Ruth Enid Zambrana. 2020. "Challenging Stereotypes: A Counter-Narrative of the Contraceptive Experiences of Low-Income Latinas." *Health Equity* 4 (1): 10–16. https://doi.org/10.1089/heq.2019.0107.

Chace, Alexandra. 2018. "Barriers to Motherhood : Biotechnology, Reproductive Justice, and Transgender Women." In *National Women's Studies Association Annual Conference*, 1–9.

Chiweshe, Malvern, and Catriona Macleod. 2018. "Cultural De-Colonization versus Liberal Approaches to Abortion in Africa : The Politics of Representation and Voice." *African Journal of Reproductive Health* 22: 49–59. https://doi.org/10 .29063/ajrh2018/v22i2.5.

Chiweshe, Malvern, Jabulile Mavuso, and Catriona Ida Macleod. 2017. "Reproductive Justice in Context: South African and Zimbabwean Women's Narratives of Their Abortion Decision." *Feminism & Psychology* 27 (2): 2013–224. https://doi.org/10 .1177/0959353517699234.

Chrisler, Joan C. 2012. *Reproductive Justice: A Global Concern*. Santa Barbara, CA: ABC-CLIO.

Cohen, Amy, and Susana Caxaj. 2018. "Bodies and Borders: Migrant Women Farmworkers and the Struggle for Sexual and Reproductive Justice in British Columbia, Canada." *Alternate Routes: A Journal of Critical Social Research* 29: 90–117. http://alternateroutes.ca/index.php/ar/article/view/22448/18242.

Collins, Patricia Hill. 1991. *Black Feminist Thought: Knowledge, Consciousness, and the Politics of Empowerment*. 2nd ed. New York: Routledge.

———. 2017. "On Violence, Intersectionality and Transversal Politics." *Ethnic and Racial Studies* 40 (9): 1460–73. https://doi.org/10.1080/01419870.2017.1317827.

Crenshaw, Kimberle. 1989. "Demarginalizing the Intersection of Race and Sex: A Black Feminist Critique of Antidiscrimination Doctrine, Feminist Theory and Antiracist Politics." *University of Chicago Legal Forum* 1989: 139–67.

Davis, Dána-Ain. 2018. "Obstetric Racism: The Racial Politics of Pregnancy, Labor, and Birthing." 38 (7): 560–73. https://doi.org/10.1080/01459740.2018.1549389.

———. 2019. *Reproductive Injustice Racism, Pregnancy, and Premature Birth.* New York: New York University Press.

———. 2020. "Reproducing While Black: The Crisis of Black Maternal Health, Obstetric Racism and Assisted Reproductive Technology." *Reproductive Biomedicine & Society Online* 11 (November): 56–64. https://doi.org/10.1016/J.RBMS.2020.10.001.

Delay, Cara, and Beth Sundstrom. 2019. "The Legacy of Symphysiotomy in Ireland: A Reproductive Justice Approach to Obstetric Violence." 20: 197–218. https://doi.org/10.1108/s1057-629020190000020017.

Eaton, Asia A., and Dionne P. Stephens. 2020. "Reproductive Justice: Moving the Margins to the Center in Social Issues Research." *Journal of Social Issues* 76 (2): 208–18. https://doi.org/10.1111/josi.12384.

Fixmer-Oraiz, Natalie. 2013. "Speaking of Solidarity: Transnational Gestational Surrogacy and the Rhetorics of Reproductive (in)Justice." *Frontiers* 34 (3): 126–63. https://doi.org/10.5250/fronjwomestud.34.3.0126.

Foulkes, Risha K. 2008. "Abstinence-Only Education and Minority Teenagers : The Importance of Race in a Question of Constitutionality." *Berkley Journal of African American Law Policy* X (1): 3–51.

Friedman, May. 2014. "Reproducing Fat-Phobia: Reproductive Technologies and Fat Women's Right to Mother." *Journal of the Motherhood Initiative for Research and Community Involvement* 5 (2): 27–41.

Friedman, May, Carla Rice, and Emily R. M. Lind. 2020. "A High-Risk Body for Whom? On Fat, Risk, Recognition and Reclamation in Restorying Reproductive Care through Digital Storytelling." *Feminist Encounters: A Journal of Critical Studies in Culture and Politics* 4 (2): 36. https://doi.org/10.20897/FEMENC/8524.

George, Marie-Amelie. 2020. "Queering Reproductive Justice." *University of Richmond Law Review* 54 (3): 671–704.

Gomez, Anu Manchikanti, and Mikaela Wapman. 2017. "Under (Implicit) Pressure: Young Black and Latina Women's Perceptions of Contraceptive Care." *Contraception* 96 (4): 221–26. https://doi.org/10.1016/j.contraception.2017.07.007.

Gomez, Anu Manchikanti, E. S. Mann, and V. Torres. 2018. "'It Would Have Control over Me Instead of Me Having Control': Intrauterine Devices and the Meaning of Reproductive Freedom." *Critical Public Health* 28 (2): 190–200. https://doi.org/10.1080/09581596.2017.1343935.

Grzanka, Patrick R., and Elena Schuch. 2020. "Reproductive Anxiety and Conditional Agency at the Intersections of Privilege: A Focus Group Study of Emerging Adults' Perception of Long-Acting Reversible Contraception." *Journal of Social Issues* 76 (2): 270–313. https://doi.org/10.1111/josi.12363.

Grzanka, Patrick R., and Keri A. Frantell. 2017. "Counseling Psychology and Reproductive Justice : A Call to Action." https://doi.org/10.1177/0011000017699871.

Hamayel, Layaly, Doaa Hammoudeh, and Lynn Welchman. 2017. "Reproductive Health and Rights in East Jerusalem: The Effects of Militarisation and Biopolitics on the Experiences of Pregnancy and Birth of Palestinians Living in the Kufr 'Aqab Neighbourhood." *Reproductive Health Matters* 25 (suppl): S87–95. https://doi.org/10.1080/09688080.2017.1378065.

Hans, Sydney L., and Barbara A. White. 2019. "Teenage Childbearing, Reproductive Justice, and Infant Mental Health." *Infant Mental Health Journal* 40: 690–709. https://doi.org/10.1002/imhj.21803.

Harris, Lisa H., and Taida Wolfe. 2014. "Stratified Reproduction, Family Planning Care and the Double Edge of History." *Current Opinion in Obstetrics and Gynecology* 26 (6): 539–44.

Hartmann, Betsy. 2016. *Reproductive Rights and Wrongs: The Global Politics of Population Control*. 3rd ed. Haymarket Books.

Heinz, Erin M., and Louise Marie Roth. 2019. "As Many as I Can Afford: Ideal Family Size in Contemporary Uganda." In *Reproductive Justice and Sexual Rights: Transnational Perspectives*, edited by Tanya Saroj Bakhru, 191–212. New York: Routledge.

Higgins, Jenny A., Renee D. Kramer, and Kristin M. Ryder. 2016. "Provider Bias in Long-Acting Reversible Contraception (LARC) Promotion and Removal: Perceptions of Young Adult Women." *American Journal of Public Health* 106 (11): 1932–37. https://doi.org/10.2105/AJPH.2016.303393.

Hillard, Paula J. Adams. 2018. "Contraception for Women with Intellectual and Developmental Disabilities: Reproductive Justice." *Obstetrics and Gynecology* 132 (3): 555–58. https://doi.org/10.1097/AOG.0000000000002814.

Ho, Szu-Ying. 2019. "Passing for Reproduction: How Lesbians in Taiwan Use Assisted Reproductive Technologies." In *Reproductive Justice and Sexual Rights: Transnational Perspectives*, edited by Tanya Saroj Bakhru, 105–24. New York: Routledge.

Holt, Kelsey, Icela Zavala, Ximena Quintero, Doroteo Mendoza, Marie C. McCormick, Christine Dehlendorf, Ellice Lieberman, and Ana Langer. 2018. "Women's Preferences for Contraceptive Counseling in Mexico: Results from a Focus Group Study." *Reproductive Health* 15 (1): 128–39. https://doi.org/10.1186/s12978-018-0569-5.

Jarman, Michelle. 2015. "Relations of Abortion: Crip Approaches to Reproductive Justice." *Feminist Formations* 27 (1): 46–66.

Jones, Cecily. 2013. "'Human Weeds, Not Fit to Breed?': African Caribbean Women and Reproductive Disparities in Britain." *Critical Public Health* 23 (1): 49–61. https://doi.org/10.1080/09581596.2012.761676.

Julian, Zoë, Diana Robles, Sara Whetstone, Jamila B. Perritt, Andrea V. Jackson, Rachel R. Hardeman, and Karen A. Scott. 2020. "Community-Informed Models of Perinatal and Reproductive Health Services Provision: A Justice-Centered Paradigm toward Equity among Black Birthing Communities." *Seminars in Perinatology* 44 (5): 151267. https://doi.org/10.1016/J.SEMPERI.2020.151267.

Kane, Nazneen. 2020. "COVID-19 and Reproductive Injustice : The Implications of Birthing Restrictions during a Global Pandemic." *COVID-19: Two Volume Set*, December, 85–93. https://doi.org/10.4324/9781003142065-9.

LaMarre, Andrea, Carla Rice, Katie Cook, and May Friedman. 2020. "Fat Reproductive Justice: Navigating the Boundaries of Reproductive Health Care." *Journal of Social Issues*, 1–25. https://doi.org/10.1111/josi.2019.00.issue-0/issuetoc.

Lorde, Audre. 1984. *Sister Outsider: Essays and Speeches*. Berkley, CA: Crossing Press.

Luna, Zakiya. 2018. "Black Celebrities, Reproductive Justice and Queering Family: An Exploration." *Reproductive Biomedicine and Society Online* 7: 91–100. https://doi.org/10.1016/j.rbms.2018.12.002.

Luna, Zakiya, and Kristin Luker. 2013. "Reproductive Justice." *Annual Review of Law and Social Science* 9: 327–52. https://doi.org/10.1146/annurev-lawsocsci-102612-134037.

Lynch, Ingrid, Tracy Morison, Catriona Ida Macleod, Magdalena Mijas, Ryan du Toit, and Seemanthini Tumkur Shivakumar. 2018. "From Deviant Choice to Feminist Issue: An Historical Analysis of Scholarship on Voluntary Childlessness (1920 to 2013)." In *Voluntary and Involuntary Childlessnes: The Joys of Otherhood*, edited by Natalie Sappleton, 11–47. Bingley, UK: Emerald Publishing Limited.

Macleod, Catriona Ida, and John Hunter Reynolds. 2021. "Reproductive Health Systems Analyses and the Reparative Reproductive Justice Approach : A Case Study of Unsafe Abortion in Lesotho." *Global Public Health*, 1–14. https://doi.org/10.1080/17441692.2021.1887317.

Macleod, Catriona, Siân Beynon-Jones, and Merran Toerien. 2016. "Articulating Reproductive Justice through Reparative Justice: Case Studies of Abortion in Great Britain and South Africa." *Culture, Health & Sexuality*, 1–5. https://doi.org/http://dx.doi.org/10.1080/13691058.2016.1257738.

Madhok, Sumi, Maya Unnithan, and Carolyn Heitmeyer. 2014. "On Reproductive Justice: 'Domestic Violence', Rights and the Law in India." *Culture, Health & Sexuality* 16 (10): 1231–44. https://doi.org/10.1080/13691058.2014.918281.

Majety, Chandramathi, and Sravani Bejugam. 2016. "Challenges and Barriers Faced by Women in Accessing Justice against Obstetric Violence." *International Journal of Reproduction, Contraception, Obstetrics and Gynecology* 5 (9): 2899–903. https://doi.org/10.18203/2320-1770.ijrcog20162968.

Mavuso, Jabulile Mary Jane Jace. 2020. "Reproductive Injustice: Forced Sterilisations in Post-Apartheid South Africa." *Feminism & Psychology Blog*, 2020. http://fap-journal.blogspot.com/2020/03/reproductive-injustice-forced.html#.YW4L5BpByHt.

Mohapatra, Seema. 2012. "Achieving Reproductive Justice in the International Surrogacy Market." *Annals of Health Law* 21 (1): 191–200.

———. 2019. "Law in the Time of Zika: Disability Rights and Reproductive Justice Collide." *Brooklyn Law Review* 84 (2): 325–64.

Morison, Tracy. 2021. "Reproductive Justice: A Radical Framework for Psychology." *Social and Personality Psychology Compass*, 1–10. https://doi.org/10.1111/spc3.12605.

Morison, Tracy, and Sarah Herbert. 2019. "Rethinking 'Risk' in Sexual and Reproductive Health Policy: The Value of the Reproductive Justice Framework."

Sexuality Research and Social Policy 16 (4): 434–45. https://doi.org/10.1007/ s13178-018-0351-z.

Morison, Tracy, Catriona Macleod, Ingrid Lynch, Magda Mijas, and Seemanthini Tumkur Shivakumar. 2016. "Stigma Resistance in Online Childfree Communities: The Limitations of Choice Rhetoric." *Psychology of Women Quarterly* 40 (2): 184–98. https://doi.org/10.1177/0361684315603657.

Nixon, Laura. 2013. "The Right to (Trans)Parent: A Reproductive Justice Approach to Reproductive Rights, Fertility, and Family-Building Issues Facing Transgender People." *William & Mary Journal of Women and the Law* 20 (1): 73–103.

Oaks, Laury. 2016. *Giving up Baby: Safe Haven Laws, Motherhood, and Reproductive Justice.* New York: New York University Press. https://doi.org/10.18574/nyu /9781479897926.001.0001.

O'Connell, Katie. 2016. "We Need to Talk about Disability as a Reproductive Justice Issue." *Reproaction.* https://reproaction.org/we-need-to-talk-about-disability-as-a -reproductive-justice-issue/.

Oluoch-Aridi, Jackline, Smith-Oka, Vania, Jessica Dailey, and Ellyn Milan. 2021. "Making Dignified Care the Norm: Examining Obstetric Violence and Reproductive Justice in Kenya." In *The Routledge Handbook of Anthropology and Reproduction*, edited by Sallie Han and Cecilia Tomori, 494–509. Oxon, UK & New York: Routledge.

Perez, Miriam Zoila. 2007. "Queering Reproductive Justice." *Rewire News*, May 31. https://doi.org/10.2307/j.ctt1pwt8jh.9.

Price, Kimala. 2010. "What Is Reproductive Justice? How Women of Color Activists Are Redefining the pro-Choice Paradigm." *Meridians* 10 (2): 42–65.

———. 2019. "Queering Reproductive Justice in the Trump Era: A Note on Political Intersectionality." *Politics & Gender* 14 (2018): 581–601. https://doi.org/10.1017 /S1743923X18000776.

Rabionet, Silvia E., Carmen D. Zorilla, Juana I. Rivera-Vinas, and Yeney Guerra-Sanchez. 2018. "Pregnancy and Zika: The Quest for Quality Care and Reproductive Justice." *Puerto Rico Health Sciences Journal* 37 (S1): S45–50.

Rebouché, Rachel. 2017. "Reproducing Rights: The Intersection of Reproductive Justice and Human Rights." *U.C. Irvine Law Review* 7: 579–609.

Riggs, Damien W., and Clare Bartholomaeus. 2019. "Toward Trans Reproductive Justice: A Qualitative Analysis of Views on Fertility Preservation for Australian Transgender and Non binary People." *Journal of Social Issues*, 1–24. https://doi .org/10.1111/josi.12364.

Rios, Elsa, and Angela Hooton. 2005. "A National Latina Agenda for Reproductive Justice." New York and London. https://www.latinainstitute.org/sites/default/files/ Natl-Latina-Agenda-for-Repro-Justice-Jan2005.pdf.

Rogers, Arneta. 2015. "How Police Brutality Harms Mothers : Linking Police Violence to the Reproductive Justice Movement." *Hastings Race & Poverty Law Journal* 12 (2): 205–34.

Ross, Loretta J. 2017. "Conceptualising Reproductive Justice Theory: A Manifesto for Activism." In *Radical Reproductiv Justice: Foundation, Theory, Practice, Critique,* edited by Loretta Ross, Erika Derkas, Whitney Peoples, Lynn Roberts, Pamela Bridgewater, and Dorothy Roberts, 170–232. New York: Feminist Press at CUNY.

Ross, Loretta J., and Rickie Solinger. 2017. *Reproductive Justice: An Introduction.* Oakland: California University Press.

Rubin, David, A. 2019. "Provincializing Intersex: U.S Intersex Activism, Human Rights, and Transnational Body Politics." *Reproductive Justice and Sexual Rights: Transnational Perspectives*, 229–53.

Salter, Cynthia L., Abisola Olaniyan, Dara D. Mendez, and Judy C. Chang. 2021. "Naming Silence and Inadequate Obstetric Care as Obstetric Violence Is a Necessary Step for Change." 27 (8): 1019–27. https://doi.org/10.1177/1077801221996443.

Saravanan, Sheela. 2016. "'Humanitarian' Thresholds of the Fundamental Feminist Ideologies: Evidence from Surrogacy Arrangements in India." *Analize-Journal of Gender and Feminist Studies* 6: 66–88.

Senderowicz, Leigh. 2019. "'I Was Obligated to Accept': A Qualitative Exploration of Contraceptive Coercion." *Social Science and Medicine* 239 (September): 112531. https://doi.org/10.1016/j.socscimed.2019.112531.

Shaw, Jessica. 2013. "Full-Spectrum Reproductive Justice : The Affinity of Abortion Rights and Birth Activism." *Studies in Social Justice* 7 (1): 143–59.

Silver, Lauren J. 2020. "Queering Reproductive Justice: Memories, Mistakes, and Motivations to Transform Kinship." *Feminist Anthropology* 1 (2): 217–30. https://doi.org/10.1002/FEA2.12019.

SisterSong. 2007. "Reproductive Justice Briefing Book: A Primer on Reproductive Justice and Social Change." *SisterSong.* https://www.law.berkeley.edu/php-programs/courses/fileDL.php?fID=4051.

Smietana, Marcin, Charis Thompson, and France Winddance Twine. 2018. "Making and Breaking Families – Reading Queer Reproductions, Stratified Reproduction and Reproductive Justice Together." *Reproductive Biomedicine and Society Online* 7: 112–30. https://doi.org/10.1016/j.rbms.2018.11.001.

Smith, Andrea. 2005. "Beyond Pro-Choice versus pro-Life : Women of Color and Reproductive Justice." *NWSA Journal* 17 (1): 119–40.

Solinger, Rickie. 2010. "The First Welfare Case: Money, Sex, Marriage, and White Supremacy in Selma, 1966, A Reproductive Justice Analysis." *Journal of Women's History* 22 (3): 13–38.

Vasquez Del Aguila, E. 2020. "Precarious Lives: Forced Sterilisation and the Struggle for Reproductive Justice in Peru." *Global Public Health.* https://doi.org/10.1080/17441692.2020.1850831.

Ward, Pamela, and Deborah Mcphail. 2019. "Fat Shame and Blame in Reproductive Care: Implications for Ethical Health Care Interactions." *Women's Reproductive Health* 6 (4): 225–41. https://doi.org/10.1080/23293691.2019.1653581.

Wu, Justine, Jianying Zhang, Monika Mitra, Susan L. Parish, and Geeth Kavya Minama Reddy. 2018. "Provision of Moderately and Highly Effective Reversible Contraception to Insuredwomen with Intellectual and Developmental Disabilities." *Obstetrics and Gynecology* 132 (3): 565–74. https://doi.org/10.1097/AOG.0000000000002777.

Yam, Shui-yin Sharon. 2020. "Visualizing Birth Stories from the Margin: Toward a Reproductive Justice Model of Rhetorical Analysis." 50 (1): 19–34. https://doi.org/10.1080/02773945.2019.1682182.

Yook, Sung Hee, and Hosu Kim. 2018. "Decolonizing Adoption Narratives for Transnatinal Reproductive Justice." *CLCWeb: Comparative Literature and Culture* 20 (6). https://doi.org/10.7771/1481-4374.3323

Zavella, Patricia. 2016. "Intersectional Praxis in the Movement for Reproductive Justice: The Respect ABQ Women Campaign." *Signs* 42 (2): 509–33.

Chapter 1

Sex Worker Narratives in Accessing Sexual and Reproductive Justice in South Africa

Marion Stevens, Dudu Dlamini,
and Lance Louskieter

It has been well documented that most of the focus on sex workers comes from a welfarist approach, most often addressing HIV prevention in "most at risk populations" (World Health Organisation 2021). This focus is often motivated by a desire to address the "contagion," "harm," or "threat" that sex workers "pose" to public health (Sultana 2015). This dominant risk focus is critiqued by sex workers and scholarship informed by their perspectives. Stabile (2020) discusses how a risk focus has become hegemonic in Western feminist discourse on sex work that focusses on the need for rescuing sex workers. This discourse has become dominant in legislation and civil society engagement in much of the world. It undermines sex workers' human dignity and reproduces racism, sex/gender binaries, and colonialism (Stabile 2020).

In contrast, Smith and Mac (2018) caution against the welfarist, liberal "saviour" response to sex work, advocating instead for harm reduction. Writing *as sex workers*, Smith and Mac's (2018) work brings a fresh perspective. They provide an in-depth analysis and critical examination of sex work realities, discussing the devastation of incarceration and the importance of labour rights for sex workers, as well as broader issues of justice and resistance to White supremacy. Their work is, however, an exception in the literature in that little published research is informed by sex workers' perspectives or experiences.

Existing research documenting sex workers' experiences illuminates the widespread sexual and reproductive injustices they face. Research on sexual and reproductive health includes Scorgie et al.'s (2013) qualitative study conducted in Kenya, Zimbabwe, Uganda, and South Africa in which sex workers reported unmet health needs (e.g., contraception and treatment of STIs), denial of care (including for injuries from violence), and hostile care. Similarly, Scheibe et al.'s (2016) research on HIV care for sex workers in South Africa highlights health system barriers and the need for legal reform. Comparatively, little research focusses on sex workers' access to and use of abortion services. A notable exception is Gerdts et al.'s (2017) study that sought to determine rates of illegal/informal abortion in South Africa with sex workers as the majority of participants. The findings suggest that because sex work is criminalised and on account of the social stigma directed at sex workers in formal healthcare settings, some women who are engaged in sex work choose to go to informal providers where abortions may be unsafe/illegal.

We identified a lack of empirical research that focusses on sexual and reproductive health and rights for sex workers, particularly sex worker mothers, and that is informed by a Reproductive Justice perspective. Indeed, the recognition that sex workers can be mothers and persons in their own right with agency is not a central assumption in funded work for sex worker programmes (e.g., Global Fund's (2019) programming) and theorisation of Reproductive Justice has, to our knowledge, not included sex workers' experiences. Thus, work that produces first-hand information about sex workers' sexual and reproductive health and rights *and* that highlights the issue of parenthood/childcare for sex workers is important.

The right to parent is articulated in the Reproductive Justice framework as are issues of gender identity, personal dignity, bodily autonomy, and sexual pleasure (Ross 2020; Ross and Solinger 2017), yet none of its foundational texts addresses the issue of sex work, including sexual and reproductive health services and parenting support. Our work seeks to address the gaps in these literatures: our research is co-produced with/by sex workers and conducted within a Reproductive Justice framework. This study is, to our knowledge, the first to consider the continuum of overlapping and interlinking areas of the social and sexual determinants of health and in particular experiences of contraception, abortion, and the criminalisation of sex work. Our overarching aim was to explore how Reproductive Justice is undermined by both the criminalisation of sex work and the denial of quality and humanising sexual and reproductive healthcare.

The focus of the research we present in this chapter is on the barriers to Sexual and Reproductive Justice experienced by sex workers, including sex worker mothers. The study was conducted in South Africa, where sex work is criminalised and involved a series of participatory workshops using body mapping to stimulate discussion. The approach we take in this chapter is one of co-production with sex workers, as discussed by Louskieter et al. (2021). We see this co-production as a political act; sex workers' marginalised voices have not simply been included; the research is driven by and foregrounds their priorities and demands.

We demonstrate how sexual and reproductive injustice is not restricted to sexual and reproductive healthcare spaces but part of the wider context in which sex workers live and work as poor and/or impoverished, Black women who perform criminalised and stigmatised labour, extending from public state entities (public health services, police) through to more private interactions with clients, family members, and others.

OUR STUDY

This study is the outcome of a collaboration between *Mothers for the Future* (M4F)[1] and the *Sexual and Reproductive Justice Coalition* (SRJC)[2] and was informed by sex worker-led processes. M4F is a group of sex worker mothers in South Africa set up using a Reproductive Justice lens to support and organise sex workers who are mothers. The group has a historical relationship with the SRJC—a South African NGO that includes sex work as a focal area. The partnership between SRJC and M4F is built on acknowledging the different structural positions of various parties involved and power as relational. As a team, identities traverse differences and similarities in relation to race, gender, class, education, language, and access to networks, knowledge, and experiences.

Beginning in 2014, Dudu Dlamini—the leader of M4F—and Marion Stevens —formerly the director of SRJC—charted a collaborative consciousness-raising programme with sex worker mothers about their sexual and reproductive rights. Monthly workshops were hosted by M4F addressing specific information requests on sexual and reproductive health topics and issues (e.g., physiology and anatomy, illnesses, health-seeking). The group subsequently developed to organise, access support, build skills, participate in research community advisory committees, and share knowledge.

In 2017, a series of workshops were held with a feminist organisation addressing violence against women, the SRJC, and M4F. As part of this, "artivism" (Jordan 2016) was employed, requiring participants to draw and name the experience of abortion access. M4F and SRJC decided to continue to explore how the lack of access to safe abortion continues and is linked to the need to decriminalise sex work. To this end, three participatory workshops conducted by Dudu and Marion were held with 15 sex workers in 3 major South African cities (Cape Town, Durban, and Johannesburg).

All 45 participants identified as women, including gender non-conforming women, and with diverse sexual identities. At the time of the study, the women had different relationship statuses (partnered, divorced, or single). Age and specific location are not neutral as to sex workers, they have currency and power. However, we did not extract this specific data within this group. Instead, we confirmed the age range and noted that the participants ranged in age from 19 to their late 50s. Race, ethnicity, and culture are also loaded and laden within South Africa. While most participants would be observed as Black, participants did not self-identify, and we did not probe this. Poverty and class were expressed by all. Participants had a range of educational backgrounds, some having primary school years while one had a professional qualification but had been deregistered as she was an alcoholic. Similarly, participants had a range of spaces they called home; one defined as a migrant, some "slept rough," and some lived in stand-alone homes, flats/apartments, and houses. Over a third of participants (14) disclosed being HIV positive and taking anti-retroviral drugs (ARVs). There was also an array of reproductive experiences among the participants, including deeply desired and unsupportable pregnancies.[3] Most women defined themselves as mothers and had biological children and some grandchildren. Many spoke of the joy of their chosen pregnancies, and proudly of their children and their ability as mothers to support them well through sex work. Some had not had children and others spoke of extended families with fostered and adopted children. For example, one woman spoke of the burden of unsupported pregnancies and not having access to contraception for herself and her daughter. She had two children and five grandchildren and a daughter who was pregnant with another child. She felt overwhelmed by having to support her family and felt unable to work as she had challenges with untreated infections. Some had stillbirths or children who had died soon after birth or as young children. Some participants had experienced sterilisation, with one recounting her experience of forced sterilisation.

Data collection, conducted by Marion and Dudu, included body mapping using a variety of media to enable narratives to be shared in the participants' own languages and at a self-determined pace (De Jager 2016). Participants were asked about their experiences of contraception and abortion and to draw these experiences on their body maps. After painting, drawing, and writing these, the maps were stuck on the wall and each group circulated and viewed them. Participants were then given a chance to tell their story in their own words. This facilitation process enabled an opt-in process where participants determined their own narrative. Multiple languages were used including English, Afrikaans, isiZulu, isiXhosa, and Sesotho. Notes were written by a rapporteur, these were augmented by notes, photographs, and observations from Marion and Dudu to compile an initial data set. This initial data set was then disassembled, reassembled, and interpreted by the research team using thematic analysis (Castleberry and Nolen 2018).

Ethical engagement with participants was informed by M4F's code of conduct regarding a dialect of participation, boundary setting, confidentiality, opting out, rules of engagement, partnerships, and ensuring personal needs are met (e.g., needing to sleep, eat, or wash if having worked the night before). The code of conduct includes the acknowledgement of working with trauma, conflict, and sensitive issues, which both Dudu and Marion have experienced as facilitators. Finally, M4F had a referral process for counselling that was used, as the process of participation evoked a need for addressing trauma and abuse. Ethics approval was provided by the Faculty of Humanities at the University of Cape Town, through the African Gender Institute (AGI). The SRJC and SWEAT (Sex Workers Education and Advocacy Task Force) (M4F) discussed confidentiality and anonymity with participants and obtained written consent from participants to take part. We have given pseudonyms to the narratives documented below, given sensitivities and to protect participants.

FINDINGS

The following central themes were generated by our analysis: (i) *navigating a world of injustice and violence*, which captures participants' narration about the contexts in which they live (experiences of rejection and abuse in primary families) and work (highlighting criminalisation as a form of systemic violence); (ii) *an unhealthy health system*, which captures sex workers' experiences with/of the health system, with a focus on contraceptive and abortion care; and finally the (iii) *mental health challenges* that sex workers in our study experience as a result of the injustices they face. Figure 1.1 provides an overview of the themes and sub-themes and we present each in turn. Anonymised extracts from sex workers' narratives are used in the analysis and some exemplars of participants' body maps appear below, with consent, to illustrate participants' experiences of sexual and reproductive injustices perpetrated by clients, the state, and participants' families and communities.

Theme 1: Navigating a World of Injustice and Violence

This section includes the sub-themes of rejection, abuse, and abandonment from primary families and communities, and criminalisation as a form of systemic violence. Abuse and violence are endemic in South Africa. Just over half of the participants described experiences of violation or abuse from their families or male partners. These experiences of violence and abuse had significant implications for participants, their health and well-being, and for their children.

Rejection, Abuse, and Abandonment
in Primary Families and Communities

Participants identified their primary birth families as unsafe spaces for them to grow up and told of insecurity and vulnerability, food insecurity and

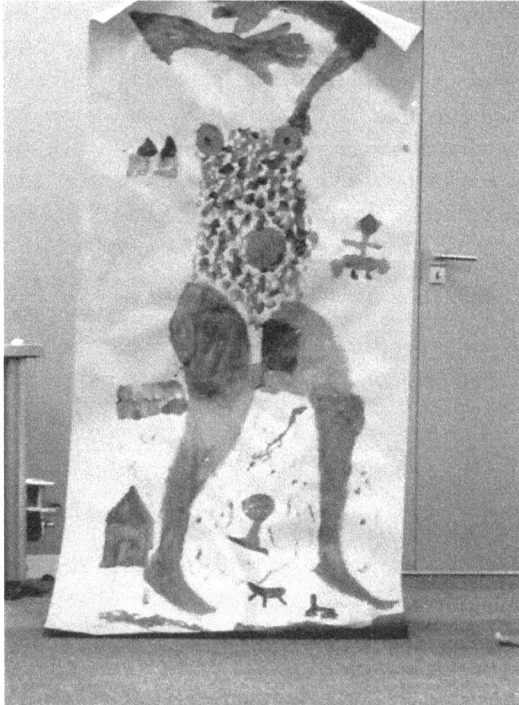

Figure 1.1   Our Bodies with Paint Telling Our Stories. *Source*: Photo by Marion Stevens.

hunger in their households. Others described childhoods characterised by power imbalances and being forced to do house labour, provide childcare, or run errands. All participants described being stolen from, violated, judged, or silenced by family members, as well as feelings of being abandoned and not having had adults to care for them when they were young. Ricky and Thoko's extracts below reflect some of the challenges many of the sex workers experienced with their families.

Ricky:
My Mom kicked me out of the house. I get abused. "Why are you so beautiful?" I am hurt. I am judged by official appearance. I am beautiful, but this beauty brings me pain. My heart is red because I have been abused a lot. People do not understand when I am hurting, and people judge me.

Thoko:
I got pregnant at 16 years while still at school. I had no support from anyone. I cannot go back home to my parents, so I ran away from home to live in the streets, this is where I learnt survival skills and where things happen. I started sex work and not knowing the work and how to protect myself. I am from a

poor background—I got pregnant when I was 16 and was forced to marry the guy who impregnated me. I was not allowed to consent to sex or not.

Two women described being sexually violated by the same man as children growing up in the same township in Cape Town. Some described being aggressive and physically abusive themselves, and how they have learnt this behaviour to cope or assert boundaries. Others described generations and relationships of violence that endure in families and communities:

Sugar:
I was repeatedly raped by my uncle at home and [by] community members, which led me to run away from home. A taxi driver wanted to kill me and I jumped out rolling, I escaped. I have a 1-year-old boy but he['s] not with me; he is with my family. I was locked up for 10 days and raped by my family. I live on the streets, because I fear my family.

Dinah:
I fell pregnant at an early age and at the time I did not use any contraception. I worked at the truck stop and went with Candy man—he gave me sweets and biscuits. At 18, he raped me and I got my baby boy. He died in prison.

Sugar and Dinah's narratives reflect the gruesome experiences over time of physical and sexual violence in participants' families and communities, and the precarious nature of their lives.

Criminalisation as a Form of Systemic Violence

We identified the theme of criminalisation of sex work as a form of systemic violence: the physical, psychological, or sexual harm people experience due to societal structures and institutions sustaining and reproducing it (De Bruyn 2002). Sexual, emotional, and physical violence experienced by sex workers, produced and sustained through the criminalisation of sex work, was reflected in some participants' narratives. They gave examples of how the criminalisation of their work limited safe access to sexual and reproductive health services, as shown in Gemma's account below (figure 1.2).

Gemma:
My tired red feet. I am tired. I walk and work every day. Clinics they refused to give me tablets, pills. I am on ARVs. I use my feet and my vagina even when I do not want to work. The police do not protect the streets. At the clinics they change our tablets sometimes and they do not ask us if the tablets are good for us [or] not but there are side effects. The tablets are not all the

same. They refuse to give me tablets because of the referral from the mobile clinic—TB/HIV care. The police harass me.

As Gemma's account illustrates, sex workers are in a precarious position because they are hyper-visible and seen as criminals by police. Participants spoke of being arrested due to petty bylaws (e.g., "loitering" in places where they should not be), a continuation of apartheid geo-spatial practices where Black persons are policed for inhabiting certain spaces (Muntingh et al. 2015). They are arbitrarily rounded up and experience abuse from police who solicit sexual acts. For example, Gina shared a regular experience: "The police arrest me—and ask me to *skom* [masturbate/fellate them]." Participants also described having their medications and personal belongings taken from them and as a result it was difficult to be adherent to ARVs and TB drugs. As a result, some described sharing drugs and working out strategies to get more ARVs in between clinic visits. In addition, most often police officers do not accept rape charges by sex workers, believing that it is expected for sex workers to be raped as part of their work.

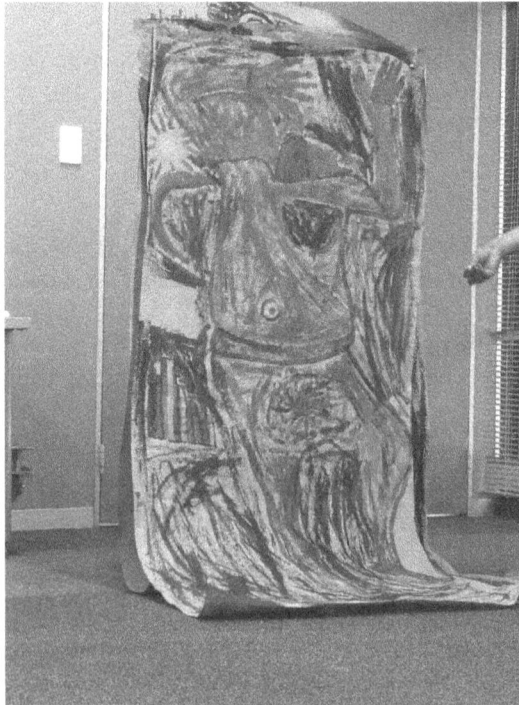

Figure 1.2   Criminalised: Hands Up and Heads Down. *Source*: Photo by Marion Stevens.

Police abuse of sex workers in South Africa has been well documented including the confiscation of condoms as evidence (Rangasami, Konstant, and Manoek 2016). Globally, Smith and Mac (2018) argue that where sex workers are criminalised, stories emerge of police inflicting beatings, rape, and extortion, noting that sex workers fear police more than anyone else. Smith and Mac (2018) argue that criminalisation forces (sex) workers to compromise on some or all their safety strategies in the hope of avoiding the police.

The women in this study could not talk to health workers freely about occupational hazards and challenges to their health as they felt judged and stigmatised. Similarly, while participants received condoms from health services (SWEAT or clinics) for their own safety and that of their clients, these were often confiscated by police. They described nurses as not being easy to talk to when they would explain having had their personal belongings (purses with medicines and condoms) confiscated while they were held in custody by the police. We elaborate on experiences in healthcare spaces in the following theme.

It is clear from the participants' experiences that not only are their sexual and reproductive health and rights undermined by not being able to access services but that those meant to protect them either exacerbate harm and vulnerability or actively contribute to it. The participants consequently argued that decriminalisation would go a long way towards enabling access to health services (including sexual and reproductive health services) and justice. They explained that they would feel freer to discuss their specific needs and hold health workers, police officers, policymakers, and state bureaucrats accountable for improved services and the actualisation of their human rights. Similarly, they would be able to report violations and non-consensual sexual encounters.

Theme 2: An Unhealthy Health System

Participants' narratives reflect experiences of a health system that is stressed and overburdened, unresponsive to their needs, unsafe and hostile, and, overall, that does not facilitate comfort and healing. They describe poor access to sexual and reproductive information, as well as dehumanising sexual and reproductive care and services. Their accounts include reports of obstetric violence, disrespectful contraceptive care with limited contraception options and provision, experiences of contraceptive and reproductive coercion, lack of access to legal and safe abortion services, poor delivery of state-funded abortion services, and judgemental treatment on the basis of being sex workers. Participants described that health workers do not know how to be responsive to the differentiated care needs of sex workers. Rather, Lulu recounted, "they treat you as criminals because what we do is illegal." Health providers appear to have little understanding of how to provide for sex workers' health needs and tend to administer services with annoyance and resentment, as the following quotations illustrate.

Lulu:

This is me. My first real experience in the clinics is represented here in the clinic. It was terrible. The nurses have bad attitudes towards people. At the public clinic when you explain to the nurses what you feel they treat you like you do not know your own body. Once a nurse asked me what do I know about a fallopian tube and what do I know about a uterus, because I am just a patient. I had a boil inside. The nurse was angry.

Bertha:

Time went on I had period pain issues and abdominal pains and at the clinic they just say its constipation. I only found out recently that I had fibroids and a cyst, which I wouldn't have known if I didn't get admitted to hospital, because at the day clinics they told me it is just constipation.

Thuli:

I had an STI and went to the clinic. The sister shouted at me. She knows where I work and I was treated as a sex worker. I left the clinic embarrassed. I felt the stigma. I went to a Zulu traditional leader and got treatment. I never went back to the clinic. I am perfectly fine.

These extracts show how public clinics were generally not a place of healing, rather illnesses more often went undiagnosed and untreated. Lulu, Bertha, and Thuli's experiences echo the blunt and inadequate care to sex workers by the health system and healthcare providers as reported by Scheibe, Richter, and Vearey (2016). As a consequence, participants avoid public health services for fear of scolding and judgement by health workers and seek assistance elsewhere. For instance, Khosi related with confidence: "I have moved on from using public health services. I now use private doctors because I feel that I can use the services without being questioned or treated with disrespect." In addition to private healthcare, some sought care from traditional healers who listened and provided privacy and acceptance.

The extracts above also show how clinics were not a source of sexual and reproductive information, which emerged as a gap for participants. Participants expressed that they had no space to discuss their health freely, including basic information about their bodies, or to feel comfortable and not judged in asking these questions. Participants felt that they should be able to ask a health provider questions about their body or illnesses. However, as shown in the extracts above, these conversations were not welcomed by health workers, and participants experienced the treatment by health workers as uncomfortable, dismissive, or judgemental.

Our findings resonate with Comins et al.'s (2019) research with sex workers in South Africa, which highlights gaps in relation to sexual and reproductive health and rights in HIV programming and the failure to address the expressed needs of sex workers. This was reflected in our study as well, as Dina explains:

Dina:
I am on ARVs [anti-retrovirals] which I collect from the local clinic. I had a boil at the mouth of the vagina, it makes me uncomfortable. I have been tested for a pap smear and the results were OK, but I still have this pain which makes me uncomfortable during intercourse.

Thus, the stand-alone programming of HIV has enabled an ARV distribution programme with little agility to provide for the comprehensive health needs of clients. Nonetheless, some participants maintained that they only really got services and attention, albeit sub-standard, because of HIV clinics. In this theme, we have focussed on participants' descriptions of the conditions that enable or limit their fertility options in being able to choose to support their pregnancy or not. As we have shown, their fertility intentions and options to have children or not were not well provided for by the health system. Their sexual and reproductive health and rights were routinely denied as were their rights to parent with dignity in safe and healthy environments or *not* to have children.

Participants' narratives describe poor quality care received, including untreated STIs, misdiagnosed and untreated conditions, and experiences of the consequences of side effects of contra-indicated treatments. This had a significant impact on their sexual health, as well as their ability and right to earn a living. These reproductive injustices are allowed by the criminal status of sex work, as evident in frequent arrests and harassment by police, as well as structural violence through the healthcare system. In the following section, we focus on the public healthcare system.

Contraceptive Services: Constrained Agency and Coercive Practices

In our study, *Depo Provera* (injectable contraceptive) was referred to by most (21) of the women as the contraceptive they used. This reflects broader patterns in South Africa as a legacy of population control when long-acting reversible contraceptives were used because health workers suggest that (certain) women cannot be "trusted" to control their fertility (Stevens 2021). (See also chapter 13 in this volume regarding the use of long-acting reversible contraceptives in South Africa.). Of those using injectables, few were able to note the difference between the three-month or six-week contraception

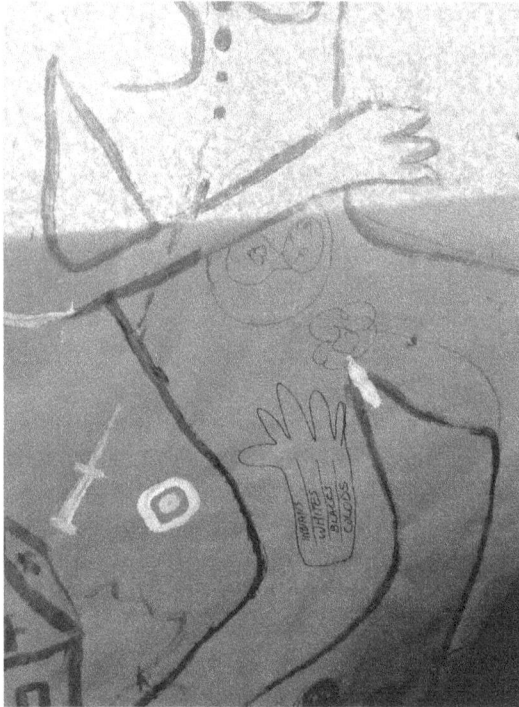

Figure 1.3   The Injection and Segregated Contraception Services. *Source*: Photo by Marion Stevens.

injectable options, reflecting a lack of information available. The remainder described using the inter-uterine device (IUD) and others oral contraceptive pills (figure 1.3).

Less than half of the participants (19 participants) confirmed using condoms. For some this reflected a lack of condoms, with participants describing using alternative methods as contraception which they believed to be protective, such as sponges, particularly kitchen sponges or the sponge from a female condom, to absorb semen. Of those who described using condoms, some described choosing only to do so with their clients but not regular partners.

As Lebo and Thumi describe below, Depo Provera was chosen for them and provided by the health worker with limited choices as to what option might suit them.

Lebo:

I use injectable as a contraceptive. The nurses choose for me at the clinic and tell me what to use.

Thumi:
I am on ARVs and I am healthy. I stopped contraceptives but after labour, you get depo [*Depo Provera*] without no questions asked. I do not know how long I will carry on condoms as contraception. I bled too much so stop and use condoms. I was HIV positive with my first pregnancy and wanted an abortion but had no choice.

In a similar vein, some participants told about how health providers acted as gatekeepers to desired contraception. Several recounted how condoms sometimes burst in the process of their work and that when they ask for emergency contraception, they are frequently discriminated against and rebuffed. Others recounted experiences where their ability to make choices about contraception—such as discontinuing or changing a method—was restricted by the limitations of contraceptive care in the public health sector. For example, Gigi, a migrant, had the implant Norplant inserted while in Zimbabwe, but South African health providers were unable to remove it:

Gigi:
I had the implant, *Norplant*, [meant to last] for five years, but I had it for 10 years. I had no sexual feelings for 6 years. I have never had an unwanted pregnancy. I have been using a 10-year implant and after I removed it got sick, started bleeding heavily. I removed the implant in June 2009.

Accounts like Gigi's reveal the neglect that patients endure in not being able to seek specific care and the lack of training of health providers. Senderowicz (2019), who conducted research on contraception services in sub-Saharan Africa, argues that such structural barriers represent mundane limits to free, full, and informed choice. This amounts to a form of subtle coercion as women are compelled to continue an undesired contraceptive method, course of action, or pregnancy. Alongside providers' coercive practices, some participants' contraceptive use was determined by clients, who paid extra to have sex without a condom.

The lack of coordination across different services and programmes for the treatment of illnesses such as HIV, TB, and fertility planning was expressed by participants in a variety of ways, demonstrating programmatic gaps in the health system related to Sexual and Reproductive Justice. For example, of two participants who described pregnancies while on contraception, Gemma noted how her ARVs had interfered with her implant, while Ricky was on TB drugs that interacted with her contraception. Nonki felt that she had not been able to discuss her fertility intentions with health providers to prevent unintended pregnancies. She described the pain of losing her child soon after birthing, as well as having another child and being unable to access treatment to prevent vertical transmission to her daughter, who is now HIV positive. Nonki was unsure how to disclose her HIV status or her daughter being infected to healthcare providers. These experiences speak to the failure of healthcare to create spaces for sex workers to discuss their comprehensive health needs, including chronic diseases and fertility intentions and planning, freely and openly.

Abortion

Inaccessible abortion has been described as reproductive injustice (Macleod, Beynon-Jones, and Toerien 2017). Twelve participants had abortions in the formal sector, mostly public sector. Delays in access were also noted as barriers to accessing care. Some women who had consulted providers described being asked to consider not having an abortion, despite going to the clinic to request this service, as described by Nonki in the following extract.

> *Nonki*:
> I slept in the hospital because I had an early pregnancy. I tested HIV positive
> and I could not breastfeed. Before this I wanted to abort, and the nurses told
> me not to have an abortion. I had a premature baby boy.

For Nonki, being denied an abortion in the public sector resulted in a forced pregnancy. Similarly, another participant described efforts to access an abortion and not being able to access one despite attempts both legally and informally. She subsequently gave her child up for adoption.

For some, fear of mistreatment at public facilities shaped their abortion-seeking experiences. One woman explained that she had had two abortions in the public sector and had to go to two different clinics far apart from each other as she wanted to avoid being shouted at by the nurses. Another woman described how she had self-induced three abortions on herself using a catheter and hot water. She would induce bleeding and then would go to the hospital and tell the health workers she was having a miscarriage and have a procedure to evacuate her uterus. She explained to fellow participants in detail how to insert the catheter to safely induce an abortion (following this, facilitators provided accurate clinical information about abortion access in the public sector). There has been at least one reported death of a group member from an unsafe abortion.

Fear of how they would be treated at facilities legally authorised to offer abortion care also led some women to turn to informal or illegal providers. Eight participants described consulting a provider outside the formal health system to access an abortion using an illegal method. This echoes Gerdts et al.'s (2017) finding that women use informal sector abortion providers because they seek privacy and fear mistreatment and stigma in public health facilities. Some participants also resorted to the informal sector when denied abortion services in the formal sector. Queenie recounted her experience of being denied abortion care in the public health service:

Queenie:
I wanted an abortion, but the clinic they refused. A friend got pills: 4 tablets
for R600. I bled and went to the hospital and the nurses laughed and were rude.

Another reason that participants used informal abortion providers was due
to the time and cost involved, due to the repeat visits required in the formal
public health sector. Participants explained that each time one must arrange
to go to the clinic, it involves costs of missed work, childcare, transport, and
security arrangements. They explained that it was much better to have a once-
off appointment with an informal provider who did not need to confirm the
pregnancy or do an ultrasound.

In contrast to the above experiences of seeking an abortion and being
denied or being unable to obtain one that had been desired, one participant
described her devastation in having her family pressurise her to have an abortion, despite her having wanted to continue the pregnancy. She lost her baby
after it was born. The right to have a child is therefore elusive for participants.

The accounts encompassed by this theme suggest that health workers do
not know how to support sex workers and to ensure that they are safe and
healthy; sex workers therefore remain vulnerable in an unhealthy health system and beyond. The final theme considers the poor mental health outcomes
resulting largely from systemic injustices and neglect.

Theme 3: Mental Health Challenges Resulting from Injustice

Mental health challenges featured as a theme with over a third (16 out of
45) of participants describing challenging mental health symptoms. These
included bouts of depression, anxiety, and sadness. The following extracts
from participants' narratives describe the mental health implications of sexual
and reproductive injustices (figure 1.4).

Lulu:
My heart bleeds because of terrible things, there is a dark cloud over me,
nothing good happens to me. I cry a lot and am stressed. There are chains
preventing me from accepting new things. I go to church when I feel lonely.

Jasmin:
This is me, ugly and sad because of the things I have been through in my
life. My eyes are crying as I had an unplanned pregnancy. I am not thinking
straight.
Lex:
There are a lot of noises in my mind. I have dots on my body [in the picture]
and this is a problem. I get judgement from partners and clients. I have been

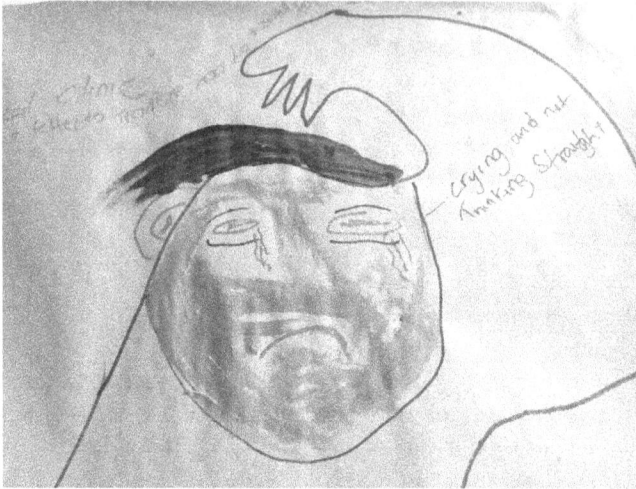

Figure 1.4   Crying and Not Thinking Straight: Mental Ill Health. *Source*: Photo by Marion Stevens.

abused. Because of poverty one must do [draw] the stomach. I have been taken advantage of by clients. I drink alcohol because of a lot of challenges.

These extracts and the body maps illustrate the impact that injustices related to sex work have on the mental health of many participants and, particularly, those who are mothers. The deep psychological distress, pain, and anguish described by Lulu, Jasmin, and Lex above are injustices carried by their bodies. Participants describe poverty and the challenge of feeding families (Lex refers to "the stomach" in the previous extract). Several participants experienced reproductive losses and the trauma of this. Several experienced miscarriages, some had experienced a stillbirth and one a neonatal death. This deep trauma regarding fertility loss was expressed as an overwhelming sadness. Participants had little recourse to care to address their devastating trauma.

To cope with their emotional challenges and hostile work contexts, many participants described using substances to self-medicate for anxiety or depression. Below, Jenny describes the ambivalence of her being confident in her lucrative work on the one hand, and noting on the other hand that this comes with depression and violence:

Jenny:
Clients come and we go, in cars. I use condoms. I am proud of my vagina; it gives me a fortune in the bush. I have a scar, the *skollies* [criminals/hooligans] stab me for my long legs. I use alcohol for depression.

Similarly, nine participants described using alcohol. Cally, for instance, disclosed, "I have been mentally ill because of the abuse I have suffered from and I am alcoholic which means I cannot work as a nurse." Facilitators referred participants to SWEAT's counselling and mental health services. However, the participants remain underserved. Meeting mental health needs for sex workers and sex worker mothers is an urgent and continuing challenge.

CONCLUDING DISCUSSION

Through body mapping and personal narratives, participants recounted painful experiences of denial of dignity and bodily autonomy in relation to sexuality and reproduction, experiences of violence in families and communities, frequently sanctioned or committed by state entities, notably the police service and health system. Overall, our findings underscore the importance of social and structural health determinants, particularly in relation to sexuality and reproduction. They show, in particular, how the criminalisation of sex work perpetuates interlinking and overlapping sexual and reproductive injustices, undermining sex workers' ability to access quality sexual and reproductive healthcare, to make decisions in line with their reproductive desires and their sexual autonomy, and to parent in supportive environments. This clearly amounts to the denial of Sexual and Reproductive Justice and citizenship for sex workers.

We have also highlighted the psychological and emotional impacts of sexual and reproductive injustices perpetrated by a range of actors, including the state (police and healthcare services), clients, and primary families, as well as physical violence. Access to mental healthcare and supportive services are thus also part of a range of participants' health needs. Based on these findings, we contend that criminalisation of sex work is a key barrier to Sexual and Reproductive Justice. As our analysis indicates, the material conditions of work, safety, and health were prominent in participants' narratives. Pleasure did not feature in our participants' accounts. Instead, it is evident that the ability to decide if and when to have sex and without pain or discomfort—including for a living—was severely constrained by state- and client-perpetrated violence and the denial of quality sexual and reproductive healthcare. We therefore advocate for a focus on labour rights and an avoidance of sex-positivity politics with its emphasis on the right to sexual pleasure.

Indeed, working class and Black sex workers have long criticised the race and class privilege of sex-positivity politics, and labour rights and safety are not the same as pleasure. As a result, the sex worker movement has moved away from a liberal feminist, sex-positive, "happy hooker" narrative—which does not capture the realities of many Black, working class, and many other sex workers—towards a Marxist-feminist and labour-centred analysis (Smith and Mac 2018).

Our use of a Reproductive Justice lens highlights the structural violences that sex workers face and that are both enabled and aggravated by the criminalisation of sex work. It also allows for a nuanced view of how criminalisation intersects with classism and racism to produce a particular range of experiences for the Black and working-class sex workers that took part in our study. Our work demonstrates that a Reproductive Justice approach, which is sex worker informed and led, can extend Marxist-feminist and labour-centred analyses, by revealing how structural violence and the denial of labour rights produce sexual and reproductive injustices. A Reproductive Justice approach further reveals the interrelated nature of sex workers' rights to economic freedom and security with sexual and reproductive rights, including rights not to have children, to have children under chosen conditions, and to parent free from intervention and violence, *including* healthcare institutions.

Ensuring that Sexual and Reproductive Justice is realised for sex workers requires various strategies and solutions. Sex workers in our study identified full decriminalisation as being an option to open health services and make it safer for sex workers to access care. In addition, we argue that sex workers should be more centrally involved in all aspects of research, scholarship, and policy related to sex work enabling the subaltern to meaningfully speak, and importantly to lead and direct recourse to Sexual and Reproductive Justice for sex workers.

ACKNOWLEDGEMENT

Amplify Change for funding this project. Grant no: 64DM-X2CT-PM.

NOTES

1. M4F is part of the Sex Workers Education and Advocacy Task Force (SWEAT)/ Sisonke formations. The SWEAT is a sex worker-led NGO with groupings such as Sisonke and Mothers for the Future allied to the mother body. See www.sweat.org.za.

2. See www.srjc.org.za for information regarding the Sexual and Reproductive Justice Coalition.

3. Definition of unsupportable pregnancy—Unsupported pregnancies take the notion of unplanned/unintended pregnancies further from a reproductive justice perspective noting that pregnancies are supported or unsupported beyond the individual

to also involve families, communities, and societies (Macleod, Beynon-Jones, and Toerien 2017).

REFERENCES

Castleberry, Ashley, and Amanda Nolen. 2018. "Thematic Analysis of Qualitative Research Data: Is it as Easy as it Sounds?" *Currents in Pharmacy Teaching and Learning* 10 (6): 807–15. https://doi.org/10.1016/j.cptl.2018.03.019.

Comins, Carly A., Sheree R. Schwartz, Katherine Young, Sharmistha Mishra, Vijayanand Guddera, Mfezi Mcingana, Deliwe R. Phetlhu, Harry Hausler, and Stefan Baral. 2019. "Contextualising the Lived Experience of Sex Workers Living with HIV in South Africa: A Call for a Human-Centred Response to Sexual and Reproductive Health and Rights." *Sexual and Reproductive Health Matters* 27 (1): 316–18. https://doi.org/10.1080/26410397.2019.1686200.

De Bruyn, Tom. 2002. "Policy, Fear and Systemic Violence: A Review of the Johannesburg Context." *Urban Forum* 13 (3): 80–98. https://doi.org/10.1007/s12132-002-0009-y.

De Jager, Adèle, Anna Tewson, Bryn Ludlow, and Katherine Boydell. 2016. "Embodied Ways of Storying the Self: A Systematic Review of Body-Mapping." *Forum Qualitative Sozialforschung/Forum: Qualitative Social Research* 17 (2). https://doi.org/10.17169/fqs-17.2.2526.

Gerdts, Caitlin, Sarah Raifman, Kristen Daskilewicz, Mariette Momberg, Sarah Roberts, and Jane Harriesl. 2017. "Women's Experiences Seeking Informal Sector Abortion Services in Cape Town, South Africa: A Descriptive Study." *BMC Women's Health* 17 (95). https://doi.org/10.1186/s12905-017-0443-6.

Global Fund. 2019. *Technical Brief on HIV and Key Populations: Programming at Scale with Sex Workers, Men Who Have Sex with Men, Transgender People, People Who Inject Drugs, and People in Prison and Other Closed Settings.* Geneva: The Global Fund. https://www.theglobalfund.org/media/4794/core_key-populations_technicalbrief_en.pdf.

Jordan, John. 2016. "Artivism—Injecting Imagination into Degrowth." In *Degrowth in Movement(s): Exploring Pathways for Transformation*, edited by Corinna Burkhart, Matt hias Schmelzer and Nina Treu, 59–72. UK: Zero Books.

Louskieter, Lance, Marion Stevens, Dudu Dlamini, Asha George, and Shanaaz Munchi. 2021. "Co-production of Research with Sex Workers as a Political Act." *The BMJ Opinion,* February 16. https://blogs.bmj.com/bmj/2021/02/16/co-produc-tion-of-research-with-sex-workers-as-a-political-act.

Macleod, Catriona Ida, Siân Beynon-Jones, and Merran Toerien. 2017. "Articulating Reproductive Justice through Reparative Justice: Case Studies of Abortion in Great Britain and South Africa." *Culture, Health & Sexuality* 19 (5): 1–15. https://doi.org/10.1080/13691058.2016.1257738.

Muntingh, Lukas, and Kristen Petersen. 2015. *Punished for Being Poor: Evidence and Arguments for the Decriminalisation and Declassification of Petty Offences.* South Africa: Dullah Omar Institute & Pan-African Lawyers Union.

Rangasami, Jerushah, Tracey Konstant, and Stacey-Leigh Manoek. 2016. *Police Abuse of Sex Workers: Data from Cases Reported to the Women's Legal Centre Between 2011 and 2015*. Women's Legal Centre.

Ross, Loretta. 2020. "ICPD Through a Lens of Reproductive Justice." *YouTube Video*, 1:30, October 14. https://youtu.be/qEma4fPUeFA.

Ross, Loretta, and Ricky Solinger. 2017. *Reproductive Justice: An Introduction*. University of California Press.

Scheibe, Andrew, Marelise Richter, and Jo Vearey. 2016. "Sex Work and South Africa's Health System: Addressing the Needs of the Underserved." *South African Health Review* 1: 165–78. https://hdl.handle.net/10520/EJC189310.

Scorgie Fiona, Daisy Nakato, Eric Harper, Marlise Richter, Sian Maseko, and Prince Nare. 2013. "'We are despised in the hospitals': Sex Workers' Experiences of Accessing Health Care in Four African Countries." *Culture, Health & Sexuality* 15 (4): 450–65. https://doi.org/10.1080/13691058.2012.763187.

Smith, Molly, and Juno Mac. 2018. *Revolting Prostitutes: The Fight for Sex Workers' Rights*. London: Verso.

Stabile, Lua Da Mota. 2020. "Sex Work Abolitionism and Hegemonic Feminisms: Implications for Gender-Diverse Sex Workers and Migrants from Brazil." *The Sociological Review Monographs* 68 (4): 852–69. https://doi.org/10.1177/0038026120934710.

Stevens, Marion. 2021. "Sexual and Reproductive Health and Rights: Where is the Progress since Beijing?" *Agenda* 35 (2): 1–13. https://doi.org/10.1080/10130950.2021.1918008.

World Health Organisation. 2021. "Percentage of Most-at-Risk Populations (MARPs) Reporting use of a Condom in their Most Recent Sex." Accessed May 2021. https://www.who.int/data/gho/indicator-metadata-registry/imr-details/3129.

Chapter 2

Indigenous Sexual and Reproductive Justice in Aotearoa (New Zealand)

Mitigating Ongoing Colonial Harm in the Revitalisation of Māori Sexual Violence Prevention Knowledge, Expertise, and Practice

Jade Le Grice, Cheryl Turner,
Linda Waimarie Nikora, and Nicola Gavey

Sexual violence victimisation remains a pervasive Sexual and Reproductive Justice issue for Indigenous women globally (UNFPA and CHIRAPAQ 2018). In Aotearoa New Zealand, Māori (Indigenous) women are twice as likely to be impacted by sexual violence than other women (Fanslow et al. 2007), and it is estimated that around one-quarter of young Māori women have experienced some form of forced sex by the age of 18 (Clark et al. 2016). Research has also noted concern about non-consensual sex experienced by takatāpui[1] and vulnerability associated with being newly "out of the closet" within wider gay networks (Aspin et al. 2009). This issue is overlooked and overshadowed by dominant blaming discourses that suggest Māori youth are "problematic" (Moewaka Barnes 2010). Psychological impacts of sexual violence are often severe, wide ranging, potentially traumatising, and shape people's lives in complex ways (Gavey and Schmidt 2011; Le Grice 2017).

   The pervasive presence and extensive impact of sexual violence on Māori occur against a backdrop of individualising and cultural deficit explanations that blame Māori culture and individual victims (Le Grice 2019). The harms of historical and ongoing colonisation are oft denied in national narratives (O'Malley and Kidman 2018) and rarely understood in contextualising Māori experiences of sexual violence (Cavino 2016; Pihama et al. 2016). If unaddressed, sexual violence is a serious public health and social issue. Yet, racism pervades support and justice systems, preventing Māori from reaching out for assistance in contexts of interpersonal harm (Le Grice 2017). Meaningful, effective, and tailored interventions to support Māori are required to not only mitigate impacts and prevent further harm but to support the development of satisfying, safe sexualities and lives unhampered by negative psychological and relational impacts of sexual violence, thereby allowing victims and survivors to reach their full educational, economic, social, and whānau[2] potential.

Indigenous (Māori) self-determination in sexual violence prevention, intervention, and healing in Aotearoa New Zealand is facilitated by specialist practitioners and wider community investment in the well-being of current and future generations. While sociocultural, institutional, and material continuities in the perpetuation of colonial harm across generations remain, the cultural principle of whakapapa (ancestral connections) affirms Māori aspirations for the well-being of future generations. In this cultural context, the amelioration of sexual violence and associated impacts upon Māori is an important Reproductive Justice praxis. In this chapter, we report on a kaupapa Māori (Māori-led) qualitative interview-based study with 23 key stakeholders in sexual violence prevention. Drawing on a pūrakau[3] approach to analysis that invited reflexive elaboration, we explore tensions associated with recent gains to push back against the dominance of Eurocentric knowledge and systems of practice, and recentre forms of practice derived from Indigenous ways of knowing, being, and healing from colonial histories and contemporary sociocultural contexts. Drawing on our context in Aotearoa New Zealand, we argue that Indigenous self-determination of knowledges, expertise, and ability to enact and practice them is a crucial issue for Sexual and Reproductive Justice for Indigenous peoples.

THE IMPACT OF COLONIALISM IN SHAPING SOCIAL CONTEXTS OF SEXUAL VIOLENCE

The impact of settler colonialism on shaping social contexts that have rendered Māori vulnerable to sexual violence cannot be overstated. As Hayley Cavino (2016) writes:

> The accumulating factors of settler patriarchy, colonial knowledge systems, and land alienation produce a form of violence which manifests as a forced separation between people of Māori descent and the "content" of what it might actually mean to be Māori, including knowledge of our whakapapa, tikanga,[4] language, and ancestors—in short, our understanding of ourselves and our place in the world. (6–7)

While colonialism has gutted Māori ways of knowing and being from the corporeal realities of many Māori living in contemporary contexts, some of the specific drivers and causes of sexual violence have been more subtly shaped. The predominance of colonial notions of nuclear family at the expense of more expansive notions of whānau held by Māori has isolated victims from intergenerational networks of support through which the values that supported tikanga and relationships would be transmitted, and a perpetrator of sexual violence held to account (Cavino 2016; Kruger et al. 2004; Pitman 2013). Fluidity in gender norms was replaced by entrenched binarised gender roles within households and domestic settings, and economic stability was undermined by stolen land bases (King and Robertson 2017). An assault on the ingenuity, innovation, and economic base of our communities, particularly in the North of New Zealand, occurred through Crown violations of the relationship established with Māori through Te Tiriti o Waitangi[5] and He Whakaputanga[6] (Johnson 1996). Māori rangatiratanga[7] and governance across all aspects of our lives continue to be undermined by the government in terms of decision-making power, inequitable access to resources and services, and inequities in health, social, and justice system outcomes.

While colonisation disrupted connections between Māori people and Māori knowledge systems (Cavino 2016), the status of mātauranga Māori[8] has not always rested comfortably in the context of Eurocentric approaches to knowledge production as legitimated within the academy (Groot, Le Grice, and Nikora 2019; Ruru and Nikora 2021; Smith 1999). Yet, gains continue to be made in situating Māori knowledge bases anchored in traditional Māori approaches—as well as new Māori innovations—on equal footing with those derived from Eurocentric traditions and innovations (e.g., see Crocket et al. 2017; Kingi et al. 2018; Nairn et al. 2012; NiaNia, Bush, and Epston 2016; Waitoki and Levy 2016). Māori knowledge forms in sexual violence prevention and intervention have also been reinvigorated by sexual violence specialist practitioners (Te Wiata and Crocket 2017). Indeed, the support and retention of Māori sexual violence specialist academic and community researchers who are consolidating a knowledge base to support, extend, and develop Māori sexual violence prevention initiatives are important to a Sexual and Reproductive Justice agenda in Aotearoa New Zealand.

Existing sexual violence research with Māori has demonstrated how in the aftermath of sexual violence, meaning-making and giving testimony are often intertwined with the harms and impacts of settler colonialism (Cavino 2016; Ngā Kaitiaki Mauri 2015). For instance, like the violence of colonialism, sexual violence can disrupt whakapapa—the connective tissue between kinship groups and a collective consciousness that moves across time from the past, present, and future. It can disrupt cultural concepts that connect the individual's spirituality to the broader collective (Pihama et al. 2016).

Māori-derived therapeutic approaches often go beyond individualising, Eurocentric mainstream approaches of working solely with a victim-survivor, to instead include working with a whānau (see Te Wiata, Smith, and Crocket 2017). Therapeutic approaches may be oriented to individuals and whānau with a view to "repatriate whānau to their mana motuhake,[9] to their own greatness" (from Te Korowai Aroha o Aotearoa, cited in Ngā Kaitiaki Mauri 2015, 34) and recognising who they are, alongside the narrative of what has happened to them (Pitman 2013). Restoring cultural constructs can also be drawn upon as practice tools when working with whānau in the context of sexual violence. Further invigoration of Māori insights may be derived from Māori language terms that lattice psychological meaning and convey the depth of cultural significance of intertwined experiences of sexual and colonial violation (Kruger et al. 2004).

MĀORI SPECIALIST SEXUAL VIOLENCE
SERVICES AND COMMUNITY ENGAGEMENT

In Aotearoa New Zealand, *Te Ohaakii a Hine: National Network Ending Sexual Violence Together* (TOAHNNEST) is an organisation comprising sexual violence specialists who maintain a relationship with government, with a view to strengthen policy, research, practice, and programme evaluation. The organisation interweaves a range of initiatives and areas of intervention in the pursuit of ending sexual violence. It includes specialist representation from people working in sexuality education, therapists working with people who sexually harm, and therapists working with victims/survivors of sexual violence and their whānau. Across these domains are further areas of specialism including ameliorating violence against women and the unique needs of migrant, Pacific, men, queer survivors, and survivors with disabilities.

TOAHNNEST operates through a Tiriti o Waitangi partnership between Māori and Tauiwi,[10] allowing distinctive priorities and initiatives to be led from each caucus, as well as scope for collaborative projects and advocacy. This structure yields a space for *Nga Kaitiaki Mauri*, the Māori caucus of TOAHNNEST, to determine aspirations, processes, and actions that directly benefit Māori people, communities, and organisational structures. *Nga Kaitiaki Mauri* is engaged in vital work to increase recognition of colonising harms, harmful social norms, and practices as forms of violence that contribute to current high rates of sexual violence. *Nga Kaitiaki Mauri* also supports community engagement and capacity building to engage in sexual violence prevention and therapeutic practices that are sourced from mātauranga, tikanga, and te reo Māori (Ngā Kaitiaki Mauri 2015).

MĀORI SEXUAL AND REPRODUCTIVE JUSTICE

Addressing sexual violence and associated impacts on Māori is vital Reproductive Justice praxis. We might imagine ways to disrupt intergenerational trauma from sexual violence and intersecting harm created by colonisation to instead create pathways for Māori to be born into the world safe from harm. We might imagine thriving communities and well-resourced services. Yet, how do aspirations for Sexual and Reproductive Justice hold in the context of ongoing struggles for Māori self-determination in the context of ongoing colonialism?

Research documents this challenge in related sectors. In mental health services, for instance, a recent report based on a government enquiry identified several challenges faced by kaupapa Māori services. These included: (1) not being recognised and considered as legitimate in the context of Eurocentric health service provision, (2) having to work around Eurocentric, individualised, deficit, and illness focussed models of practice, (3) inequitable financial investment, and (4) existing service mechanisms constructing barriers to service access (Russell, Levy, and Cherrington 2018).

Similar issues are documented in services working with children and youth. Research has explored how sociocultural tensions impacting young Māori men coalesce in coercive and punitive engagements with health or forensic systems, rather than pathways that facilitate their self-determination into services that support them to well-being (Hamley and Le Grice 2021). Research into the state removal of Māori children from their whānau following assessed risk of harm highlights how removal exacerbates intergenerational colonial harm, is predicated on assessment tools far removed from Māori cultural contexts, *and* places children at risk of abuse in care (Tupaea 2020). Tupaea (2020, 46) points to "appropriations of mātauranga and tikanga Māori in state sanctioned practices, under the guise of biculturalism": the effect of invisible colonial norms that result in selective, strategic, and shallow utilisation of mātauranga Māori in structures of state care. The rhetoric of an equitable bicultural relationship between Māori and the Crown is merely a façade that pivots Māori people, knowledge, and culture on a Eurocentric axis.

Eradicating sexual violence is important Sexual and Reproductive Justice praxis that requires engaging with layered issues of colonisation, intergenerational trauma, and systemic bias against Māori who seek support for sexual violence. There are known tensions legitimating Māori knowledge in academic and institutional contexts, but what challenges are encountered by Māori sexual violence specialist practitioners and community engaged in sexual violence prevention?

METHODS

In this chapter, we report on data generated from a larger project supported by Cheryl Turner from Pakanae marae, funded by the *Health Research Council of New Zealand*. The project has progressed across three phases: (1) interviews with 23 key stakeholders, (2) interviews with 30 young Māori, and (3) development of a set of educational resources for Māori youth (underway) that addresses themes raised across each set of interviews. This chapter is based on data generated in the interviews with key stakeholders who were recruited through Jade's and Cheryl's networks in the Northland region of Aotearoa New Zealand.

A kaupapa Māori research methodology (Smith 1999) was utilised in the research conceptualisation and design, relational engagement with participants, and analyses of the study. This methodology informed an approach that sought to situate the issue of sexual violence within a colonial sociocultural context and to identify barriers and strategies for Māori self-determination in sexual violence prevention. Further, as kaupapa Māori research is Māori-led, the architecture of the research is informed by those who have been subject to colonisation, have been nurtured in Māori sociocultural contexts, and have lived experience of being Māori.

We sought views from a range of different people working in community settings who were involved in primary prevention of sexual violence through sexuality education and secondary and tertiary prevention through their work in supporting victims and survivors of sexual violence, their whānau, and the rehabilitation of those who had sexually violated or harmed another person. Interviews included nine clinicians, eight kaumātua,[11] two educators, three public servants, and five community volunteers; some participants had more than one role. The average participant age was 61 years, ranging from 35 to 80 years of age. Sixteen women and seven men were interviewed. Twenty-one of the participants were Māori and two were non-Māori who had been recommended by Māori in the community. However, all extracts reported in this article are from Māori participants.

Participants were engaged in the research through manaakitanga,[12] utilising a qualitative interview design, allowing dialog between an interviewer and participant to generate rich and detailed descriptions of participants' lived experiences and the meanings attributed to them (Denzin and Lincoln 2005). Semi-structured interviews allowed us to explore textures of possibilities, challenges, tensions, and opportunities derived from the sociocultural context the participants were speaking from across different topics of interest. We also note the potential for dialog to inform deeper conversation, where knowledge exchange can occur between researcher and participant, rather than a one-sided exchange. All the interviews were conducted between 2018 and 2019 by Jade who is Māori, from the tribes Ngāpuhi and Te Rarawa in the far North of New Zealand. She is a survivor of intergenerational trauma, childhood sexual abuse, rape, and intimate partner violence as a teenager (see Le Grice 2017). She is a member of *Nga Kaitiaki Mauri*, invested in improving outcomes for Māori victims of sexual violence, and preventing the occurrence of sexual violence, particularly for those in rural areas that are difficult to access.

A pūrakau approach was utilised in assembling and analysing the data (Lee 2009). The analysis was informed by Māori epistemology and ontology, as a kaupapa Māori project that takes Māori ways of knowing as the normative starting point for analysis (Moewaka Barnes 2000). Kaupapa Māori research may also be informed by critical theory (Hoskins and Jones 2017) that aims to delineate how colonisation and other vectors of marginality shape and constrain Māori agency (Le Grice 2017). Sociocultural contexts informed by Indigeneity and Coloniality are explored in the interpretation and analysis of stakeholders' contributions. Each participant's interview was analysed independent of the broader dataset by the first author, with analytic insights presented alongside selected extracts to participants in a summary report for their review (Nikora, Masters Awatere, and Te Awekotuku 2012). Participants were given the option to be named in relation to quoted extracts and contacted to confirm their approval after sighting quoted material in narrative context of the chapter. Participants whose interview extracts appear in this chapter are noted in order of appearance, in table 2.1.

In preparing the summary reports, participant interviews were transcribed verbatim, extracts relevant to sexual violence prevention selected and edited for readability, and checked for integrity in a holistic appraisal of their interview. These were structured by initial analytic codes that indicated how they might be utilised in analysis, and participants were given an option to review their summary report to ensure they were comfortable with the researcher's interpretations, and to allow reflexive elaboration (Tracy 2010). Through initial inductive analyses of participants' summary reports a clear thread became apparent about *how* participants' professional practice was often

Table 2.1   Participant Extracts, Names, and Details

Extract number	Name	Role	Gender
1	Phillipa Pehi	Clinician	Woman
2	Lorene Royal	Community volunteer	Woman
3	Penni Norman	Clinician and kaumātua	Woman
4	Sheree George	Educator	Woman
5	Kare (pseudonym)	Community volunteer	Woman
6	Penni Norman	Clinician and kaumātua	Woman
7	Michael Norman	Clinician and kaumātua	Man

curtailed in various ways. This initial insight shaped an abductive basis for the research question explored in this chapter, namely, how are the efforts of an Indigenous community engaged in sexual violence prevention marginalised or curtailed in a colonial context? How might academic knowledge production be complicit in this process?

RESULTS

This pūrakau (Māori narrative) outlines three broad areas where Indigenous approaches to sexual violence prevention are undermined: (1) curtailing Māori community agency in responding to sexual violence, (2) overlooking Māori innovators and expertise, and (3) disconnecting Māori ingenuity from originating people and place.

Curtailing Māori Community Agency in Responding to Sexual Violence

Under-resourcing of kaupapa Māori services was an issue in sexual violence specialist services, as also identified in mental health services (Russell, Levy, and Cherrington 2018). Phillipa Te Paea Pehi, a clinician, spoke about issues with workforce capacity to support people affected by sexual violence.

Extract 1, Phillipa Pehi (clinician, woman)
Up here, there's very few of us who are qualified and are accepted as qualified by ACC[13] to work with people. I feel, there's a lot more in our community, like [name of mutual connection]. You know? She'd be great! Does she have the qualifications to do the ACC work? No. [Pause] But those are the sort of people that have access, love, and care, and understand the cultural milieu and everything else. And they're the ones that get missed out all the time, because they don't have these bits of paper. And there's the burnout for those of us that are in it. So, there's so many levels of work, when you talk about prevention.

Speaking of issues with a lack of sexual violence specialist practitioners in a rural area, Phillipa also points to the capacity within the community: Māori with excellent skills could be supported by receiving further specialist training. Public funding for counselling for victims and survivors of sexual violence is available but contingent on the availability of specialised practitioners to deliver therapeutic approaches of this kind. While pathways have been recently created from iwi[14] practice-based qualifications to full accreditation, there remains further work to build capacity of the Māori specialist sexual violence practitioner workforce. Demand for sexual violence specialist practitioners in rural Northland remains, and access to important services may be hampered by long travel distances. Community members step into support roles and bear witness to narratives of sexual violence disclosures out of necessity or mahi aroha (work that is done for love) but are not often compensated and must manage this work alongside other responsibilities.

Like Phillipa quoted above (see extract 1), several participants spoke of the burden placed on the few sexual violence specialist practitioners in the area. This burden may result in burnout, compounded in contexts with few people in connecting support services and underfunded volunteer services. As stated by another participant, "The resources we have up there are very bloody limited without a doubt" (Woman, clinician). Another outcome is vicarious trauma resulting from the complexity of working with intergenerational colonial harm and the effects of sexual abuse and victimisation. This trauma may be intensified when understaffing means that practitioners have whānau connections to those they are working with.

Despite difficult, under-resourced contexts and limits imposed by Eurocentric approaches to sexual violence victim support, Māori self-determination in specialist and community approaches to sexual violence prevention is nevertheless forged. Meanwhile, broader national conversations about sexual violence can create further barriers to Māori self-determination. This is illustrated in the following quote in which Lorene Royal, a community volunteer, refers to the role played by the wider sociocultural context in which conversations about sexual violence occur.

Extract 2, Lorene Royal (community volunteer, woman)

An impact (perhaps intentional and indirect) of colonialism is that Māori are disenfranchised from ownership of the conversations and solutions in addressing sexual violation—at the heart of it is perhaps a "cultural" conflict and [the] hegemony of Western beliefs based on revenge and tepid, if anything, attempts at rehabilitation with the dominant society acting like there is no redemption—once a paedophile, always a paedophile.

Here, Lorene describes the politics of knowledge production and the privileging of dominant Eurocentric approaches in ways that overlook approaches preferred by Māori. For instance, she describes how the dominant retributive approach favoured by Eurocentric interventions often forecloses possibilities for rehabilitation. Māori sexual violence specialists and communities are often required to advocate for approaches that go beyond what is normatively considered realistic or desirable in mainstream discourse. Māori community agency and self-determination become critical to intervention and forging new pathways and possibilities that serve the needs of their communities.

While Sexual and Reproductive Justice foregrounds the importance of ensuring safe, violence-free lives, this extends to supporting Indigenous people's agency to lead the development and innovation of therapeutic approaches, knowledges, and policies that are responsive to the realities, concerns, and contexts of Indigenous people's lives.

Māori Innovators and Experts Overlooked

Despite being in high demand, thin on the ground, and facing demanding workloads, Māori specialist sexual violence clinicians described instances where their expertise was overlooked. This included specialists holding dual roles as kaumātua, with specialism in a clinical role alongside expertise and proficiency in mātauranga, tikanga, and te reo Māori.[15] Māori psychological models of practice are often invalidated in mental health settings in favour of individualised, deficit, and illness focussed models (Russell, Levy, and Cherrington 2018), which privileges a non-Indigenous workforce through a focus on clinical expertise (Pihama et al. 2018). This is also true within the context of specialist sexual violence practice, as indicated by clinician Penni Norman, in the following quote.

> *Extract 3*, Penni Norman (clinician, kaumātua, woman)
> That's something we're battling. Being Māori and working with Māori, we have different ways of working. We have different tools and models. Who defines what's best for Māori? Who determines what an expert is when you're working with Māori? That's my biggest gripe. Because you have all these psychiatrists, psychologists, psychotherapists who are not Māori . . . I think the biggest thing is not acknowledging Māori practitioners in the field, who are using our own therapeutic models. These are not really recognised.

Penni describes the prioritisation of non-Māori clinicians' assessment and evaluation of a Māori sexual violence survivor, as shaped by the complexities of colonisation, over and above a Māori clinician and kaumātua who has lived experience of this social context. In a similar vein, other participants spoke of requiring sign-off for work by a non-Māori clinical psychologist. Frequently, these clinicians had no training in Aotearoa New Zealand and were ignorant of Māori culture, knowledge, and colonisation, yet their decisions carried weight in ways that overrode the work of the Indigenous sexual violence specialist.

Similar issues arose for Māori specialist sexuality educators whose expertise (and specialist training overseas) was often overlooked in favour of outside and overseas colleagues, as described by educator, Sheree George, quoted below.

Extract 4, Sheree George (educator, woman)

There have been multiple occasions where my skillset has been overlooked in favour of others regarded as having more "expertise." For instance, I visited [an] institution to learn from a senior psychology advisor—yet the [workplace] then paid a woman from overseas with "expertise" to run a workshop, rather than recognise my knowledge to train colleagues. . . . I'm often not seen in relation to my full skillset, but rather, a particular skillset that fits a defined role. It seems like it isn't enough to prove you have skills in te ao Pākehā[16] but also te ao Māori,[17] and you can be overlooked for selection to senior management roles without fluency in te reo Māori.

Not only are Māori models of practice overlooked, but participants described how those with expertise and skills to develop and innovate these from a broader basis of mātauranga Māori are denied recognition of their talents in shaping positive therapeutic outcomes by colleagues and managers. While imported programmes are often valorised over locally derived initiatives (Pihama et al. 2018), even Māori who have been trained in these international modalities can have their "expertise" overlooked. This can have further intersectional implications. For instance, managers deny opportunities in organisations to Māori not fluent in te reo Māori. Yet, even those who are fluent and want to innovate therapeutic approaches on the basis of mātauranga, tikanga, and te reo Māori can be curbed by Eurocentric policies and decision-making that do not recognise the value in Māori work.

In this vein, some participants described how a marae setting was not endorsed as a space for therapeutic work with clients, curtailing the possibilities for working in an innovative and multidimensional way that carries deep and important cultural resonance and insights. Alongside this invalidation of Māori-informed practice to group-based facilitation, one participant, Kare (pseudonym), described how an outside sexual violence prevention service was funded to run a restorative justice programme that overrode prior kaupapa Māori work with a whānau.

Extract 5, Kare (community volunteer, woman)

I was involved as an observer as part of the group that I was working with at the time, this would have been about 4 years ago in a case were a young boy violated a young girl at a marae. At the time, they brought in sexual violence services from outside of the area to deal with the offender and the victim. And the kaupapa Maori services were still emerging here. So part of the group that I was working with, with the kuia,[18] had been working with the young man and his family over a period of time, and also the young girl's family, 'cause they were well known from the same community. The kuia made the comment at the end of the hui,[19] that we basically had non-Māori people coming in and not fully understanding the dynamics and the contexts we were working in and imposing a style of mediation or an attempt at restorative justice. And the kuia made the statement, if he [the boy] wasn't a paedophile before this, he certainly would become one if this continued. So, it was a complete and utter insensitivity or ineptness of the facilitator to see the relationships between the two families and who the key players were to effect healing. . . . It felt to me like it was a new industry about to break into the area and it was going to have a white face.

Kare contrasts the depth of the kuia's knowledge about the dynamics of a particular whānau and wider community and a healing-focussed approach, with the outside experts contracted to deliver an intervention without engaging her or others in a position to offer guidance. Living in a community across generations brings familiarity and understanding of whānau members, having seen children grow and become parents themselves. Here, an investment in the future well-being of these children goes beyond a service contract, moving from an awareness and memory of relatives who have passed on, and extending out into the whakapapa forever. Sexual and Reproductive Justice takes on new meanings in these complex, intergenerational whānau dynamics—and extends towards the capacity to hold space for Indigenous people to heal, individually, intergenerationally, and collectively.

Māori Ingenuity Disconnected from Originating People and Place through Cultural Appropriation

When Māori expertise and innovation were acknowledged by government or others, participants reported how this created further risks, worsening existing issues related to under-resourcing, and curtailing Māori agency. For instance:

Extract 6, Penni Norman (clinician, kaumātua, woman)
I think we're quite cautious too because of when we (Penni, husband Mike and Mere Naera) set up the idea of a One Stop Shop in the Hokianga [Northland], in the mid-90s. We called it that because we had all the services coming in, because there is no public transport out this way and people were getting fines. We knew the trends that were happening in our community, so we set up all these organisations. We had legal services, we had Māori land courts, we had WINZ [Work and Income New Zealand], we had *Child Youth and Family*, we had *Housing New Zealand*. So, we had all these organisations coming in on certain days for families to make appointments. Then the government heard about it, they came up and saw what we were doing and how well it was working. Well one of those people went back and set up *Heartlands* services and took all those services out of here and put them in places like Dargaville [Northland], under *Heartlands* service. That's why we don't like passing anything on to anybody.

While the success and positive outcomes of the work by Penni and her partner were acknowledged—such that it drew attention of the government—the net effect was the removal of the services for the community where the programme was developed. While some might consider national acclaim as an endorsement of capacity, standing, and ingenuity, the success and accolades were never able to be fully enjoyed by the innovators and their community. Their knowledge was simply transported to other contexts and the material reminder of their work abandoned and neglected by the government. This follows a historical pattern of Crown abandonment and neglect of Māori in rural Northland following Māori contestation of the Crown's violation of Te Tiriti o Waitangi and He Whakaputanga agreements (Johnson 1996) to support Māori rangatiratanga. It also raises issues of appropriation and theft of Māori intellectual property by the government and, as noted by Penni, curbs possibilities for wider collaboration that prioritises community needs in under-resourced contexts.

Penni's partner, Michael, describes another such incident. A school-based intervention in mātauranga Māori that he developed to support Māori youths' well-being was appropriated by an assessor from the Ministry of Education and adapted in ways that decontextualised it from its Indigenous foundations. Below he describes speaking to one of the assessors about what had happened.

Extract 7, Michael Norman (clinician, kaumātua, man)
They had these people there, including a Pākehā fulla [fellow/man] who was one of the assessors. I said to him, "I'll put it like this. I had my car stolen. The one who stole it, did it up, painted it, sold it on to someone else. They did the motor, painted it up, reconditioned it. About seven owners later it's a classic car, goes to shows and that." I said, "Now tell me, who owns that car?" He said, "Oh I knew you were going to say that." I said, "Who owns that car?" [pause] He knew. I own it.

Māori are able to create, initiate, and innovate. We are people with capability and potential. However, appropriation or *theft* of Māori property is a cornerstone of the colonial process and Crown assumption of sovereignty over Māori. National narratives continue to justify and excuse the violation of Māori in the development of the nation as we know it, denying the extent of harm, and labelling Māori "troublemakers" for seeking restoration of their status as afforded by Te Tiriti o Waitangi (Wetherell et al. 2015). While the appropriation of land, demographic swamping[20] (see Robson and White 1980 for an account of the first author's whānau), and warfare between Māori and the Crown (see Northern Wars, Johnson 1996) speak to issues related to historical and ongoing intergenerational impact, the legitimacy of Māori

concerns and dynamics of this relational violation remain present and enduring in the present day.

The appropriation of Indigenous knowledge, in ways that decontextual-
ise and remove it from those by/for whom it was developed, conforms to
Eurocentric engagement with Indigenous knowledge more generally. Value
is ascribed on the basis of how well this knowledge can be applied to an (in
this case New Zealand) assumed European subject. The ingenuity of Māori
practitioners is disregarded as is the genuine need for Māori people to have
approaches designed with and for them. The process of academic knowledge
production and journal articles that attribute expertise to academic authors
rather than shared among community further devalue the expertise and role
of Māori sexual violence specialist practitioners. This also entrenches power
in non-Indigenous expertise, particularly in professions of psychologists
and psychiatrists. Non-Indigenous clinicians are authorised to work with
Indigenous people over and above Māori sexual violence specialist practitioners, simply by claiming to have read about Indigenous knowledge, rather
than living and breathing the experience of *being* Indigenous. A key issue
for Sexual and Reproductive Justice for Indigenous peoples remains the self-
determination of their knowledges, expertise, and ability to enact and practice
them.

DISCUSSION

This article has presented a pūrakau, or Māori narrative, of the pressures and
challenges faced by Māori sexual violence specialist practitioners working
in a rural Northland community in New Zealand. While community services were generally under-resourced, and Māori sexual violence specialist
practitioners were thin on the ground, participants spoke to the untapped
potential for local Māori who had important and relevant skills, to be supported and trained or resourced to be part of the sexual violence prevention
workforce. Māori self-determination in this context is critical to mobilising
approaches and interventions that centre the validity and innovation of Māori
approaches to sexual violence prevention. Yet, Māori practitioners were
often undermined and overlooked in favour of those whose methods aligned
with Eurocentric understandings of expertise and knowledge. Despite local
insights, te reo, mātauranga, and tikanga Māori, Māori practitioners were
often side-lined in favour of overseas experts and those with titles such as
psychiatrists, psychologists, and psychotherapists by workplaces, and government policies.

Failing to value Māori specialists for who they are and the knowledge
they have innovated and developed risks appropriation and abstraction of

meaning from the people and communities who the knowledge genuinely belongs to. The abstraction of Indigenous knowledge from lived experience of Indigenous life has implications for the ways that it is written about, interpreted, analysed, and applied. In these situations, Indigenous expert practitioners who developed this knowledge may be overlooked or mistaken for "recipients" of the knowledge that the government holds itself as the "authority" over. The abstraction of Māori words from Māori people, communities, and land further exacerbates a sense that we Indigenous people are interchangeable in the eyes of the Crown; this is particularly risky when the specific domains and skillsets for sexual violence prevention become subsumed across broad domains of health, education, social, or justice systems.

To avoid the dangers of appropriation, it is crucial to attribute and situate Indigenous knowledge in relation to the people and places it originates, and by whom this is innovated. The methodology of the present study, located within a specific region of Aotearoa New Zealand, offers a process that *can be* attentive to protecting and safeguarding written accounts of Indigenous knowledge. However, how do we ensure Indigenous rangatiratanga (chieftainship/authority) over these knowledges and theories in policy and practice? How do we understand and genuinely honour Indigenous expertise? While there has been a recent "turn" to situate mātauranga Māori as a core aspect of being and doing research and therapeutic practice in Aotearoa New Zealand, there remains further work to dismantle existing colonial tensions that undermine Māori agency and self-determination in regard to how this is put into practice to further Sexual and Reproductive Justice. We may see initiatives that appear to be a step in the right direction on the surface—but how do we ensure this progress does not become easily deployed in ways that go against any semblance of the intent? How are the government's standards for engaging with mātauranga Māori evaluated? Who evaluates the government on their ability to honour their relationship as a Tiriti partner to Māori? With an ongoing denial and minimisation of the government's own complicity in the marginalisation of Māori, what kind of message does that send for those working to alleviate the harms of sexual violence in a colonised world? While colonial histories and ongoing harms are uniquely situated and configured across different global contexts, Reproductive Justice demands that we take Indigenous leadership and self-determination seriously in the pursuit of protecting future generations of Indigenous people from sexual violence.

NOTES

1. Māori who identify with diverse genders, sexes, and sexualities.
2. Extended family, networks aligned by kin, friendship, or purpose.

3. Māori narrative approach.

4. Traditional practices.

5. Te Tiriti o Waitangi was signed in 1840 by Māori leaders and representatives of the British Crown. This guaranteed Māori undisturbed rights to access resources and sovereignty over their own people. See Healy, Huygens, Murphy (2012) *Ngāpuhi Speaks* for a fuller account.

6. The Declaration of Independence of the United Tribes of New Zealand was signed between 1835 and 1839 by Māori leaders, asserting Māori sovereign power and authority over land in Aotearoa New Zealand.

7. Māori collective self-determination.

8. Māori approaches to knowledge, situated in terms of people and place.

9. Sovereign authority.

10. Non-Māori.

11. Esteemed Māori elders who hold important roles and responsibilities within the Māori world.

12. Practices that enhance the mana of another person or people, such as hospitality and care practices.

13. Accident Compensation Corporation funds counselling for those affected by sexual violence.

14. Large kin-based grouping across a geographical region.

15. Māori language.

16. The world of New Zealand European people.

17. The Māori world.

18. Woman elder.

19. Gathering, meeting.

20. This occurs when one or more cultural groups reproduce individuals faster than other groups in the region.

REFERENCES

Aspin, Clive, Paul Reynolds, Keren Lehavot, and Jacob Taiapa. 2009. "An Investigation of the Phenomenon of Non Consensual Sex among Māori Men who have Sex with Men." *Culture, Health & Sexuality* 11 (1): 35–49. https://doi.org/10.1080/13691050802483711.

Cavino, Hayley M. 2016. "Intergenerational Sexual Violence and Whānau in Aotearoa/New Zealand: Pedagogies of Contextualisation and Transformation." *Sexual Abuse in Australia and New Zealand* 7 (1): 4–17. https://search.informit.org/doi/10.3316/informit.201458129469255.

Clark, Terryann C., Mathijs F. G. Lucassen, Theresa Fleming, Roshini Peiris-John, Amio Ikihele, Tasileta Teevale, Elizabeth Robinson, and Sue Crengle. 2016. "Changes in the Sexual Health Behaviours of New Zealand Secondary School Students, 2001–2012: Findings from a National Survey Series." *Australian and New Zealand Journal of Public Health* 40 (4): 329–36. https:// doi.org/10.1111/1753-6405.12543.

Crocket, Kathie, Eugene Davis, Elmarie Kotzé, Brent Swann, and Huia Swann, eds. 2017. *Moemoeā: Māori Counselling Journeys*. Auckland: Dunmore Publishing Ltd.

Denzin, Norman, and Yvonna Sessions Lincoln, eds. 2005. *The Sage Handbook of Qualitative Research*, 3rd ed. London: Sage.

Fanslow, Janet, Elizabeth E. Robinson, Sue Crengle, and Lana Perese. 2007. "Prevalence of Child Sexual Abuse Reported by a Cross-Sectional Sample of New Zealand Women." *Child Abuse & Neglect* 31 (9): 935–45. https://doi.org/10.1016 /j.chiabu.2007.02.009.

Gavey, Nicola, and Johanna Schmidt. 2011. "'Trauma of Rape' Discourse: A Double-Edged Template for Everyday Understandings of the Impact of Rape?" *Violence Against Women* 17 (4): 433–56. https:// doi.org/10.1177/10778012114 0419.

Groot, Shiloh, Jade Le Grice and Linda Waimarie Nikora. 2019. "Māori psychology, Aotearoa New Zealand." In *Asia-Pacific Perspectives on Intercultural Psychology*, edited by W. Li., K. H. Foo, and D. Hodgetts, 198–217. London: Routledge.

Hamley, Logan, and Jade Le Grice. 2021. "He Kākano Ahau – Identity, Indigeneity and Wellbeing for Young Māori (Indigenous) Men in Aotearoa/ New Zealand." *Feminism and Psychology* 31 (1): 62–80. https://doi.org/10.1177 /0959353520973568.

Healy, Susan, Ingrid Huygens, and Takawai Murphy. 2012. *Ngāpuhi Speaks: He Whakaputanga and Te Tiriti o Waitangi: Independent Report on Ngāpuhi Nui Tonu Claim*. Kaitaia: Te Kawariki.

Hoskins, Te Kawehau, and Alison Jones, eds. 2017. *Critical Conversations in Kaupapa Māori*. Auckland: Huia Publishers.

Johnson, Ralph. 1996. *The Northern War 1844-1846*. An Overview Report Commissioned by the Crown Forestry Rental Trust.

King, Pita, and Neville Robertson. 2017. "Māori Men, Relationships, and Everyday Practices: Towards Broadening Domestic Violence Research." *AlterNative: An International Journal of Indigenous Peoples* 13 (4): 210–17. https://doi.org/10 .1177/1177180117729850.

Kingi, Te Kani, Mason Durie, Hinemoa Elder, Rees Tapsell, Mark Lawrence, and Simon Bennet. 2018. *Maea te Toi Ora: Māori Health Transformations*. Wellington: Huia.

Kruger, Tāmati, Mereana Pitman, Di Grennell, Tahuaroa McDonald, Dennis Mariu, Alva Pomare, Teina Mita, Matehaere Maihi, and Keri Lawson-Te Aho. 2004. *Transforming Whānau Violence: A Conceptual Framework, Second Edition*. Wellington: Second Māori Taskforce on Whānau Violence.

Le Grice, Jade. 2017. "Exotic Dancing and Relationship Violence: Exploring Indigeneity, Gender and Agency." *Culture, Health & Sexuality* 20 (4): 367–80. https://doi.org/10.1080/13691058.2017.1347962.

———. 2019. "Indigenous Stakeholder Narratives of Sexual Violence in Colonial Contexts: Deconstructing Ongoing Suppression and Silence in an era of #Metoo." Presentation at the 13th Biennial Conference of the Asian Association of Social Psychology, Academia Sinica, Taipei, Taiwan, July 12.

Lee, Jenny. 2009. "Decolonising Māori Narratives: Pūrākau as a Method." *MAI Review* 2 (3): 1–12. http://www.review.mai.ac.nz/mrindex/MR/article/download /242/242-1618-1-PB.pdf.

Moewaka Barnes, Helen. 2000. "Kaupapa Māori: Explaining the Ordinary." *Pacific Health Dialog* 7 (1): 13–16. http://pacifichealthdialog.org.fj/Volume207/No1 20Maori20Health20in20New20Zealand/Original20Papers/Kaupapa20maori20exp laining20the20ordinary.pdf.

———. 2010. *Sexual Coercion, Resilience and Young Māori: A Scoping Review*. Auckland: SHORE and Whariki Research Centre, Massey University.

Nairn, Raymond, Phillipa Pehi, Roseanne Black, and Waikaremoana Waitoki, eds. 2012. *Ka Tu Ka Oho: Visions of a Bicultural Partnership in Psychology*. Wellington: New Zealand Psychological Society.

Ngā Kaitiaki Mauri. 2015. *Ngā Kaitiaki Mauri Primary Prevention Programme*. Wellington: Te Ohaakii A Hine: National Network Ending Sexual Violence Together.

NiaNia, Wiremu, Allister Bush, and David Epston. 2016. *Collaborative and Indigenous Mental Health Therapy: Tātaihono – Stories of Māori Healing in Psychiatry*. New York: Routledge.

Nikora, Linda Waimarie, Bridgette Masters Awatere, and Ngahuia Te Awekotuku. 2012. "Final Arrangements Following Death: Māori Indigenous Decision Making and Tangi." *Journal of Community and Applied Social Psychology* 22 (5): 400–13. https:// doi.org/10.1002/casp.2112.

O'Malley, Vincent, and Joanna Kidman. 2018. "Settler Colonial History, Commemoration and White Backlash: Remembering the New Zealand Wars." *Settler Colonial Studies* 8 (3): 298–313. https://doi.org/10.1080/2201473X.2017 .1279831.

Pihama, Leonie, Linda Tuhiwai Smith, Ngaropi Cameron, Tania Mataki, Hinewirangi Kohu, and Rihi Te Nana. 2018. "He Oranga Ngākau: Māori Approaches to Trauma Informed Care." Presentation at the 8th Biennial International Indigenous Research Conference, Auckland, New Zealand, November 16.

Pihama, Leonie, Rihi Te Nana, Ngaropi Cameron, Cherryl Smith, John Reid, and Kim Southey. 2016. "Māori Cultural Definitions of Sexual Violence." *Sexual Abuse in Australia and New Zealand: An Interdisciplinary Journal* 7 (1): 43–51. https:// search.informit.org/doi/10.3316/informit.20155129432556.

Pitman, Mereana. 2013. "2013 Symposium: Mereana Pitman." Presentation at Fostering Te Pā Harakeke: Health and Prosperous Families of Mana, Tauranga Moana, New Zealand, November 25-26.

Robson, Reitu and Paul White. 1980. *Te Whānau Harris*. Auckland: Direct Multi Print.

Ruru, Jacinta, and Linda Waimarie Nikora. 2021. *Ngā Kete Mātauranga. Māori Scholars at the Research Interface*. Dunedin: Otago University Press.

Russell, Lynne, Michelle Levy, and Lisa Cherrington. 2018. *Whakamanawa: Honouring the Voices and Stories of Māori who Submitted to the 2018 Government Inquiry into Mental Health and Addiction in Aotearoa*. Wellington: Unpublished report.

Smith, Linda Tuhiwai. 1999. *Decolonizing Methodologies: Research and Indigenous Peoples*. London: Zed Books.

Te Wiata, Joy, and Kathy Crocket. 2017. "Mana Wahine." In *Moemoeā: Māori Counselling Journeys*, edited by Kathie Crocket, Eugene Davis, Elmarie Kotzé, Brent Swann, and Huia Swann, 71–79. Auckland: Dunmore Press.

Te Wiata, Joy, Russell Smith, and Kathy Crockett. 2017. "Pūrakau Old and New, in the Context of Harm." In *Moemoeā: Māori Counselling Journeys*, edited by Kathie Crocket, Eugene Davis, Elmarie Kotzé, Brent Swann, and Huia Swann, 162–70. Auckland: Dunmore Press.

Tracy, Sarah. J. 2010. "Qualitative Quality: Eight 'Big-Tent' Criteria for Excellent Qualitative Research." *Qualitative Inquiry* 16 (10): 837–51. https://doi.org/10.1177/1077800410383121.

Tupaea, Morgan. 2020. *He Kaitiakitanga, He Māiatanga: Colonial Exclusion of Mātauranga Māori in the Care and Protection of Tamaiti Atawhai*. Unpublished Master's thesis, The University of Auckland, New Zealand.

United Nations Population Fund and Centre for Indigenous Cultures of Peru. 2018. *Recommendations of the UN Permanent Forum on Indigenous Issues Regarding Sexual and Reproductive Health and Rights and Gender Based Violence: Report on Progress and Challenges*. New York: United Nations.

Waitoki, Waikaremoana, and Michelle Levy, eds. 2016. *Te Manu Kai i te Mātauranga*: *Indigenous Psychology in Aotearoa*. Wellington: New Zealand Psychological Society.

Wetherell, Margaret, Tim McCreanor, Alex McConville, Helen Moewaka Barnes, and Jade Le Grice. 2015. "Settling Space and Covering the Nation: Some Conceptual Considerations in Analysing Affect and Discourse." *Emotion, Space and Society* 16, 56–64. https:// doi.org/10.1016/j.emospa.2015.07.005.

Chapter 3

Sexual and Reproductive Justice for Adolescents with Intellectual Disabilities

A Qualitative Study with Residential Facility Care Workers

Busisiwe Nkala-Dlamini and Sanele Twala

In 1994, the notion of reproductive rights as human rights entered the global agenda at the International Conference on Population and Development (ICPD). The definition of reproductive healthcare and its provisions by the World Health Organisation (WHO) has also broadened its focus from fertility control through access to contraception and abortion. These developments signify a fundamental shift away from the focus on population control, specifically, regulations concerning women's fertility, to acknowledging the importance of people's reproductive autonomy and human rights (WHO, 1995). Building on the momentum of this conceptualisation of reproductive rights, Reproductive Justice proponents advocated for the right not to have a child, to have a child under conditions of one's choosing, and to parent in safe and healthy environments (Ross 2017).

Understandings of sexual health have also undergone a significant shift. Thus, understandings of sexual rights and policies on healthcare provision have broadened beyond the prevention of negative outcomes of sexual interaction and sexual dysfunction, to include the recognition of sexual autonomy (being able to decide if and when sex takes place), access to sexuality information and education, and the notion that sexual experiences should be pleasurable, and free from coercion, discrimination, and violence (Armas 2007).

Despite these advancements, however, serious concerns regarding the implementation of these policies and the provision of certain sexual and reproductive health services (SRHS) remain. Globally, marginalised groups continue to face barriers to the realisation of their sexual and reproductive rights, including being denied access to sexual and reproductive healthcare. Thus, despite the recognition of adolescents' sexual and reproductive health rights at the 1994 ICPD conference and that concerted efforts are needed to ensure their sexual and reproductive health, adolescents continue to face a range of obstacles to attaining sexual and reproductive health, including societal beliefs that continue to stigmatise adolescents' sexuality and reproduction (Braeken and Rondinelli 2012). Similarly, research on the sexual and reproductive healthcare experiences of persons with disabilities reveals that disabled people are marginalised in the design and implementation of sexual and reproductive health programmes and service delivery (Mohamed and Shefer 2015), despite the United Nations Convention on the Rights of Persons with Disabilities recognising the sexual and reproductive health needs and rights of persons with disabilities (UN 2006). This marginalisation is the result of societal beliefs about disability that fail to recognise disabled people's sexual and reproductive rights.

SEXUAL AND REPRODUCTIVE HEALTH IN SOUTH AFRICA: ADOLESCENTS AND PEOPLE WITH DISABILITIES

The Constitution of the Republic of South Africa (1996) has been hailed for its principles of non-discrimination based on disability, gender, or age; gender equality; equality of opportunity; accessibility; respect for diversity; and full inclusion in society. Efforts to achieve this with regard to disabled persons include a specific focus by the Ministry of Women, Children, and Persons with Disabilities on the promotion of inclusivity, as described in the National Disability Strategy (Department of Social Development (DSD) 2015a, 2015b). The National Adolescent Sexual and Reproductive Health and Rights Framework Strategy provides that adolescents can access SRHS independently (DSD 2015c).

Yet, significant health inequities persist in democratic South Africa, despite the equal rights assigned to all citizens and despite constitutional provisions for ensuring non-discrimination and inclusion. Indeed, South African research on adolescents' and persons living with disabilities' access to and experiences of sexual and reproductive healthcare align with international trends. This was indicated in a mixed-methods study by Hunt et al. (2017) which found that non-disabled people perceived persons with physical disabilities as having fewer sexual and reproductive rights and gaining less benefit from sexual and reproductive services than persons without disabilities. For youth with disabilities, this may be compounded by the widespread stigmatising of teenage sexuality that leads to adolescents being denied SRHS (Wood & Jewkes, 2006).

South African studies have identified the stigmatisation of adolescents and adult women with intellectual disabilities (Meer & Combrimck, 2015). In their study with caregivers, Kahonde, McKenzie, and Wilson (2019) identified that stigmatisation is influenced by caregivers' protectionist stance. Thus, in the caregivers' endeavour to protect persons within their care, they may prioritise security and well-being over the sexual and reproductive rights of adults with intellectual disabilities (Kahonde, McKenzie, and Wilson 2019; McKenzie, McConkey, and Adnams 2014).

Adding to the aforementioned literature that focusses on the rights of adults with intellectual disabilities in their family's care or in residential care facilities, our chapter uses data collected from healthcare providers working with adolescents with intellectual disabilities in a residential care facility in South Africa to demonstrate the multiple barriers to sexual and reproductive healthcare and services and the realisation of sexual and reproductive rights faced by adolescents with disabilities. We argue that to uphold the inherent dignity of persons with intellectual disabilities, their fundamental freedoms and their right to enjoy equal access to sexual and reproductive rights, and, importantly, their self-determination in whether and when to exercise these rights, must be supported. We conclude with recommendations for how this can be achieved in residential care facilities for persons with intellectual disabilities in South Africa.

Defining Disability

Despite tendencies to group disabled persons into a homogenous category, disabilities vary and include visual, physical, hearing, emotional, communication, and intellectual/learning disabilities (DSD, DWCPD, and UNICEF 2012) (STATSSA 2014). People's sexual and reproductive experiences may differ according to their disability and the different social meanings attached to their disabilities (Mohamed and Shefer 2015). For example, while people with physical disabilities are often understood as asexual, those with intellectual disabilities are believed to be pathologically "hypersexual" and/or asexual.

Different ways of understanding disability also impact the treatment and experiences of disabled persons. These models include human rights (alluded to earlier), diversity, charity, medical, and social models. In the charity model, disabled people are understood as vulnerable and in need of protective caretaking (from non-disabled people) but may also be understood as a threat from which others must be protected (Jackson 2018).

The medical model constructs disability as a pathology to be treated through medical interventions. This model is evident in the common practice of persons with intellectual disabilities, especially in residential placements, being identified and diagnosed using the Diagnostic and Statistical Manual of Mental Disorder's (DSM-5) diagnostic criteria for intellectual disability (American Psychiatric Association 2013).

The social model understands the manner in which society responds to persons with disabilities as the disabling factor (Swartz 2012). Therefore, as Burns-Lynch, Salzer, and Baron (2011) maintain, the impairment alone is not sufficient for disablement to occur. The social model aims to transform society by creating conditions that are necessary for people with disabilities to be included and participate in society (Mohamed and Shefer 2015). Extensions of the social model understand that both societies and disabilities may be disabling and/or enabling (Shakespear 2013). In analysing the data from our study and current literature, we believe that using a human rights lens can positively transform societal attitudes towards young people with intellectual disabilities and contribute to creating the conditions necessary to meet their reproductive and health needs in residential care facilities.

Below, we describe the study on which this chapter is based. In the subsequent section, we present our findings where we show that providers' understandings and practices related to sexual and reproductive healthcare provision for residential care-based adolescents with intellectual disabilities are informed by societal meanings attached to adolescence and intellectual disability. We argue that providers' understandings and practices suppress the sexuality and reproductive freedom of the adolescents with intellectual disabilities in their care.

OUR STUDY

Our study sought to explore the perceptions and practices of healthcare providers in the provision of sexual and reproductive healthcare services to adolescents with intellectual disabilities in a residential care facility in Johannesburg, South Africa. As non-disabled researchers, our engagement in the study was influenced by our passion for the sexual and reproductive rights of young people and our social work conviction to respect the rights of individuals to self-determination irrespective of their dis/ability or social status. The first author has been involved in SRHS provision for young people and has a strong conviction that there is a need to change the existing social injustices within the society by disrupting the societal norms which hinder the rights of young people to have enjoyable sexual and reproductive lives, and this includes adolescents with intellectual disabilities.

To be eligible to participate in the study, volunteers had to have worked at the facility for at least a year and be over 18 years old (the majority age in

South Africa). The 10 participants include medical and non-medical person-nel aged between 29 and 59 and who, at the time of the study, had worked in the facility from 18 months up to 18 years. The participants' work involved providing residential or home-based care for persons with intellectual dis-abilities—which includes assisting with daily tasks such as bathing, dressing, and meals—and/or doing administrative work (e.g., oversight, coordination). Seven participants were female and three were male, nine identified as Black and one identified as Coloured.

Ethics approval was granted by the Human Research Ethics Committee (Non-Medical) of the University of the Witwatersrand prior to commence-ment of data collection. Data were collected via semi-structured interviews conducted by the second author, Sanele. The interviews were conducted in English, in which all participants were conversant as their second or third language. The data were analysed using the six phases of thematic analysis outlined by Braun and Clarke (2006).

FINDINGS

The following themes were generated in our analysis: (1) "They are disabled so they can't decide": choosing on behalf of young people, (2) "There is no need for information because they do not have an understanding": regulating sexual and reproductive information, and (3) "We do not allow that here at the home": coercive contraceptive provision and sterilisation. We discuss each of these in turn.

(1) "They are disabled so they can't decide": Making Decisions on Behalf of Young People with Intellectual Disabilities.

Self-determination is related to freedom and autonomy. Akbar (2011) adds that it denotes that individuals qualify to make their own decisions. In social work practice, self-determination emphasises a collaboration of cli-ent's choices and decisions by empowering clients through identifying their strengths (Taylor 2006). In residential care facilities, it is common for deci-sions to be taken on behalf of persons with intellectual disabilities. Some residents are either orphaned or abandoned, and the residential care facility functions as their legal guardian, making decisions concerning their well-being. Residents whose families have placed them in residential facilities are still under the care of the facility and may still have decisions made on their behalf.

In our study, healthcare providers' data point to the ways in which they make decisions on residents' behalf. Although care providers understood

their practices as the result of good intentions, contextualised by the victimisation that people with disabilities face, providers' practices may also
be shaped by negative perceptions of intellectually disabled adolescents as
unable to act in their own interests. Thus, in our data, care providers take
control of the sexual and reproductive health of the adolescents with intellectual disabilities in their residential care, while excluding them from decision-
making. The following are examples of the justifications healthcare providers
gave for their interventions.

> *Extract 1*, *Participant #2* (female, 31 years old, Black, 1 year as healthcare
> provider)
> Remember they are disabled so they can't decide.

> *Extract 2*, *Participant #4* (female, 57 years old, Black, 30 years as healthcare
> provider) We have mentally and physically handicapped children. So, what we
> do is just give them medication just to control their behaviour.

> *Extract 3*, *Participant #2* (female, 31 years old, Black, 1 year as healthcare pro-
> vider) They are together in the dining hall only, where there is the kitchen and
> they eat. As for when it is time to sleep there's a boys' side and a girls' side. So,
> they are safe. Cameras all over. Housemother and staff is there 24/7.

In extracts 1 and 2 the care providers claim that the adolescents in their care
are not capable of making their own decisions about their sexual health needs.
In addition to the individual care providers' own understanding and practices,
of importance are the policies and living arrangements that enforce provider's
understandings that adolescents with intellectual disabilities in this residential
care facility on the one hand are not capable of safely self-directing their sexuality and on the other hand need to be protected from sexual victimisation.
Hence, decisions are taken on their behalf, making the residential care facility a protective space that nevertheless controls the freedom of adolescents
with disabilities and reinforces the existing perceptions and practices by care
providers, as shown by reference to gender-segregated facilities.

According to the care providers, the structural arrangement serves to keep
the adolescents with intellectual disabilities "*safe.*" Here the participants construct the sexuality of youth with intellectual disabilities as a source of vulnerability on the one hand and a potential threat on the other, thereby requiring
protection from (sexual) harm. By making reference to the adolescents as
"children," providers' use of language correlates with how they view the adolescents in their care and already poses a barrier to them providing adequate
services. By constructing youth with intellectual disabilities as vulnerable,
providers are able to frame their practices within a charity model where,
as non-disabled adults, they protect the adolescents with intellectual disabilities. Thus, understandings of young people and people with intellectual

disabilities as needing protection and as incapable of self-determination are here heightened for adolescents with intellectual disabilities.

Over the past few years, in line with the Declaration of Alma-Ata (WHO 1978) to transform service delivery to people living with disabilities, to enhance their quality of life, and to ensure inclusion in sectors of society and participation (WHO 2011), there has been a call for persons with intellectual disabilities to have a normalised life experience. This includes their integration into the broader community.

In contrast to this, the placing of people with disabilities in institutional care has been argued as justified due to the prospect for protection that these institutions may offer from physical, sexual, and other kinds of abuse (WHO and United Nations Population Fund 2009). Indeed, disabled people are abused (including sexually) at rates higher than non-disabled people (Mohamed and Shefer 2015).

At the same time, persons with intellectual disabilities are often denied or restricted from actively making their own decisions regarding their life, health, sexual, and reproductive health, and the use of related services (Bleazard 2010). While this may in part be a protective measure, it is also made possible by the construction of intellectually disabled persons as asexual on the one hand and on the other as hypersexual and their sexual desires and expression as "dangerous," "threatening," and needing to be externally controlled (Mohamed and Shefer 2015). These practices and constructions may be evident in the policies of residential facilities themselves.

In the following extract, one of the care workers participating in this study relates how a parent challenged these practices and beliefs.

Extract 4, *Participant #4* (female, 57 years old, Black, 30 years as healthcare provider). So there was once a resident whom the parents felt that he must have a relationship. So, we thought okay, it's fine if you think this is not the place to be . . . it means that you must take your child out. And that mother did that because she thinks that her child needs to fall in love. She took her child out.

In the above extract, a mother who is a primary caregiver of an adolescent boy had a different approach to the protection of her son, one which was based on an understanding of her son as having sexual and romantic needs (although whether these needs were expressed by her son himself is unclear), and by positively viewing his sexuality. Furthermore, the mother's approach appears to be informed by an understanding of her son's agency. In contrast, the institution and care providers overlook these needs as well as the agency of adolescents with intellectual disabilities within their care to be self-directive regarding their sexual and reproductive health. Thus, in this instance, the mother understands the residential environment as negatively impacting adolescents with intellectual disabilities, rather than perceiving adolescents with intellectual disabilities as negatively impacting the environment. While the care provider does not openly disagree with the mother on the sexual needs of the adolescent in their care, she takes the position as per the policy of the institution.

Extract 5, Participant #3 (female, 41 years old, Black, 5 years as healthcare provider). He is a human being and he is active like everyone, like you and me. The only difference is that he is not allowed to do that here.

In the above quote, the healthcare provider acknowledges that adolescents with intellectual disabilities in their residential care are human beings, and subtly acknowledges that they are sexually active, but insists that adolescents with intellectual disabilities cannot be allowed to be sexually active in their care. Despite the care providers' recognition of the fact that adolescents with disabilities are sexual beings, residential policy was restrictive and informed by healthcare providers' own interpretation of the sexual needs, or lack thereof, of adolescents with intellectual disabilities. This demonstrates that a lack of engagement with the experiences of persons with disabilities leads to decisions about persons with disabilities being sought from experts who inform legislation (Bazzo et al. 2007) and not from adolescents with disabilities themselves (Jackson 2018).

Finally, healthcare providers explained that they availed themselves to make decisions on the residents' behalf, in order to protect the residents, as illustrated in the following quote.

Extract 6, Participant #9 (female, 35 years old, Black, 9 years as healthcare provider) You know what, because they are vulnerable, they are most vulnerable because people can take chances with them.

The care providers believe that their actions are meant to protect the intellectually disabled adolescents from (sexual) harm and victimisation. The practice of the care providers may therefore be shaped by the charity model as, through the practices they describe and their perceptions, they are positioned as non-disabled with a responsibility to protect the adolescents with intellectual disabilities in their care (Jackson 2018). While this is in part a protective measure against the targeted victimisation of disabled persons, by not respecting the adolescents' autonomy, right to self-determination, and right to privacy, they are inadvertently making intellectually disabled adolescents vulnerable and are themselves causing harm, as the next theme demonstrates.

(2)　"There is no need for information because they do not have an understanding": Regulating Sexual and Reproductive Information and Education

In accordance with their belief that adolescents with intellectual disabilities are incapable as earlier demonstrated, some care providers reported not providing any sexual and reproductive education to the residents, thus denying the right to education and information: "No, there is no need for education because they do not have an understanding." (Participant #4, female, 57 years old, Black, 30 years as healthcare provider). This is despite the fact that the Convention on the Rights of Persons with Disabilities gives individuals with intellectual disabilities the same rights to good sexual and reproductive health, as people without disabilities (UN 2006). These rights include the right to retain fertility, to relationships, family, and parenthood, and to education on reproduction and family planning in an age—and development—appropriate manner.

Healthcare providers participating in our study who reported that they *did* provide sexual and reproductive information and education suggested that whatever information they conveyed to the residents was limited and had to be carefully worded and "simplified." Furthermore, only information deemed to be "safe" was shared with the residents.

Extract 7, Participant #2 (female, 31 years old, Black, 1 year as healthcare provider)
No well, there needs to be a way that you approach them because their mind is not the same as mine. So even his understanding is not the same as mine. So, there is supposed to be a way of how I will approach the situation. I need to have a reason as to why I am telling him this

Extract 8, Participant #1 (male, 47 years old, Black, 9 years as healthcare provider). You know sometimes it's like what I said when you talk about it you need to be very cautious because to some of the residents it might happen that, OK, I am teaching them not to do this. To others, it's like you are preparing them

In extracts 7 and 8 above, it is notable that healthcare workers refer to sexual activity as "it," which may convey reluctance and awkwardness, even with the researcher, around discussing the sexual activity of adolescents with intellectual disabilities. Research conducted by Muserwa and Kasiram (2019) with people with disabilities and their care providers in two residential care facilities in South Africa demonstrated similar awkwardness by the care providers.

Providers' responses and practices rely on a medical discourse of understanding intellectual disability as deficit. This discourse does not recognise the capacities of disabled persons nor that the environment may be a disabler. Thus, providers in our own study did not seem to recognise their practices as hindering the inclusion and participation of adolescents with intellectual disabilities, *as* sexual beings, through the denial of access to sexual and reproductive information. Such information could have the potential of enabling residents to make informed decisions, including around their right to a safe and pleasurable sex life.

Although providers may believe that persons with intellectual disability are incapable of understanding sexual and reproductive information, a study conducted by Scheepers et al. (2005) revealed that one of the disparities in sexual and reproductive healthcare provision for persons with intellectual disabilities relates to communication. When a person with an intellectual disability communicates in ways that are not socially recognised or valued, staff untrained in alternative modes of communication may not be able to effectively impart information, nor understand what is being communicated (Scheepers et al. 2005). Therefore, barriers are created by society.

(3) "We do not allow that here at the home": Coercive Contraceptive Provision and Sterilisation

Persons with intellectual disabilities have been, and continue to be, subjected to practices to prevent and restrict childbearing, including compulsory and non-voluntary sterilisation and segregated institutionalisation (Ćwirynkało, Byra, and Żyta 2017).

In our study, participants reported that the main types of contraceptives used in the residential care facility were the injectable long-acting contraceptive *Depo-Provera* (a synthetic progestin used for numerous purposes, of which the most known is for pregnancy prevention) and the oral contraceptive pill. However, they were not voluntarily utilised by residents to prevent conception, but rather imposed for the coercive suppression and control of sexual behaviour and to coercively manage the residents' menstrual cycles, as described by one study participant.

Extract 9, Participant #1 (male, 47 years old, Black, 16 years as healthcare provider) So we refer the child to the sisters [professional nurses], and it is the sisters who will sit them down and counsel them and give them something. Whether it can be a depo [Depo-Provera] or whatever for prevention that they want to give to that particular child or maybe to reduce the sensation, you understand, so that they can calm down. The sisters are able to make the decision as to what they should give the children.

Extract 10, Participant #4 (female, 57 years old, Black, 30 years as healthcare provider)

Yes some are worse than others, so even those that are mild, they know the rule that we do not allow that here at the home. Anyway, depo is in our policy. Each and every resident, once we see you masturbating, we just put you on depo, then it suppresses it.

In extract 9, the care provider states that adolescents with intellectual disabilities are given Depo-Provera to reduce sexual desire. In the second quote the healthcare provider mentions that depo is given to inhibit masturbation. In both extracts, the care providers have constructed intellectually disabled adolescents' sexuality as a threat, out of control, and inappropriate, echoing research findings by Muswera and Kasiram (2019). In Muserwa and Kasiram's study, residents reported receiving contraceptives but may not have had full knowledge on why these were being administered, nor was it clear that they had a choice on whether to use them. Importantly, Carlson and Wilson (2000) draw attention to the fact that the ethical implications of non-consensual use of Depo-Provera on men are often disregarded. In contrast, coercive administering of Depo-Provera to non-disabled (cis) women has been challenged.

Persons with intellectual disabilities are often regarded as asexual as their sexuality is either overlooked or actively suppressed (Bleazard 2010). In Mavuso's (2013) study, individuals with disabilities reported that healthcare workers would often advise them to be sterilised instead of supporting them to explore other available contraceptive methods. Similarly, participants in our study described the coercive sterilisation of adolescents with intellectual disabilities, as shown below.

Extract 11, Participant #8 (male, 50 years old, 15 years as healthcare provider)
There are some of the girls who are sterilised. And it is their parents who decide for them. Many parents prefer their child to be sterilised. But many doctors will say no to do that because it is the child who needs to take that decision. What is done the day they want children?

In the quotation above, and in contrast to Mavuso's (2013) study, the participant describes how healthcare professionals refuse to coercively sterilise adolescents with intellectual disabilities. This refusal is due to considering the long-term consequence of coercively administering the intervention. Here, parents' attempts to coercively sterilise their adolescent girls with intellectual disabilities deny them the choice to ever have a child, a point alluded to by the participant in the extract above. Indeed, during interviews some of the residents in Muserwa and Kasiram's (2019) study expressed their desires to have children one day.

CONCLUDING DISCUSSION

This study explored residential care workers' perceptions and organisational policy and practices related to the sexual and reproductive health needs of adolescents with intellectual disabilities. The findings of our study map two broad categories of barriers to accessing SRHS and rights for adolescents with intellectual disabilities living in a residential care facility. Our findings identified a gap between providers' perceptions of the needs of persons with intellectual disabilities versus what these needs may be, the services available in residential facilities, and their rights to access these services. Thus, residential care facility policies around surveillance monitoring by cameras, the separation of male and female dormitories, policy on injecting Depo-Provera to suppress sexual behaviour, and withholding of information on sexual and reproductive health, together with the healthcare providers' coercive practices were implicated in this gap. The study suggests that healthcare providers lack the knowledge (and perhaps may also lack the necessary support) to provide adequate SRHS to persons with intellectual disabilities. We argue that the guiding policies and the norms and the practices by healthcare providers are all examples of sexual and reproductive injustice.

Ćwirynkało, Byra, and Żyta (2017) note that healthcare providers' language and beliefs towards persons with intellectual disability and their sexuality can either act as a barrier or a facilitator to accessing SRHS. In our study, the healthcare providers' communication and beliefs regarding adolescents with intellectual disabilities and seeing residents as "children" instead of services users present a barrier to adequate sexual and reproductive healthcare provision.

Our data point to healthcare providers' failure to recognise and uphold residents' right to self-determination, demonstrated by undermining the capacity of adolescents with intellectual disabilities to have control over and to direct their own lives (Servais 2006). This is despite the fact that the right to self-determination is a key tenet of human rights treaties, policies, and legislation, such as the Constitution of the Republic of South Africa (1996). However, despite the progressive nature of these instruments, adolescents with intellectual disabilities in this residential facility remain vulnerable to systemic inequality and oppressive practices in terms of SRHS and decision-making. Parents and guardians often decide to sterilise without their consent and without informing the person concerned. Although a common reason provided for the sterilisation of persons with disabilities is to better manage menstruation (Servais 2006), this stance may promote ignorance in society and does not take into consideration the right of persons with intellectual disabilities to self-determination.

In addition, our findings reveal how normative constructions of intellectual disabilities underpinned and affected the provision of SRHS to adolescents with intellectual disabilities. Thus, in providers' own understandings of disability, and their practices and residential care policies, their description of disability was largely understood through a medical perspective which ignores the interaction of people with their environment, constructing disability as necessarily disabling, and adolescents with intellectual disability as incapable of safely expressing their sexuality. Thus, the residential care facility environment has been structured such that boys' and girls' dormitories are separated. This creates a physical barrier to freedom of association which forms part of sexual and reproductive health, as sexual and reproductive health involves relationships and interaction among people. As stated by (Swartz 2012), impairment alone is not sufficient for disablement to occur, but social exclusion can be disabling as well (Shakespear 2013). Indeed, the response of society, which has constructed normalcy as non-disability and disability as pathology and abnormality, contributes to disablement (Davis 2017).

On the one hand, myths and stigmatisation of the sexuality and reproduction of adolescents with intellectual disabilities informed practices and policies at the residential care facility. Thus, in our study, young adolescents with intellectual disabilities were constructed as asexual and incapable of understanding sexuality information. Their sexual desires and expression were also constructed as a threat and needed to be tightly and forcibly controlled and inhibited. Where the young persons with intellectual disabilities did express their sexual desires, they were construed as hypersexual and the healthcare workers described their role as necessarily including the coercive administering of Depo-Provera, with the intention of suppressing residents' sexual feelings and expression thereof. Thus, these normative understandings of intellectual disabilities and adolescence systematically categorise adolescents with intellectual disabilities as not deserving the right to sexual and reproductive health or to be educated, enabling a gross violation of their human rights and sexual and reproductive justice.

On the other hand, some of the organisational policy and practices, and providers' perceptions of residents in their care, may also have been informed by knowledge of the victimisation experienced by disabled persons. Thus, it must be acknowledged that policy and practice may, through protective measures, have in part served to uphold residents' rights to freedom from sexual violence. And since sexual violence may result in undesired pregnancy, healthcare providers may also have been acting to ensure intellectually disabled adolescents' right to *not* have children, which may be undermined through this violence. Societal changes are therefore needed to stop these patterns of victimisation and denial of rights. At the same time, residential care providers must be supported to uphold the *full* sexual and reproductive rights of those in their care, guided by residents' own desires and their right to self-determination.

Research has demonstrated that access to sexual and reproductive health-care services is stalled mainly by the marginalisation of persons with intellectual disabilities (Hunt et al. 2017). For example, research conducted elsewhere in South Africa shows persons with disabilities' lack of access to sexuality education, which, in addition to beliefs about adolescence and disability may also be due to facilities' lack of access to funding and resources. Indeed, McKenzie, McConkey, and Adnams' (2014) case study of residential care facilities for adults with intellectual disabilities in the Western Cape found that sexuality education programs were available upon referral only at 19 (of 37) facilities and that managers reported minimal availability on a daily, weekly, or monthly basis. Our own findings show how at the residential care facility, persons with intellectual disabilities were subjected to intervention strategies that look to increase compliance and/or eliminate perceived "undesirable" behaviours, rather than intervention strategies that seek to educate residents with intellectual disabilities and support their self-determination, thus promoting sexual and reproductive justice. Addressing barriers faced by persons with intellectual disabilities in accessing SRHS will contribute to the fulfilment of their sexual and reproductive rights by supporting the self-fulfilment of their individual sexual and reproductive health needs.

The rights-based approach focusses on the human rights of adolescents with intellectual disabilities. Sexual and reproductive health is a human right and concerns the right to make decisions about one's life, including the right to sexual health, sexuality information, the choice of whether to have sex, the right to safe and pleasurable sex, freedom from sexual violence, and to choose whether to have children. Unmet sexual and reproductive rights of adolescents in residential care, therefore, equate to the denial of human rights.

The rights-based approach places the responsibility on duty bearers to fulfil their obligations (Ife 2012). Consequently, healthcare workers, as duty bearers, are responsible for fulfilling their obligations to young persons with intellectual disabilities, who are rights holders. It is also the obligation of government and society to ensure suitable conditions for one to implement one's sexual and reproductive decisions (Ross 2017a).

The rights-based approach also looks at the interplay between influences that could hamper equal access to and provision of services. Thus, the approach recognises that obstacles to sexual and reproductive health have major consequences that need to be effectively addressed. Our study demonstrates that this is evident in the treatment of young persons with intellectual disabilities who, in terms of their rights and utilisation of SRHS, are often overlooked or inhibited in residential care facilities.

Based on our findings, we recommend training and sensitisation of care providers around the sexual and reproductive health needs and rights of adolescents with intellectual disabilities. According to Lee et al. (2015), awareness and sensitisation training would challenge current service providers' misconceptions about sexuality and disability. Training should also include education about the communication styles and patterns to use with persons with intellectual disabilities. Changes in the language used to describe persons with intellectual disabilities may also strengthen healthcare providers' capacity to provide better quality SRHS to persons with intellectual disabilities (Lee et al. 2015). Furthermore, we propose including values clarification workshops to assist healthcare providers to interrogate their own values on embracing diversity and ensuring sexual and reproductive justice for the people they provide services and care to.

Lastly, the promotion of educational programmes is critical in supporting adolescents with intellectual disabilities in their right to make their own decisions regarding their sexual and reproductive health. It is a right that, throughout the years, has been denied by society to both young people and people with disabilities. And the denial of this right is a social injustice that should not be tolerated and should not be business as usual.

REFERENCES

Akbar, Ginneh L. 2011. "Child Welfare Social Work and The Promotion of Client Self Determination." DSW diss., University of Pensylvania. https://repository.upenn.edu/edissertations_sp2/28/.

American Psychiatric Association. 2013. *Diagnostic and Statistical Manual of Mental Disorders*. Washington: American Psychiatric Association. https://doi.org/10.1176/app.books.9780890425596.

Armas, Henry. 2007. *Whose Sexuality Counts? Poverty, Participation and Sexual Rights*. Institute of Development Studies Working Paper 294. Chichester: RPM Print & Design. https://opendocs.ids.ac.uk/opendocs/handle/20.500.12413/4150.

Bazzo, Giuseppe, Laura Nota, Salvatore Soresi, Lea Ferrari, and Patricia Minnes. 2007. "Attitudes of Social Service Providers Towards the Sexuality of Individuals with Intellectual Disability." *Journal of Applied Research in Intellectual Disabilities* 20 (2): 110–15. https://doi.org/10.1111/j.1468-3148.2006.00308.x.

Bleazard, Adele Venitia. 2010. "Sexuality and Intellectual Disability: Perspectives of Young Women with Disabilities." PhD diss., Cape Town: Univeristy of Stellenbosch. https://scholar.sun.ac.za/handle/10019.1/4006.

Braeken, Doortje, and Ilka Rondinelli. 2012. "Sexual and Reproductive Health Needs of Young People: Matching Needs with Systems." *International Journal of Gynecology & Obstetrics* 119 (S1): S60–S63. https://doi.org/10.1016/j.ijgo.2012.03.019.

Braun, Virgina, and Victoria Clarke. 2006. "Using Thematic Analysis in Psychology." *Qualitative Research in Psychology* 3 (2): 77–101. https://doi.org/10.1191 /1478088706qp063oa.

Burns-Lynch, Bill, Mark S. Salzer, and Richard Baron. 2011. *Managing Risk in Community Integration: Promoting the Dignity of Risk and Supporting Personal Choice.* Philadelphia: Temple University Collaborative on Community Inclusion of Individuals with Psychiatric Disabilities. http://tucollaborative.org/wp-content/uploads/2017/05/Managing-Risk-in-Community-Integration-Promoting-the -Dignity-of-Risk-and-Supporting-Personal-Choice.pdf.

Carlson, Glenys, Miriam Taylor, and Jill Wilson. 2000. "Sterilisation, Drugs Which Suppress Sexual Drive, and Young Men Who Have Intellectual Disability." *Journal of Intellectual and Developmental Disability* 25 (2): 91–104. https://doi .org/10.1080/13269780050033517.

Ćwirynkało, Katarzyna, Stanislawa Byra, and Agnieszka Żyta. 2017. "Sexuality of Adults with Intellectual Disabilities as Described by Support Staff Workers." *Hrvatska Revija Za Rehabilitacijska Istrazivanja* 53: 77–87. https://depot.ceon.pl/ handle/123456789/18561.

Davis, Lennard. J. 2017. *The Disability Studies Reader.* New York: Routledge: Taylor and Francis.

DSD. 2015a. *White Paper On The Rights Of Persons With Disabilities Official Publication And Gazetting Of The White Paper On The Rights Of Persons With Disabilities.* No. 39792. Pretoria: South African Government. https://www.gov.za/ sites/default/files/gcis_document/201603/39792gon230.pdf.

———. 2015b. *National Disability Strategy.* Pretoria, South Africa: Department of Social Development. https://static.pmg.org.za/150216bationaldisabilityrig htspolicy.

———. 2015c. *National Adolescent Sexual and Reproductive Health and Rights Framework Strategy 2014-2019.* Pretoria: Department of Social Development. http://www.dsd.gov.za/index2.php.

DSD, DWCPD, and UNICEF. 2012. *Children With Disabilities in South Africa: A Situational Analysis 2001–2011.* Pretoria, South Africa: Department of Social Development, Department of Women, Children and People with Disabilities, and UNICEF. https://www.unicef.org/southafrica/media/1336/file/ZAF-Children-with -disabilities-in%20South-Africa-2001-11-situation-analysis.pdf.

Hunt, Xanthe, Stine Hellum Braathen, Leslie Swartz, Mark Thomas Carew, and Poul Rohleder. 2017. "Intimacy, Intercourse and Adjustments: Experiences of Sexual Life of A Group of People With Physical Disabilities in South Africa." *Journal of Health Pschology* 23 (2): 289–305. https://doi.org/10.1177 /1359105317741761.

Ife, Jim. 2012. *Human Rights and Social Work: Towards Right-Based Practice*, 3rd ed. Cambridge: Cambridge University Press. http://handle.westernsydney.edu.au :8081/1959.7/uws:39495.

Jackson, Mary Ann. 2018. "Models of Disability and Human Rights: Informing The Improvement of Built Environment Accessibility for People With Disability at Neighborhood Scale?" *Laws* 7 (1): 1–21. https://doi.org/10.3390/laws7010010.

Kahonde, Callista K., Judith Mckenzie, and Nathan J. Wilson. 2019. "Discourse of Needs Versus Discourse of Rights: Family Caregivers Responding to Sexuality of Young South African Adults With Intellectual Disability." *Culture, Health & Society* 21 (3): 278–92. https://doi.org/10.1080/13691058.2018.1465202.

Lee, Kira, Alexandra Devine, Ma. Jesusa Marco, Jerome Zayas, Liz Gill-Atkinson, and Cathy Vaughan. 2015. "Sexual and Reproductive Health Services for Women With Disability: A Qualitative Study With Service Providers in the Philippines." *BMC Women's Health* 15 (87): 1–11. https://doi.org/10.1186/s12905-015-0244-8.

Mavuso, Sibusisiwe Siphelele. 2013. "Access to Sexual and Reproductive Health Service for Persons With Disabilities: A Case Study of Clarendon Home for Persons With Disabilities, Durban, KwaZulu-Natal." Masters diss., University of KwaZulu-Natal. https://researchspace.ukzn.ac.za/handle/10413/11408.

McKenzie, Judith, Roy McConkey, and Colleen Adnams. 2014. "Residential Facilities for Adults Wth Intellectual Disability In A Development Country: A Case Study From South Africa." *Journal of Intellectual and Developmental Disability* 39 (1): 45–54. https://doi.org/10.3109/13668250.2013.865157.

Meer, Talia, and Helene Combrinck. 2015. "Invisible Intersections: Understanding The Complex Stigmatisation of Women With Intellectual Disabilities in Their Vulnerability to Gender-Based Violence." *Agenda: Empowering Women for Gender Equity* 29 (2): 14–23. https://doi.org/10.1080/10130950.2015.1939307.

Mohamed, Kharnita, and Tamara Shefer. 2015. "Gendering Disability and Disabling Gender: Critical Reflections On Intersections of Gender and Disability." *Agenda: Empowering Women for Gender Equity* 29 (2): 2–13. https//doi.org/10.1080/10130950.2015.1055878.

Muserwa, Tapiwa, and Madhu Kasiram. 2019. "Understanding The Sexuality of Persons With Intellectual Disability in Residential Facilities: Perceptions of Service Providers and People With Disabilities." *Social Work/Maatskaplike Werk* 55 (1): 196–204. http://dx.doi.org/10.15270/52-2-715.

Ross, Loretta J. 2017. "Reproductive Justice As Intersectional Feminist Activism." *Souls: A Critical Journal of Black Politics, Culture, and Society* 19 (3): 286–314. doi:10.1080/10999948.2017.1389634.

Scheepers, M., M. Kerr, D. O'Hara, D. Bainbridge, S.-A. Cooper, R. Davis, G. Fujiura, et al. 2005. "Reducing Health Disparity in People with Intellectual Disabilities: A Report from Health Issues Special Interest Research Group of the International Association for the Scientific Study of Intellectual Disabilities." *Journal of Policy and Practice in Intellectual Disabilities* 2 (3–4): 249–55. http://doi.org/10.1111/j.1741-1130.2005.00037.x.

Servais, Laurent. 2006. "Sexual Health Care in Persons with Intellectual Disabilities." *Mental Retardation and Developmental Disabilities Research Reviews* 12: 48–56. https://doi.org/10.1002/mrdd.20093.

Shakespear, Tom. 2013. "The Social Model of Disability." In *The Disabilty Studies Reader,* edited by Lennard J. Davis, 214–21. New York: Routledge.

STATSSA. 2014. *Census 2011: Profile of Persons with Disabilities in South Africa.* Cataloguing in-Publication (CIP), Pretoria: Statistics SA. http://www.statssa.gov.za/publications/Report-03-01-59/Report-03-01-592011.pdf.

Swartz, Leslie. 2012. "Able-Bodied: Scenes From A Curious Life." *Culture, Medicine, and Psychiatry* 36 (3): 571–73. https://doi.org/10.1007/s11013-012 -9272-0.

Taylor, Melissa. F. 2006. "Is Self-Determination Still Important? What Seasoned Social Workers Are Saying." *Journal of Social Work Values and Ethics* 3 (1). https://libres.uncg.edu/ir/uncg/f/M_Floyd-Pickard_Is_2006.pdf.

UN. 2006. *Convention on the Rights of Persons with Disabilities.* New York: United Nations. http://www.un.org/esa/socdev/enable/rights/convtexte.htm.

WHO. 1978. "Declaration of Alma-Ata." International Conference on Primary Health Care. Alma-Ata, USSR: World Health Organization. 6-12 September. www.who .int/hpr/NPH/doc/declaration almaata.

———. 1995. *Achieving Reproductive Health for All: The Role of WHO.* Geneva: WHO, FHE, GPA, and HRP. https://apps.who.int/iris/handle/10665/63717.

———. 2011. *World Report on Disability.* Library Cataloguing, Malta: World Health Organization. https://www.who.int/about/licensing/copyright_form/en/index.htm.

WHO, and United Nations Population Fund. 2009. *Promoting Sexual and Reproductive Health for Persons With Disabilities.* WHO/UNFPA Guidance Note. Geneva: WHO and United Nations Population Fund. https://www.who.int/reproductivehe-alth/publications/general/9789241598682/en/ check legal doc referncing.

Wood, Kate, and Rachel Jewkes. 2006. "Blood Blockages and Scolding Nurses: Barriers to Adolescent Contraceptive Use in South Africa." *Reproductive Health Matters* 14 (27): 109–18. https://doi.org/10.1016/S0968-8080(06)27231-8.

Chapter 4

Sexual Injustice

(In)access to Gender Affirming Medical Care for Transgender and Gender Diverse South Africans

Landa Mabenge

In this chapter, I explore limited access to sexual and reproductive health (SRH) and rights in the form of gender affirming care (GAC) for individuals who are transgender and gender diverse and are seeking alignment through psychosocial, hormone, and/or surgical therapies. GAC includes a range of SRH services catering to the needs of transgender and gender diverse people. Individual needs will vary depending on one's sexual and gender identity. A transgender or gender diverse man might require GAC in the form of testosterone hormone therapy and surgical therapies that might include a mastectomy, hysterectomy, and genital reconstruction surgeries. A transgender or gender diverse woman might require GAC in the form of oestrogen hormone therapy and breast and genital reconstruction therapies. Finally, respecting the right of all whether or not to have children means ensuring that transgender and gender diverse people seeking GAC also have equitable access to fertility treatment, in the form of freezing their gametes, before undergoing gender alignment surgical procedures (Zali 2020).

Unrestricted access to SRH services forms part of the World Health Organisation's (WHO 2004) reproductive health strategy that, among other goals, seeks to fulfil international development goals linked to the understanding of human sexuality and health. These goals highlight, among others, the sexual and reproductive needs of individuals as a form of sexual justice and prioritise the need to recognise individual autonomy in making "informed decisions and to achieve the highest standard of sexual and reproductive health and reproductive justice" (Waldman and Stevens 2015, 94; WHO 2017). While many countries across the globe have made gains in ensuring the establishment of policies that seek to realise access to SRH services, many individuals experience inequitable and insufficient access, due to the lack of priority afforded to "neglected issues, such as adolescent sexuality, gender-based violence, abortion, and diversity in sexual orientations and gender identities" (Starrs et al. 2018, 2642).

In South Africa, advancements in SRH policies have seen a shift from the pre-democratic draconian Apartheid laws in service provision, which limited a suite of maternal and child services to the country's minority White population. To limit population growth, these policies placed significant emphasis on the provision of contraceptives to the majority Black population, through a poorly developed and inaccessible primary healthcare system (Cooper et al. 2004). There is no literature detailing the existence of Apartheid-era (1948–1994) SRH policies for individuals who embodied diverse sexual orientations and gender identities. What exists are accounts of lived experiences by individuals who experienced gross human rights violations and bodily oppressions through the Aversion Project, which was carried out by clinicians in the country's National Defence Force. This project entailed electroshock therapy and forced sex reassignment surgeries on homosexual conscripts as a form of punitive treatment, aimed at enforcing patriarchal constructions of sex, gender, and sexuality (van Zyl et al. 1999; Kaplan 2001).

With South Africa's transition to democracy, came a global model of constitutionalism, through a promissory note detailing human rights guarantees promising access to SRH rights and protections for all citizens, including those marginalised under Apartheid due to their sexual orientation or gender identity and expression. The constitution of South Africa (1996) clearly positions the right to non-discrimination based on sex and gender identity, among others, as inalienable through section 9, also known as the equality clause. The equality clause is a guarantee of equal treatment, protection, and benefit for all citizens before the law and avows that the state and its citizens may not discriminate against any person on this basis. Complementary to this is the right of access to health care services as a fundamental and basic human rights guarantee according to section 27 of the same constitution. This right extends to reproductive care services and makes it a violation of the constitution for any healthcare provider to refuse to provide services.

For many transgender and gender diverse people, there remains a big disconnect between these judicial promises and the envisioned guarantees. Both individuals and institutions persistently violate transgender and gender diverse people's bodily autonomy and safety, right to non-discrimination, and access to health resources and medical interventions. The Civil Union Act 17 (2006) and Alteration of Sex Description and Status Act 49 (2003) have been developed to ensure the implementation of these guarantees. Respectively, these legislative policies are acts of parliament that legalise all unions regardless of gender and allow individuals who are transgender and gender diverse to amend their sex description and status in the country's births and deaths register.

The Alteration of Sex Description and Status Act (2003), hereinafter referred to as Act 49, is a necessary step towards the legal recognition of transgender and gender diverse individuals' self-recognition. However, it has been critiqued for not specifically including gender identity; the focus of Act 49 is on sex description and does not include gender identity or gender markers. This results in the continued limitation of agency due to the pathologisation of identity, which is viewed by administrators of policies and healthcare through the binary of sex, and a "change" from one sex description to another.

For transgender and gender diverse individuals who would like to change their gender markers and are *not* seeking any surgical alignment interventions, the focus on sex description could lead to intense gatekeeping by health providers, due to the non-inclusion of gender identity in Act 49. This could also result in a denial of gender marker changes in the country's births and deaths register, as healthcare providers who would provide documentation in support of this would be operating within a narrow view of a transgender and gender diverse person as seeking an alteration of sex description. This is not only a limitation on individual rights and access to services, but it is also a deviation from international human rights laws applicable to gender identity and sexual orientation through the Yogyakarta Principles (2006), which prioritise the right to self-determination through the amendment of gender markers on identification documents based solely on gender identity (Strand and Smit 2020; Klein 2012; Theron and Kgositau 2015).

While the Civil Union Act and Act 49 have been implemented to drive the recognition of guarantees contained in the country's constitution, discrimination continues to drive elevated rates of gender and sexual violence, including homophobic and transphobic violence, across multiple intersectional levels in the country (Shefer 2019). This is especially true for individuals who seek gender alignment interventions, as they are constantly met with barriers to access due to the binary classification of gender and sex in public health and administrative facilities (Nduna 2013). Added to this is the violence of limited to no access to gender affirming medical interventions due to the exclusionary and discretionary nature of care provided by healthcare practitioners in the country (Spencer et al. 2017). This results in many transgender and gender diverse people's continued marginalisation when seeking access to SRH services (among other healthcare services), which constitutes sexual injustice.

My aim in this chapter is to link racial, class, and gender injustice to the experience of sexual injustice brought about by inaccessible GAC in South Africa. To do this, I draw on an intersectional framework and illustrate how restrictions to GAC for this population group are a denial of sexual justice. By way of background, I begin with an exploration of the existing health system in South Africa, drawing on relevant research to show how access is bed-rocked on the gender/sex binary. I then explicate how intersectionality, as a social justice framework, can be applied to transgender and gender diverse individuals as of bodies with intersectional needs in terms of access to specific GAC and go on to demonstrate how race, class, and gender politics shape the ways that sexual injustice is experienced by transgender and gender diverse people in South Africa. I conclude with commentary on the denial of GAC as sexual injustice for transgender and gender diverse individuals. The South African situation of in/access to GAC is of course shaped by the country's unique sociopolitical history. However, this case study illuminates how the intersectional nature of this issue can be similarly parsed out in other contexts.

SOUTH AFRICA'S BINARY HEALTH SYSTEM: TRANSGENDER AND GENDER DIVERSE PEOPLE'S ACCESS TO HEALTHCARE

South Africa has a two-tiered healthcare system: public and private. The majority of the population accesses care at government funded public facilities, while 16% of the country's 58.56 million citizens can afford private healthcare through medical aid (health insurance) (Müller 2017). The public sector is characterised by scarcity in the form of inadequate human resourcing due to poor administration and under resourcing (Coovadia et al. 2009). This is exacerbated by the challenge of an unequal society premised on varying socioeconomic statuses and social identities, all vying for healthcare access (Mbunge 2020; Staunton et al. 2020). Thus, while public spending in healthcare has increased since the dawn of democracy, there continues to be an increase in income and social inequality and this results in inadequate health resources for the majority of the population reliant on public services (Nattrass and Seekings 2001).

Transgender and gender diverse individuals face additional barriers navigating this unequal healthcare system. These include limited policies addressing their health needs beyond HIV care.[1]

Apart from inadequate policies for transgender and gender diverse individuals seeking access to gender affirming health interventions, the main barrier is the entrenchment of the gender binary in the healthcare system. While there is a paucity of South African research into these experiences, existing literature shows that transgender and gender diverse individuals either avoid seeking health interventions or experience violence and/or rejection on the basis of their non-conforming gender identity (Maesela 2019). This is largely rooted in the taken-for-granted assumption of a cisgender and heterosexual patient whose body is presumed to exhibit physical characteristics reflecting the male/female binary construction of the body in which gender is assigned at birth based on physical sex characteristics. This hetero-gendered assumption results in the disregard of experiences and personal constructions of identity in favour of rigid and restrictive either/or cisnormative classifications, as guidelines and protocol in care provision exclude gender diversity as a factor in healthcare (Nagoshi and Bruzy 2010; Müller 2016).

In South Africa, there are no specific guidelines or policies for GAC or the provision thereof for transgender and gender diverse individuals in the public health system. Despite this, there are three (out of twenty one) tertiary public health facilities in South Africa that provide psychosocial, hormonal, and surgical care specifically for transgender and gender diverse individuals. This care is reliant on provider willingness and acumen. This limited care has been the result of focussed research foregrounded by civil society organisations like GenderDynamix (GDX) and Transgender Intersex Africa (TIA), among others, lobbying for inclusion and diversity in the public healthcare space (Müller 2017; Spencer et al. 2017).

Evidence also exists suggesting that transgender and gender diverse individuals, who have the means to access care, elect to "avoid/delay receiving healthcare or engage in selective disclosure about their transgender identity to health providers in order to avoid discrimination" by healthcare providers (Kcomt et al. 2020, 2). Consequently, those who avoid/delay receiving care carry a heavy mental health burden, finding it difficult to navigate terrains that delegitimise their identity and gender autonomy (Benjamins and Whitman 2014; Seelman et al. 2017). This occurs against the backdrop of a scarcity of providers who are knowledgeable and willing to provide the required care (Luvuno et al. 2019).

Where access is not possible or is prevented by prior or expected discrimination, transgender and gender diverse individuals are left navigating intersecting forms of stigma that, in most cases, can result in suicide attempts related to persistent dysphoria (Kcomt et al. 2020). According to Hughto et al. (2015), stigma is a form of social control through labelling, stereotyping, and marginalisation operating at a structural, interpersonal, and individual level. At a structural level, providers with limited or no relevant training, and without clinical guidelines, may perpetrate behaviours upholding cisnormative care practices. For example, provider assumptions about how an individual's needs are based on biological sex may be enforced by providers through interpersonal dynamics (e.g., threats of violence and verbal abuse) which could exacerbate patients' poor mental health outcomes. Thus, while South African research into these specific incidents remains limited, studies have shown that transgender individuals in South Africa do "experience significant health disparities and . . . discrimination and systemic biases that decrease access to care, as well as . . . health professionals' ignorance" (de Vries et al. 2020, 2; Luvuno et al. 2019).

Most studies with a specific SRH approach in South Africa are focussed on the HIV/AIDS SRH needs of lesbian, gay, bisexual, transgender, and intersex (LGBTI) individuals in public healthcare spaces. For instance, a 2016 systematic review of research on responses to homophobic attacks assessed the inclusive participation of LGBT groups in the country's HIV/AIDS response. The study also sought to determine what interventions would be needed to coordinate effective care for the HIV/AIDS needs of this demographic (Mprah 2016). The results showed that greater participation by LGBT individuals is necessary to develop policy guidelines and programmes, to improve specific healthcare interventions and access at public facilities. This participation would encourage greater research into the socioeconomic experiences of these individuals as contributors to HIV/AIDS transmission, and thus the development of appropriate prevention and care strategies (Mprah 2016).

As regard transgender and gender diverse people's experiences of accessing GAC, South African research is incredibly scarce. One notable exception is a 2019 ethnographic study of transgender people's experiences accessing reproductive care, including GAC, in KwaZulu Natal Province. The study found that the prevalence of scarce resources and inadequate provider acumen resulted in adverse experiences for the transgender population (Luvuno et al. 2019). All 16 participants had undergone a process of self-discovery and disclosed feelings of being in the wrong body and a desire to achieve congruence between gender identity and physical bodies.

A key finding was the exclusionary nature of the deeply cisgender healthcare system (Luvuno et al. 2019). Participants who sought sexual health care were left feeling like spectacles. They experienced discomfort, hostility from healthcare workers, and violations to privacy and autonomy, largely due to provider ignorance and a lack of acumen. Participants were treated as mentally unstable and held responsible for any health issues they might have. Furthermore, some participants described how providers would link their gender identity to their health issues, even if their health needs were unrelated to their gender identity. To avoid such transphobic experiences, some participants would choose not to disclose their transgender identity. Where participants chose to inquire about GAC,

> They were met with confusion from health care workers who were unable to offer care, advice or appropriate referral . . . and were sent from pillar to post and seen by numerous health care workers without success, much to their personal distress and frustration. (Luvuno et al. 2019, 6)

These findings point to the difficulty transgender patients experience in finding knowledgeable providers who provide appropriate GAC and how they risk stigma and discrimination in doing so. Accordingly, Luvano et al. (2019) highlight the need for training and policies on transgender specific care in the public health sector and "to include transgender health in the pre-service training curriculum for health care workers, coupled with in-service training and sensitisation" (Luvuno et al. 2019, 9). Thus, the entrenchment of the gender binary in healthcare settings continues to hinder access to GAC for many transgender and gender diverse individuals, despite formal legal and social rights. Current legal protections in South Africa promote equality and the right to non-discrimination, including access to general and SRH care.

Having provided a background to the South African context, which will resonate with other countries, in the following section I seek to examine more closely the challenges in access to GAC that have been documented. To do this, I take a social justice perspective to analyse the various intersecting aspects of continued obstruction to GAC (Pelletan 2019; Müller 2016). Taking an intersectional approach, I seek to unpack and illuminate the quagmire of intersecting struggles faced by gender diverse people of colour in a country marred by "unequal distribution of wealth and income" (Müller 2016, 200). This is the focus of the next section.

LIMITATIONS TO GAC: THE INTERSECTION OF CISNORMATIVITY WITH RACE, CLASS, AND GENDER INJUSTICE

The term "intersectionality" was coined by Kimberlé Crenshaw to emphasise the importance of power "relationships between and within the social categories of race and gender" (Wesp et al. 2019, 288) in enquiries about oppression and social justice. The concept is rooted in Women of Colour resistance movements from the early 19th to 20th centuries (Bowleg 2012). As a critical social framework, intersectionality allows for an analytical enquiry and understanding of how multiple social identities "intersect at the micro-level of individual experience" (Lacombe-Duncan 2016, 128) to reflect "interlocking systems of privilege and oppression at the macro social structural level" (Bowleg 2012, 1267).

Intersectional enquiry into transgender and gender diverse healthcare access usually engages with the themes of cisnormativity and provider discrimination as oppressions on the macrolevel which facilitate exclusion and serve as barriers to required inclusive and specific transgender healthcare (Müller 2016; Wesp et al. 2019). An intersectional analysis of race, class, and gender, among many other social identities, can enhance understandings about systematic social exclusions underpinned by intersecting oppressions faced by transgender and gender diverse individuals seeking specific care in South Africa and elsewhere. Doing so will satisfy the need to "account for multiple grounds of identity" (Crenshaw 1991, 1245) when analysing the oppressive exclusion of, and harms perpetrated against, transgender and gender diverse individuals in healthcare.

Most South African research focussed on transgender and gender diverse people is foregrounded by civic organisations advocating for diversity and inclusion in the healthcare space. However, there is a body of research on broader LGBT experiences and sparse literature focussing specifically on the transgender experience. This research primarily explores the health disparities experienced by transgender and gender diverse individuals compared to their heterosexual, cisgender, socioeconomically matched peers (Müller 2017). The findings show a clear bias against transgender inclusive healthcare based on, among others, provider prejudice, limited health facilities specific to transgender and gender diverse needs, and a denial of care based on Western colonial constructions of gender. The result is a normative perception of transgender and gender diverse peoples as "unAfrican" and as "defying nature" and the "natural construction" of the body (Theron and Kgositau 2015).

In the remainder of this section, I highlight how race, class, and gender injustices in South Africa play out within the cisnormative healthcare system. Although I deal with race, class, and gender in turn, struggles for race, class, and gender justice overlap, as my discussion shows.

Racial Injustice

The development of race categories and correlating relations in South Africa is rooted in the history of Apartheid, which severely institutionalised segregation to ensure a suppression of economic growth for Black South Africans through race discrimination and socioeconomic disempowerment (Onwuzurike 1987). Against this backdrop, the transition into a democratic, rights-based approach to social justice in the country is still marred by inadequate access for this demographic and a reliance on a poorly funded and managed public healthcare system. Comprehensive analyses and studies into the impact of race and identity politics on transgender and gender diverse healthcare access remain limited nationally. However, a recent study at seven public institutions of higher learning linked discrimination and poor access to campus healthcare facilities to cisgender heteropatriarchal norms and the exclusion of Black transgender and gender diverse individuals in key decision-making structures (Ndelu 2017).

It is important to note also that those facilities that do provide some or other form of transgender and gender diverse inclusive and/or specific care are located in urban areas. These are beyond the reach of most Black transgender and gender diverse individuals who are either not aware of their existence, cannot get to these spaces, or cannot be referred due to prevailing attitudes and racial prejudice, among other reasons. Structural exclusions from healthcare, rooted in race- and class-based politics, locate Black transgender and gender diverse individuals outside the reservoir of available GAC (Müller 2017).

For transgender and gender diverse individuals located in majority Black rural areas, an absence of language linked to their gender identity constitutes initial experiences of a lack of access to GAC. Rural healthcare practitioners, who rely on Western cisnormative understandings of gender, often misconceive transgender and gender diversity as a sexual orientation, not a gender identity (Strand and Smit 2020). Like their urban counterparts, rural health providers lack "access to adequate knowledge about fluidity and diversity of gender identities" (Strand and Smit 2020, 48), but the lack of access to information, education, and resources is more pronounced in rural settings. Moreover, "the racialised divide . . . [means that] there are no specific LGBTI health centres or service providers available" (Strand and Smit 2020, 37) in rural areas. The narrow cisnormative view of gender and sex, coupled with limitations to access, information, and resources, results in experiences of marginalisation in majority Black rural communities (Strand and Smit 2020).

Class-Based Exclusions

The class struggle in South Africa continues to mirror the country's racially and economically segregated history. This manifests in socioeconomic categorisations that perpetuate an unequal society, with disparities in healthcare access and affordability of healthcare evident between racial groups. Thus, Black people carry the greatest burden of unemployment, at four times the rate of fellow White citizens, while receiving the lowest wages nationally (Jones 2020). For Black transgender and gender diverse individuals, these socioeconomic marginalisations and economic barriers intersect on multiple fronts, including lower income, homelessness, and a lack of healthcare affordability (Lacombe-Duncan 2016).

In addition, the class and economic status of Black transgender and gender diverse individuals makes it "virtually impossible . . . to access comprehensive gender affirming care in South Africa" (van der Merwe 2017, 93). Transgender and gender diverse individuals face insurmountable costs when seeking GAC healthcare. Hormone therapy or gender alignment surgical procedures are classified as cosmetic and are therefore not covered by health insurers in the private health sector. In the public health sector, there is a waiting period of 25 years for gender affirming surgery due to institutionalised policies that do not allocate enough resources for transgender and gender diverse surgical procedures (Ao 2016). Furthermore, this healthcare is located in select urban tertiary facilities and dependent on provider awareness, knowledge, and willingness. Thus, for Black transgender and gender diverse individuals in South Africa, a class struggle is simultaneously a struggle for accessible and inclusive healthcare (Koch et al. 2020; Wilson et al. 2014).

Gender Injustice

The absence of national guidelines for transgender and gender diverse specific care and the cisnormative nature of South Africa's healthcare system result in facilities becoming hostile environments that render gender diverse identities invisible (Morison and Lynch 2016) or "abnormal." The existence of a national HIV/AIDS framework for SRH for LGBTI individuals in public healthcare alongside the absence of other policies and guidelines for healthcare provision for LGBTI individuals results in a limited conceptual view of healthcare facilities that ought to be available to this demographic. As such, understandings of LGBTI groups' health needs tend to be limited to HIV/AIDS, which does not encompass the full scope of healthcare services they are entitled to and ought to be able to access. Furthermore, the existence of this HIV/AIDS framework has not translated into visible HIV/AIDS healthcare service delivery for this population due to the cisnormative nature of the health system and is limited to provide training or willingness to cater to the needs of transgender and gender diverse individuals. Indeed, the construction and implementation of health policies and procedures continues along a cis-heteronormative delivery plan, leading to experiences of discrimination as discussed earlier (Spencer et al. 2017).

For Black transgender and gender diverse individuals, who depend on public healthcare, the over-burdened system and the scarcity of resources result in greater discrimination rooted in providers' personal value judgements and prejudices (Meer and Müller 2017). This reality is also perpetuated by the invisibility and exclusion of the health needs of transgender and gender diverse individuals in medical school curricula. The absence of gender-inclusive medical school curricula makes healthcare environments a fertile ground for anti-trans hostility and prejudicial attitudes that result in a deprivation of care once a patient's identity is presented as transgender or gender diverse (Lacombe-Duncan 2016).

The above analysis shows the persistent struggle for race, class, and gender justice in South Africa's cis-heteronormative healthcare system. It also highlights the intersecting nature of these struggles. For Black transgender and gender diverse individuals, experiences of exclusion and prejudice persist as a point of (in)access to required humanising healthcare, including sexual and reproductive care, which *should* be easily and widely accessible and provided by the state, given the guarantees in the country's constitution.

DENIAL OF ACCESS TO GENDER AFFIRMING CARE AS A DENIAL OF SEXUAL AND REPRODUCTIVE JUSTICE

Sexual rights encompass the right to freedom from discrimination and the right to healthcare (Armas 2007). LGBTI and HIV/AIDS activists have advocated for the expansion of sexual rights to include respect for sexual diversity (Garcia and Parker 2006). From a Sexual and Reproductive Justice perspective, this includes recognising sexual freedom and bodily autonomy (Ross 2017). For transgender and gender diverse individuals, sexual freedom and bodily autonomy entail unrestricted access to GAC. Furthermore, the reproductive right of whether to have children necessarily entails unfettered access to fertility treatments prior to receiving GAC. However, the continued imposition of gender binaried health-care results in the development and implementation of healthcare policies that prescribe adherence to hetero-gendered logics in order to access healthcare. A transgender or gender diverse individual who does not adhere to these logics is thus relegated to the margins of care, and subjected to dehumanising care, as there is no socially recognised category for their required healthcare needs.

The exclusion of gender affirming services in healthcare policies and practices results in a denial of care. While South Africa has made significant strides by offering constitutional affirmation of, and protection to, all citizens' right to healthcare—including transgender and gender diverse individuals—this does not translate into reality for this demographic. This is not only a violation of a constitutional right, but from a Sexual and Reproductive Justice perspective, (in)access to SRH resources (such as psychosocial, hormone, and surgical therapies, as well as fertility treatments) for those seeking GAC must, I argue, be understood as a denial of sexual justice.

GLOSSARY OF TERMS[2]

The below is a non-exhaustive list of terms and definitions linked to gender identity used in the chapter.

Cisgender: People who identify with the gender they were assigned at birth, that is, people who are not transgender.

Cisnormative: Describes the worldview based on ideas and beliefs that cisgender and heterosexual people are the norm.

Gender identity: How an individual views himself/herself/themselves in terms of characteristics traditionally identified in society as male or female. A person may self-identify as purely male, purely female, or as possessing characteristics of both, or neither.

Gender diversity: An umbrella term used to describe gender identities that demonstrate a diversity of expression beyond the binary heterosexual male and female framework.

Gender non-conforming: Behaviour or expression by individuals that depict nonconformity to the gender roles linked to the binary heterosexual male and female conventions of behaviour/expression.

LGBTIAQ+/LGBTI: A sociopolitical acronym for the community composed of Lesbians, Gay Men, Bisexuals, Transgender, Intersex, Asexual, and Queer individuals. The recent addition of a "Q+" at the end refers to individuals who may affiliate with the community and are "questioning" some aspect of their gender or sexuality. Also used to include those who identify as Queer. The plus symbol refers to those who identify as a sexual orientation or gender identity other than LGBTIAQ.

Transition: A process of physical and psychosocial adjustment undertaken by some persons who are transgender and gender diverse to achieve greater congruence between the natal sex and their experienced gender.

Transgender: Individuals whose assigned sex at birth does not match their gender identity and who may or may not seek to change their physical body to match their gender identity through gender alignment surgery and hormone treatments, or in other ways as discussed under "Transition" above. In this chapter, the focus is on transgender individuals who want to align their bodies to their identity in some form. Transgender individuals' sexual orientation can be heterosexual, homosexual, bisexual, or anywhere on the continuum.

NOTES

1. Indeed, advocacy by civic organisations brought about a change in the country's HIV/AIDS national framework, which has been a milestone in care response. For example, the introduction of the 2017–2022 South African National LGBTI HIV Plan (South African National AIDS Council 2017) was the result of multi-sectoral efforts to ensure the development and implementation of inclusive HIV programming in the country, through a focussed attention on policies that address the HIV/AIDS vulnerabilities that burden this demographic (Mprah 2016).

2. These terms and definitions have been compiled from the following resources: (Ndelu 2017, 5–9; Wilson et al. 2014, 449).

REFERENCES

Ao, Bethany. 2016. "Transgender Clinic's 25-Year Waiting List." *Independent Online*, May 22, 2017. https://www.iol.co.za/news/south-africa/western-cape/transgender-clinics-25-year-waiting-list-2024496.

Armas, Henry. 2007. *Working Paper 294: Whose Sexuality Counts? Poverty, Participation and Sexual Rights*. Brighton: Institute of Development Studies, University of Sussex.

Benjamins, Maureen R., and Steven Whitman. 2014. "Relationships Between Discrimination in Health Care and Health Care Outcomes Among Four Race/Ethnic Groups." *Journal of Behavioral Medicine* 37 (3): 402–13. https://doi.org/0.1007/s10865-013-9496-7.

Bowleg, Lisa. 2012. "The Problem with the Phrase Women and Minorities: Intersectionality—an Important Theoretical Framework for Public Health." *American Journal of Public Health* 102 (7): 1267–73. https://doi.org/10.2105/AJPH.2012.300750.

Cooper, Diane, Chelsea Morroni, Phyllis Orner, Jennifer Moodley, Jane Harries, Lee Cullingworth, and Margaret Hoffman. 2004. "Ten Years of Democracy in South Africa: Documenting Transformation in Reproductive Health Policy and Status." *Reproductive Health Matters* 12 (24): 70–85. https://doi.org/10.1016/S0968-8080(04)24143-X.

Coovadia, Hoosen, Rachel Jewkes, Peter Barron, David Sanders, and Diane McIntyre. 2009. "The Health and Health System of South Africa: Historical Roots of Current Public Health Challenges." *The Lancet* 374 (9692): 817–34. https://doi.org/10.1016/S0140-6736(09)60951-X.

Crenshaw, Kimberlé. 1991. "Mapping the Margins: Intersectionality, Identity Politics, and Violence against Women of Color." *Stanford Law Review* 43 (6): 1241–99. https://doi.org/10.2307/1229039.

Garcia, Jonathan, and Richard G. Parker. 2006. "From Global Discourse to Local Action: The Makings of a Sexual Rights Movement?" *Horizontes Antropológicos* 12 (26): 13–41.

Hughto, Jaclyn M., Sari L. Reisner White, and John E. Pachankis. 2015. "Transgender Stigma and Health: A Critical Review of Stigma Determinants, Mechanisms, and Interventions." *Social Science & Medicine* 147: 222–31. https://doi.org/10.1016/j.socscimed.2015.11.010.

Jones, Alexander. 2020. "Unemployment in South Africa: Urgent Attention Required." *International Banker*, January 21. https://internationalbanker.com/finance/unemployment-in-south-africa-urgent-attention-required/.

Kaplan, Robert M. 2001. "The Aversion Project-Psychiatric Abuses in the South African Defence Force during the Apartheid Era." *South African Medical Journal* 91 (3): 216–17.

Kcomt, Luisa, Kevin M. Gorey, Betty Jo Barrett, and Sean Esteban McCabe. 2020. "Healthcare Avoidance due to Anticipated Discrimination Among Transgender People: A Call to Create Trans-Affirmative Environments." *SSM-Population Health* 11 (100608). https://doi.org/10.1016/j.ssmph.2020.100608.

Klein, Thamar. 2012. "Necessity is the Mother of Invention: Access Inequalities to Medical Technologies Faced by Transgendered South Africans." *Technology and Innovation* 15: 165–79. https://doi.org/10.3727/194982413X13650843069077.

Koch, Julie M., Cristine McLachlan, Cornelius J. Victor, Jess Westcott, and Christina Yager. 2020. "The Cost of Being transgender: Where Socioeconomic Status, Global Health Care Systems, and Gender Identity Intersect." *Psychology & Sexuality* 11 (1-2): 103–19. https:// doi.org/10.1080/19419899.2019.1660705.

Lacombe-Duncan, Ashley. 2016. "An Intersectional Perspective on Access to HIV-Related Healthcare for Transgender Women." *Transgender health* 1 (1): 137–41. https://doi.org/10.1089/trgh.2016.0018.

Luvuno, Zamasomi P., Busisiwe Ncama, and Gugu Mchunu. 2019. "Transgender Population's Experiences with Regard to Accessing Reproductive Health Care in Kwazulu-Natal, South Africa: A Qualitative Study." *African Journal of Primary Health Care & Family Medicine* 11 (1): 1–9. https://doi.org/10.4102/phcfm.v11i1.1933.

Maesela, Nickita. 2019. "Transgender-Inclusive Healthcare Ensures Access For The Marginalised." *Citypress*, November 6. https://www.news24.com/citypress/news/transgender-inclusive-healthcare-ensures-access-for-the-marginalised-20191106.

Mbunge, Elliot. 2020. "Effects of COVID-19 in South African Health System and Society: An Explanatory Study." *Diabetes & Metabolic Syndrome: Clinical Research & Reviews* 14 (6): 1809–14. https:// doi.org/10.1016/j.dsx.2020.09.016.

Meer, Talia, and Alex Müller. 2017. "They Treat Us Like We're Not There: Queer Bodies and the Social Production of Healthcare Spaces." *Health & Place* 45: 92–98.https://doi.org/10.1016/j.healthplace.2017.03.010.

Morison, Tracy, and Ingrid Lynch. 2016. "We Can't Help You Here': The discursive Erasure of Sexual Minorities in South African Public Sexual and Reproductive Health Services." *Psychology of Sexualities Review* 7 (2): 7–25.

Mprah, Andy. 2016. "Sexual and Reproductive Health Needs of LGBT." *African Journal of Reproductive Health/La Revue Africaine de la Santé Reproductive* 20 (1): 16–20. https:// doi.org/10.29063/ajrh2016/v20i1.1.

Müller, Alexandra. 2016. "Health for All? Sexual Orientation, Gender Identity, and the Implementation of the Right to Access to Health Care in South Africa." *Health and Human Rights* 18 (2): 195–208. https://www.ncbi.nlm.nih.gov/pmc/articles/PMC5395001/.

Müller, Alex. 2017. "Scrambling for Access: Availability, Accessibility, Acceptability and Quality of Healthcare for Lesbian, Gay, Bisexual and Transgender People in South Africa." *BMC International Health and Human Rights* 17 (1): 1–20. https:// doi.org/10.1186/s12914-017-0124-4.

Nagoshi, Julie L., and Stephanie Brzuzy. 2010. "Transgender Theory: Embodying Research and Practice." *Affilia* 25 (4): 431–43. https:// doi.org/10.1177/0886109910384068.

Nattrass, Nicoli, and Jeremy Seekings. 2001. "Democracy and Distribution in Highly Unequal Economies: the Case of South Africa." *Journal of Modern African Studies* 39 (3): 471–98. https://10.1017/S0022278X01003688.

Ndelu, Sandile. 2017. *In Their Own Voices: Being (Trans) Gender Diverse at a South African University.* Cape Town: Hlanganisa Institute for Development in Southern

Africa. http://www.hlanganisa.org.za/wp-content/uploads/2018/08/In-their-voices_
-Being-transgender-diverse-at-a-South-African-university_2nd-Draft.pdf.

Nduna, Mzikazi. 2013. "Alteration of Sex Description and Sex Status Act and Access to Services for Transgender People in South Africa." *New Voices in Psychology* 9 (1-2): 50–62. https://hdl.handle.net/10520/EJC146097.

Onwuzurike, Chris Ama. 1987. "Black People and Apartheid Conflict." *Journal of Black Studies* 18 (2): 215–29. https:// doi.org/10.1177/002193478701800206.

Pelletan, Charlotte. 2019. "How To "Talk Left and Walk Right" in South Africa: Access to Medicines in the Neoliberal Era. An Insight into the Public Market of Antiretroviral Treatments in South Africa." *Angles. New Perspectives on the Anglophone World* 1 (8): 1–20. https:// doi.org/10.4000/angles.613.

Ross, Loretta J. 2017. "Reproductive Justice as Intersectional Feminist Activism." *Souls: A Critical Journal of Black Politics, Culture, and Society* 19 (3): 286–314. https://doi.org/10.1080/10999949.2017.1389634.

Seelman, Kristie L., Matthew J. P. Colón-Diaz, Rebecca H. LeCroix, Marik Xavier-Brier, and Leonardo Kattari. 2017. "Transgender Noninclusive Healthcare and Delaying Care Because of Fear: Connections to General Health and Mental Health Among Transgender Adults." *Transgender Health* 2 (1): 17–28. https://doi.org/10 .1089/trgh.2016.0024.

Shefer, Tamara. 2019. "Activist Performance and Performative Activism Towards Intersectional Gender and Sexual Justice in Contemporary South Africa." *International Sociology* 34 (4): 418–34. https://doi.org/10.1177/0268580919851430.

South African National AIDS Council. 2017. "The South African national LGBTI HIV Plan, 2017–2022." South African National AIDS Council. https://sanac.org .za/wpcontent/uploads/2017/06/LGBTI-HIV-Plan-Final.pdf.

Spencer, Sarah, Talia Meer, and Alex Müller. 2017. "'The Care is the Best You Can Give at the Time': Health Care Professionals' Experiences in Providing Gender Affirming Care in South Africa." *PloS ONE* 12 (7): e0181132. https://doi.org/10 .1371/journal.pone.0181132.

Starrs, Ann M., Alex C. Ezeh, Gary Barker, Alaka Basu, Jane T. Bertrand, Robert Blum, Awa M. Coll-Seck et al. 2018. "Accelerate Progress—Sexual and Reproductive Health and Rights for All: Report of the Guttmacher–Lancet Commission." *The Lancet* 391 (10140): 2642–92. https:// doi.org/10.1016/S0140 -6736(18)30293-9.

Staunton, Ciara, Carmen Swanepoel, and Melodie Labuschaigne. 2020. "Between a Rock and a Hard Place: COVID-19 and South Africa's response." *Journal of Law and the Biosciences* 7 (1): 1–12. https:// doi.org/10.1093/jlb/lsaa052.

Strand, Mia, and Estian Smit. 2020. *Trans Rural Narratives: Perspectives on the Experiences of Rural-Based Trans and Gender Diverse Persons in South Africa-Addressing Issues of Recognition, Belonging and Access.* Gender DynamiX.

Theron, Liesl, and Tshepo Ricki Kgositau. 2015. "The Emergence of a Grassroots African Trans Archive." *Transgender Studies Quarterly* 2 (4): 578–83. https://doi .or/10.1215/23289252-3151502.

van der Merwe, Leigh Ann. 2017. "Transfeminism (s) from the Global South: Experiences from South Africa." *Development* 60: 90–95. https:// doi.org/10.1057 /s41301-017-0140-7.

Vries, Kylan Mattias de. 2015. "Transgender People of Color at the Center: Conceptualising a New Intersectional Model." *Ethnicities* 15 (1): 3–27. https://doi .org/10.1177/1468796814547058.

Waldman, Linda, and Marion Stevens. 2015. "Sexual and Reproductive Health and Rights and mHealth in Policy and Practice in South Africa." *Reproductive Health Matters* 23 (45): 93–102. https://doi.org/10.1016/j.rhm.2015.06.009.

Wesp, Linda M., Lorraine Halinka Malcoe, Ayana Elliott, and Tonia Poteat. 2019. "Intersectionality Research for Transgender Health Justice: A Theory-Driven Conceptual Framework for Structural Analysis of Transgender Health Inequities." *Transgender Health* 4 (1): 287–96. https://doi.org/10.1089/trgh.2019 .0039.

Wilson, Don, Adele Marais, Anniza de Villiers, Ronald Addinall, and Megan M. Campbell. 2014. "Transgender issues in South Africa, with Particular Reference to the Groote Schuur Hospital Transgender Unit." *South African Medical Journal* 106 (6): 449–51. https://doi.org/10.7196/SAMJ.8392.

World Health Organisation. 2004. *Reproductive Health Strategy to Accelerate Progress Towards the Attainment of International Development Goals and Targets.* WHO/RHR/04.8. World Health Organisation. https://www.who.int/repro-ductivehealth/publications/general/RHR_04_8/en/.

———. 2017. *Sexual Health and its Linkages to Reproductive Health: An Operational Approach.* World Health Organisation. https://www.who.int/repro-ductivehealth/publications/sexual_health/sh-linkages-rh/en/.

Zali, Marcia. 2020. "Transgender Healthcare Is a Matter of Human Dignity." *Health-E News*, March 30. https://health-e.org.za/2020/03/31/transgender-health-care-is-a-matter-of-human-dignity/.

Zyl, Mikki van, Jeanelle de Gruchy, Sheila Lapinsky, Simon Lewin, and Graeme Reid. 1999. *The Aversion Project: Human Rights Abuses of Gays and Lesbians in the South African Defence Force by Health Workers During the Apartheid Era.* Cape Town: Simply Said and Done.

Chapter 5

Paving the Way to Gender Affirming Mental Health Services Using a Sexual and Reproductive Justice Approach

A South African Case Study

Aneeqa Abrahams

Psychology's privileged position of speaking authoritatively on topics of human behaviour has too often been from a Euro-American perspective that centres the experiences of White, heterosexual, middle-upper class, able-bodied, cisgender male experiences. This marginalises and pathologises the experiences of "others" and reproduces dominant cis-centric and heteronormative theories (Kessi and Boonzaier 2018). Therefore, as a student of psychology concerned about the lack of inclusivity and diversity of the discourse, it is necessary that we engage with psychology critically and reflexively. In a South African context, this means reckoning with the discipline's racist and anti-queer origins and bringing to the forefront the current exclusionary practices of psychology which make mental health services inaccessible for Black, poor, and working-class LGBTQIA+ persons. As a marginalised group, the experiences of LGBTQIA+ persons in South Africa and elsewhere are intertwined by political, cultural, and economic injustices (Fraser 2005) which need to be amended to achieve justice (Stormhøj 2015). Using the principles of Sexual and Reproductive Justice (S/RJ), I argue that the discipline of psychology can and should be an agent of social change and that one possibility for doing so is through the development of an identity-affirmative approach to mental healthcare provision for LGBTQIA+ persons.

Matebeni and Msibi (2015) note that "language, naming and words can be deeply political" (3). Acknowledging this, the aim of this chapter is not to further exclude individuals from psychology, for example, by reproducing the ways in which identities, such as transgender and intersex, have been pathologised in the discipline (Husakouskaya 2013). Therefore, I use the acronym "LGBTQIA+" only when the literature being discussed in this chapter does so. Otherwise, I will be using "sexually and gender diverse" throughout the chapter.

While mainstream sexual and reproductive activism and scholarship have centred the positionalities of White, middle class, cis heterosexual womxn[1] as the generally normative experience (Kessi and Boonzaier 2018; Ross 2017; Stormhøj 2015), the Sexual and Reproductive Justice framework engages an anti-essentialist intersectional framework addressing the intersections of race, class, and gender in sexual and reproductive experiences. This framework highlights that there is no dominant experience that can account for the plurality and diverse subjectivities of different groups of people. It therefore critiques the essentialism of "gender-specific" accounts that homogenise experiences and, in addition, recognise that sexuality is often constructed in racialised and misogynistic ways (Ross 2017).

Though Reproductive Justice principles have been the primary focus, the Sexual and Reproductive Justice "includes sexual freedom and bodily autonomy" (Ross 2017, 291) and the right to be treated as equal regardless of sexual identity (Nussbaum 2010; Morison 2021). A Sexual and Reproductive Justice approach is therefore useful for interrogating the discipline of psychology that assumes a cis-heteronormative subject and for developing LGBTQIA+ affirming mental health practices and service provision in psychology, necessary for the support of LGBTQIA+ communities' sexual freedoms, bodily integrity, and mental health (Stormhøj 2015).

In this chapter, I focus on South Africa, presenting the Psychological Society of South Africa's (PsySSA) 2017 guidelines (McLachlan et al. 2019), which is well grounded in the tenets of Sexual and Reproductive Justice, as an exemplar for providing psychological care to LGBTQIA+ communities. Though each context will have unique local sociocultural and political considerations, the PsySSA guidelines make a useful case study for psychologists and other practitioners and scholars seeking to develop affirmative care in other locations. Before I discuss the guidelines, I provide some background to the provision of psychological care in the South African context, which will have resonances with other countries that have protection for sexual and gender minority groups on paper but fail in practice.

PSYCHOLOGY IN SOUTH AFRICA: A LEGACY OF PATHOLOGISATION AND ERASURE

To understand the current situation faced by gender and sexually diverse people in South Africa, it is necessary to consider the history of psychology in this context. The discipline of psychology in South Africa is rooted in colonisation and apartheid as well as the preservation of the interests of dominant groups and the maintenance of power relations and ideologies of White supremacy and cis-heteropatriarchy (Kessi and Boonzaier 2018). Psychology has both actively and implicitly drawn on, perpetuated, and lent legitimacy to eugenics and other philosophies grounded in the hierarchical categorisation of race. For example, during apartheid, psychology played an important part in the production of race science that constructed, validated, and supported the pathologisation of African people. This legacy continues to shape the way we are seen across the globe (Kessi and Boonzaier 2018).

In addition to validating and justifying racist beliefs about people of colour, African people specifically, South African psychology has contributed to and legitimised racist, classist, and gendered policies, educational programmes, and generalised racist beliefs about people of colour. A contemporary example of this is the infamous, since retracted, article written by Stellenbosch University students in 2019 regarding the "lower" cognitive function of "coloured" womxn. The article was underpinned by colonial and racist ideals and epistemological narratives that shaped the study's methodology, enabled it to be regarded as "scientific," and to generalise its finding to all "coloured" womxn (O'Connor, Ress, and Joffe 2012; Shange 2019). "Scientific" conclusions such as this are not only racist but also contribute to oppressive and racist implementations, and further ingrains "common sense" racist discourse.

The global politics of knowledge production have also played a part in this, as Euro-American psychology is often regarded as an authority that guides and rules over psychological research and knowledge production. This position reproduces the idea that the ability to perform relevant theorisation is only possible from a Euro-American standpoint (Connell 2014), leaving African psychological scholars to produce knowledge in their postcolonial contexts but compelled by geopolitical relations on knowledge production to cite Euro-American scholarship about their own contexts and lived realities (Daoust and Dyvik 2020). Then, to be recognised in their respective fields of psychology, they are compelled to publish in Euro-American journals—furthering the cycle of cultural westernisation in Africa (Connell 2014; Daoust and Dyvik 2020). However, African scholars have resisted and developed alternative psychological philosophies such as the Black consciousness movements in South Africa and recently African psychology that reassembles the "psychology of the oppressed" (Kessi and Boonzaier 2018, 301) as a standpoint for scientific enquiry in the name of social justice (Carolissen, Shefer, and Smit 2015).

As mentioned, the discipline of psychology's androcentricity ensures that psychological experiences are situated within a White, middle class, able-bodied, cisgendered, and heterosexual male standpoint. As such, psychology continues to silence and reduce space for experiences that defy the "norm" and challenge "common sense." This can be seen, for example, in the lack of psychological research concerning gender and sexual diversity. This research gap is partially due to the fact that prior to the 1980s, all research concerning non-normative sexualities was directed at "conversion therapy" and maintaining a heteronormative position in mainstream psychology (Victor and Nel 2016; Kessi and Boonzaier 2018).

The way in which the discipline has controlled and regulated human behaviour and constructed ideas of normality cannot be underemphasised as this has significantly contributed to the pathologisation and invisibilising of identities and experiences of poor womxn, Black womxn, and the LGBTQIA+ population in psychological research and practice. As a consequence, poor, Black, and queer communities lack access to mental health services (Shefer, Boonzaier, and Kiguwa 2006). In the next section, I turn to consider the psychological needs of LGBTQIA+ people in South Africa and their access to mental healthcare that is affirming of their sexual and gender identities.

SEXUAL AND GENDER DIVERSE COMMUNITIES AND MENTAL HEALTHCARE IN SOUTH AFRICA

Psychology's pathologisation and erasure of marginalised groups have been a topic of discussion on the African continent for some time now. This discussion has occurred as a form of resistance psychology to make space for marginalised peoples, such as LGBTQIA+ communities, to address their needs and health concerns. The discipline of psychology has helped support cishetero-centric systems of oppression by providing legitimation for negative views of sexual and gender minorities. For instance, "conversion therapies" to change the identities of sexually and gender diverse individuals were and still are practiced today in some mental healthcare services in South Africa and elsewhere.

The lives of many sexually and gender diverse individuals on the African continent are shaped by discrimination, prosecution, and violent persecution. For example, over 30 countries in Africa categorise homosexuality as a crime punishable by imprisonment. In others, such as Mauritania and Sudan and parts of Somalia and Nigeria, the punishment is execution (Ewing et al. 2020). In contrast, South Africa's constitution is regarded to be one of the most progressive legal documents that protect the rights of sexual and gender diverse communities (Victor et al. 2014). For example, Section 27 of the Constitution states that everyone has the right to access healthcare services, including reproductive healthcare, while Section 9 of the Constitution notes that the state cannot discriminate against anyone on one or more grounds of race, gender, sex, and sexual orientation, among others. Together, these provisions seek to ensure that sexually and gender diverse individuals have the right to access various necessities such as healthcare and mental health services.

Despite these legal provisions, discrimination, stigmatisation, and violence against sexual and gender diverse people are common in South Africa. For example, most recently on South African Twitter, the hashtag #QueerLivesMatter has been trending in response to the brutal murders of at least three LGBTQIA+ people during pride month. Another example of homophobia in South Africa was the recent incident that occurred at DF Malan high school in Cape Town. The high school administration rejected a request by students to celebrate pride month at school. Students were banned from expressing pro-pride sentiments such as having the pride flag on school premises. Some of the DF Malan high school students staged a sit-in the following week. The situation escalated as other students took it among themselves to intimidate and harass their fellow students who participated in the sit-in. The administration has said that they rejected the request in fear that it would cause "division" among the student body (Victor et al. 2014; Rakhetsi 2021; Nefdt 2021). Research also documents a broad spectrum of harm and violence resulting from cishetero-centric discrimination that exacerbates the psychological harm that sexual and gender diverse individuals experience (e.g., most prominent is homophobic rape).

The discrimination prevalent in everyday South African society is reflected in and perpetuated by the health sector. The health sector is based on the premise of *sameness*. Healthcare users and their needs are assumed to reflect dominant groups. These assumptions disempower marginalised clients when they interact with healthcare providers. These assumptions also prevent providers from reflecting on how systems of power influence access to services for different groups, shape their needs, and shape the design and delivery of healthcare services (Nel 2007; Klein 2008).

The disempowering experience sexually and gender diverse individuals face in accessing appropriate general healthcare is reflected in attempts to access mental healthcare that affirms their identities. The use of psychological methods and research to prioritise cisnormative sociocultural assumptions has provided clinicians with the space to exercise their power through diagnoses and knowledge of the discipline.

This has negatively influenced how sexually and gender diverse individuals are perceived in health spaces. For example, the clinician's utilisation and operation of "sexual disorders" (sexual dysfunction and gender identities) have only just been revised in the Diagnostic and Statistical Manual of

Mental Disorders (DSM-5) and revisions of the International Classification of Disease and Related Health Problems (ICD-11) (Marrow and Wasser 2012; Campbell and Stein 2014; McLachlan et al. 2019). In addition, South African research has demonstrated how colonialism, racism, and social inequality mediated by the discipline have affected the mental health of gender and sexually diverse individuals in a manner that has either caused distress or has exacerbated existing stressors (Marrow and Wasser 2012; Victor and Nel 2016). Similarly, critical psychological scholarship has for some time recognised that queerphobia and cis-heteronormativity have similar negative consequences for the mental health of sexual and gender diverse people (Victor et al. 2014).

There is a vast amount of international research that has demonstrated that exclusion from and prejudice received while accessing mental healthcare services can directly affect the well-being and mental health of sexually and gender diverse persons. These include a range of mental health concerns experienced by sexually and gender diverse individuals, such as internalised homophobia, fragmented identity and living a double life, social isolation, and rejection, to name a few (Harper 2005). This scholarship indicates that sexually and gender diverse individuals are more likely to experience significant psychological distress compared to their cisgender counterparts as their gender identities, and expression are often disregarded or pathologised including in healthcare spaces. Sexually and gender diverse people are therefore in an even more vulnerable position, at risk of depression, self-harm, suicide (including ideations and attempts), post-traumatic stress, and substance abuse (Lefevor et al. 2019).

South African research echoes these findings and includes research correlating prejudice, stigma, and discrimination with anxiety, depression, and substance use disorder among sexually and gender diverse persons (Victor and Nel 2016; Polders et al. 2008). Research also shows individuals from these groups may experience post-traumatic stress disorder (PTSD) and suicidal ideations (Theuninck 2000; Wells 2006). Their vulnerability can be further exacerbated due to the intersecting oppressions based on race, class, and other identity markers; for instance, they may experience challenges getting employment or access to education (Clarke et al. 2010).

Taken together, the local and international research underscores the need for identity affirming mental health services that affirm sexual and gender diverse individuals' identities, space where healing can take place, free from the fear of rejection, dismissal, and further harm.

Instead, in South Africa (as elsewhere), economic resources mediate access to mental healthcare on numerous levels. Structural and systematic barriers to accessing mental health services include the scarcity of facilities and a lack of skilled mental health practitioners catering to gender and sexually diverse groups' needs (Luvuno et al. 2019). The deep-rooted cis-heteronormative assumptions underpinning psychology create this lack of competent health-care providers and, ultimately, result in the delay or denial of mental health services as healthcare providers act as gatekeepers to these services. It is also documented that these barriers erase gender and sexually diverse individuals of colour from the mental healthcare system due to insufficient practice guidelines, and non-existent policies around providing mental health care to sexually and gender diverse individuals.

Furthermore, mental health services and facilities often group sex and gender diverse individuals together, despite the fact that individuals from these groups may have different mental health concerns as intersecting systems of power impact them in different ways (Nel, Rich, and Joubert 2007). In doing so, mental health practitioners risk disregarding the importance of identity, experience, and voice for sex and gender diverse persons, even more so when practitioners are uninformed about the harmful ways in which cis-heteropatriarchal mainstream psychology affects these individuals' mental health.

Gender and sexually diverse people who do access mental healthcare experience services as unsafe spaces and have negative experiences of the ways that mental health practitioners address matters concerning their sexual orientation, gender/sexual identity, and/or expression. For example, participants in a recent South African study talked about counsellors viewing their (i.e., the participants') sexual orientation as "abnormal" and coercing them to "choose" a gender/sexual identity (Victor and Nel 2016). These experiences suggest difficulty or inability on the part of practitioners to foster safety, security, and normalisation or self-acceptance for clients. The inability to be identity affirming can cause further harm to sexual and gender diverse individuals and continue to make mental health services inaccessible to them (Nel, Rich, and Joubert 2007). Providers' lack of sufficient understanding, knowledge, and experience is a common theme in the literature and can partially be attributed to the absence of psychology curricula advocating for affirming therapeutic approaches (Sutherland et al. 2016; Brown and Njoko 2006).

The need for affirming psychological curricula is evident in Brown and Njoko's (2006) South African study on educational psychology students' ability to counsel sexually and gender diverse individuals. The study found that the students were aware of individuals who were sexually and gender diverse but held negative views of them. The authors point to the importance of practitioners' being able to reflect on and recognise their negative attitudes, prejudice, and discrimination. The psychological curriculum and training should provide a space for psychology students to critically analyse their viewpoints and the systematic and institutional oppression at play. Failure to do so has consequences for the clients' well-being and will continue to make mental health services inaccessible to sexual and gender diverse communities in South Africa (Brown and Njoko 2006).

In the next section, I discuss the PsySSA 2017 guidelines for providing psychological healthcare to LGBTQIA+ communities (McLachlan et al. 2019). I argue that, first, it is an example of an identity affirming approach to mental healthcare provision and, second, that it exhibits the tenets of Reproductive Justice.

WORKING TOWARDS AN AFFIRMATIVE APPROACH AND SEXUAL REPRODUCTIVE JUSTICE FRAMEWORK

Psychology's failure to critically reflect on its own assumptions, knowledge production, and practice perpetuates social oppression. Instead, psychology can and should be used as an agent of social change (Grzanka and Frantell 2017). The Sexual and Reproductive Justice framework, with its intersectional social justice foundation, is useful to apply to psychological enquiry and practice with the aim of promoting a more comprehensive and inclusive understanding of mental health that recognises the impact of intersecting systems of oppression. This includes psychology's role in perpetuating normative discourse and practices regarding sexuality and gender.

The principles of Sexual and Reproductive Justice outlined at the beginning of the chapter are evident in PsySSA's 2017 position statement and practice guidelines (McLachlan et al. 2019). The position statement and practice guidelines will help practitioners navigate therapeutic spaces with sexually and gender diverse persons and ensure that sexually and gender diverse communities feel safe and protected, as well as seen and heard, in therapeutic spaces. These guidelines are the first of its kind on the continent of Africa and in South Africa and are an example of the use of psychology for social change. Situating the practice guidelines within a Sexual and Reproductive Justice framework may enable psychology professionals to respond appropriately to diverse and complex contexts, such as those in which South African practitioners often find themselves (Victor et al. 2014). These practice guidelines link sex and gender discrimination created by patriarchy and cis-heteronormativity with intersectional factors that affect well-being (Nel 2014; Victor et al. 2014). PsySSA's position statement and practice guidelines can provide mental health practitioners with the knowledge and vocabulary to respond appropriately to the unique challenges faced by sex and gender diverse communities in South Africa and elsewhere. They can help practitioners navigate therapeutic spaces with sexually and gender diverse clients to ensure that they feel safe and protected, as well as seen and heard.

The guidelines "engage with issues related to sexual orientation, gender identity, gender expression and sex characteristics" (PsySSA 2017, 6) and are extensive and detailed in nature. PsySSA's guidelines stress the importance of producing psychology professionals who are critically aware of the privilege that cis-heteronormativity affords cis-gendered and heterosexual individuals, and who analyse the social worlds in which sexually and gender diverse individuals exist. In this way, the guidelines echo the Sexual and Reproductive Justice framework's stance on bodily autonomy and oppression. The guidelines aim to support mental healthcare practitioners to address these needs and deconstruct the essentialism of psychological discourse through their practices (Woulfe and Goodman 2018; PsySSA 2017).

There are 12 guidelines, but given space constraints, I highlight guidelines 1 to 5. Guideline 1, "Non-discrimination," notes that practitioners should not assume that clients' sexual and gender diversity is the most impacting stressor as there are numerous factors that can influence the stress experienced by sexually and gender diverse persons. These should be addressed holistically as clients' sex, gender, and sexual orientation/identity may not even be of concern to clients. Instead, concern around clients' sex and gender identities may be a preconceived notion of the practitioner, which may itself have stigmatising effects (PsySSA 2017). Similarly, Guideline 2, "Individual Self-Determination," makes room for acknowledging the different experiences that sexually and gender diverse persons may face, instead of providers assuming that clients' experiences will be homogenous. For example, South Africa faces high levels of social and economic inequality which is structured by social location, including race and class. These systems of oppression distinctively influence life experiences and indirectly the mental health needs of the individual.

Taking a step back to look at the discipline and profession itself, Guideline 3, "Enhancing Professional Understanding," and Guideline 4, "Awareness of Normative Social Contexts," emphasise the need to debunk essentialist perspectives in psychology. Psychology professionals may be unaware of or may not have encountered critical literature concerning gender and sexuality and therefore may find it "abnormal" when a client's sex that they were assigned at birth does not reflect their identity, orientation, and behaviour. The practice guidelines developed by PsySSA directly challenge the pathologisation of sexually and gender diverse identities, experiences, and communities by acknowledging and recognising sexual and gender diversity. Thus, the guidelines understand that psychological difficulties must be situated within an oppressive social context that may compound or worsen pre-existing mental health concerns (Victor et al. 2014; PsySSA 2017).

Guideline 5, "Intersecting Discriminations," explicitly draws attention to intersectionality by highlighting the structural positions that situate individuals within social systems, impacting how they take up space and which spaces are safe. As such, it is useful for psychology practitioners to be familiar with the framework of intersectionality. Acknowledging the existence of various forms of oppression and discrimination, and their intersections in society, will better help psychology professionals to assist sexually and gender diverse individuals. PsySSA's Practice Guideline 5 is useful under the framework of Sexual and Reproductive Justice scholarship as advocate for the acknowledgement of these systems (PsySSA 2017). As such, Guideline 5 emphasises the need for psychology professionals to be privy to the ways in which marginalised identities may intersect within the same individual, causing compounding psychological stress. For example, the racial discrimination faced by a person of colour may be made worse by discrimination they face for being gender non-conforming or they may experience gendered discrimination from other people of colour. Thus, Guideline 5 highlights that practitioners should be aware of such intersections. Psychology professionals can understand and work to address the many effects of oppressive systems that clients may experience, including how stigmatisation of marginalised identities may result in self-loathing and self-hatred as well as the harmful effects of various forms of violence perpetrated against sexually and gender diverse individuals.

CONCLUDING DISCUSSION

Psychology can be an agent of social change by providing spaces to critically reflect and analyse social interactions and phenomenon, such as race and gender, in ways that do not require a sole reliance on quantitative measurements or pathology. In doing so, psychology can scrutinise and help to dismantle systematic and institutionalised forms of social oppression that place fault wholly within individuals while ignoring the role of context and the system itself. The discipline of psychology has roots in colonial and apartheid oppression and marginalisation of various groups of people in South Africa. However, contemporary South African psychology has drawn attention to this injustice and has set out to reconstruct a psychology that instead acts as an agent for social justice. Thus, there are various forms of resistance psychology in South Africa, one of which concerns sexually and gender diverse individuals' access to mental health services. In this respect, PsySSA has seen to the development of practice guidelines that will ensure mental health practitioners are appropriately equipped with the correct tools and knowledge to counsel sexually and gender diverse individuals in ways that affirm their identities. This is one way in which the discipline engages in acts of social change and can become an agent of change.

It may seem strange to consider Sexual and Reproductive Justice scholarship and psychology under the same banner. However, psychology is a humanities discipline and should therefore branch into these arenas to ensure it remains relevant and well informed to appropriately address and represent the mental health needs of our diverse population. By including Sexual and Reproductive Justice scholarship, psychology will further contribute towards a more progressive and inclusive social world effecting social change.

NOTE

1. I am using "womxn" to represent different groups of marginalised womxn.

REFERENCES

Brown, Annie, and Sakhile Njoko. 2019. "They are demon possessed": Educational Psychology Student Responses to Gender and Sexual Diversity at a South African University." *Gender & Behaviour* 17 (4): 14014–25. https://journals.co.za/doi/abs/10.10520/EJC-1b1678e185.

Campbell, Megan, and Stein Dan. 2014. "Sexual Health in the South African Context." *South African Medical Journal* 104(6): 493. http://www.scielo.org.za/pdf/samj/v104n6/24.pdf.

Carolissen, Ronelle, Tamara Shefer, and Estian Smit. 2015. "A Critical Review of Practices of Inclusion and Exclusion in the Psychology Curriculum in Higher Education." *PINS* 49: 7–24. http://www.scielo.org.za/scielo.php?script=sci_arttext&pid=S1015-60462015000200002.

Clarke, Victoria, Sonja Ellis, Elizabeth Peel, and Damien Riggs. 2010. *Lesbian, Gay, Bisexual, Trans and Queer Psychology: An Introduction.* United Kingdom: Cambridge University Press. https://10.1017/CBO9780511810121.

Connell, Raewyn. 2014. "The Sociology of Gender in Southern Perspective." *Current Sociology* 62: 550–67. https://doi.org/10.1177/0011392114524510.

Daoust, Gabrielle, and Synne Dyvik. 2020. *Knowing Safeguarding: The Geopolitics of Knowledge Production in the Humanitarian and Development Sector.* United Kingdom: University of Sussex.

Ewing, Deborah, Anthony Brown, Nonhlanhla Mkhize, and Thabo Msibi. 2020. "Sexual and Gender Identities: Violating Norms." *Agenda* 34 (2): 1–6. https://10.1080/10130950.2020.1756629.

Fraser, Nancy. 2005. "Reframing Justice in a Globalizing World." *New Left Review* 36: 1–10. https://10.4324/9780203085981.

Grzanka, Patrick, and Keri Frantell. 2017. "Counselling Psychology and Reproductive Justice: A Call to Action." *South African Journal of Psychology* 45 (3): 326–52. https://10.1177/0011000017699871.

Harper, Shaun. 2005. "A Journey Towards Liberation: Confronting Heterosexism and the Oppression of Lesbian, Gay, Bisexual and Transgendered People." In

Community psychology: In pursuit of liberation and wellbeing, edited by G. Nelson and I. Prilleltensky, 382–404. New York: Palgrave Macmillan.

Husakouskaya, Nadzeya. 2013. "Rethinking Gender and Human Rights Through Transgender and Intersex Experiences in South Africa." *Agenda* 27 (4): 10–24. htt ps://10.1080/10130950.2013.860268.

Kessi, Shose, and Floretta Boonzaier. 2018. "Centre/ing Decolonial Feminist Psychology in Africa." *South African Journal of Psychology* 48 (3): 299–309. http s://10.1177/0081246318784507.

Klein, Thamar. 2008. "Querying Medical and Legal Discourses of Queer Sexes and Genders in South Africa." *Anthropology Matters Journal* 10 (2): 1–17. https://10.22582/am.v10i2.37.

Lefevor, Tyler, Rebecca Janis, Alexis Franklin, and William-Michael Stone. 2019. "Distress and Therapeutic Outcomes among Transgender and Gender Nonconforming People of Color." *The Counselling Psychologist* 47 (1): 34–58. ht tps://10.1177/0011000019827210.

Luvuno, Zamasomi, Gugu Mchunu, Busisiwe Ncama, Hlolisile Ngidi, and Tivani Mashamba-Thompson. 2019. "Evidence of Interventions for Improving Healthcare Access for Lesbian, Gay, Bisexual and Transgender People in South Africa: A Scoping Review." *African Journal of Primary Health Care & Family Medicine* 11 (1): 1–10. https://10.4102/phcfm.v11i1.1367.

Marrow, Marina, and Julia Weisser. 2012. "Towards a Social Justice Framework of Mental Health Recovery." *Studies in Social Justice* 6 (1): 27–43. https://10.26522/ ssj.v6i1.1067.

Matebeni, Zethu, and Thabo Msibi. 2015. "Vocabularies of the Non-normative." *Agenda* 29 (1): 3–9. https://10.1080/10130950.2015.1025500.

McLachlan, Chris/tine, Juan Nel, Suntosh Pillay, and Cornelius Victor. 2019. "The Psychological Society of South Africa's Guidelines for Psychology Professionals Working with Sexually and Gender-Diverse People: Towards Inclusive and Affirmative Practice." *South African Journal of Psychology* 49 (3): 314–24. https:// doi.org/10.1177/0081246319853423.

Nefdt, Ashleigh. 2021. "DF Malan High School vs Pride Month: Queerphobic Incident Causes Fury." *Cape{town}Etc*, June 10. https://www.capetownetc.com/ news/df-malan-high-school-vs-pride-month-queerphobic-incident-causes-fury/.

Nel, Juan. 2007. "'Towards the 'Good Society': Healthcare Provision for Victims of Hate Crime from Periphery to Centre Stage." Unpublished Doctoral Thesis, University of South Africa.

———. 2014. "South African Psychology Can and Should Provide Leadership in Advancing Understanding of Sexual and Gender Diversity on the African Continent." *South African Journal of Psychology* 44 (2): 145–48. https://10.1177/ 0081246314530834.

Nel, Juan, Eileen Rich, and Kevin Joubert. 2007. "Lifting the Veil: Experiences of Gay Men in a Therapy Group." *South African Journal of Psychology* 37 (2): 284–306. https://10.1177/008124630703700205.

Nussbaum, Martha. 2010. *From Disgust to Humanity: Sexual Orientation and Constitutional Law*. United Kingdom: Oxford University Press.

O'Connor, Cliodhna, Geraint Rees, and Helene Joffe. 2012. "Neuroscience in the Public Sphere." *Neuron* 74: 220–26. https://10.1016/j.neuron.2012.04.004.

Polders, Louise, Juan Nel, Piet Kruger, and Helen Wells. 2008. "Factors Affecting Vulnerability to Depression Among Gay Men and Lesbian Women in Gauteng, South Africa." *South African Journal of Psychology* 38 (4): 673–87. https://10.11 77/008124630803800407.

Psychological Society of South Africa. 2017. "Practice Guidelines for Psychology Professionals Working with Sexually and Gender-Diverse People." Accessed June 2021. https://cyberleninka.ru/article/n/developing-an-affirmative-position-statement -on-sexual-and-gender-diversity-for-psychology-professionals-in-south-africa.

Rakhetsi, Aaron. 2021. "Hear Our Cry': South Africa's LGBTQ+ Activists Demand Action Amid Homophobic Attacks." *Global Citizen,* April 31. https://www.global-citizen.org/en/content/lgbtq-violence-homophobia-south-africa-action/.

Ross, Loretta. 2017. "Reproductive Justice as Intersectional Feminist Activism." *Souls: A Critical Journal of Black Politics, Culture, and Society* 19 (3): 286–314. https://doi.org/10.1080/10999949.2017.1389634.

Shange, Naledi. 2019. "Study on Coloured Women's Intelligence Scientifically Flawed, says Professor." *Sunday Times,* April 25. https://www.timeslive.co.za /news/south-africa/2019-04-25-study-on-coloured-womens-intelligence-scientifi-cally-flawed-says-professor/.

Shefer, Tamara, Floretta Boonzaier, and Peace Kiguwa eds. 2006. *The Gender of Psychology*. Cape Town: UCT Press.

Stormhøj, Christel. 2015. "Crippling Sexual Justice." *Nordic Journal of Feminist and Gender Research* 23 (2): 79–92. https://doi.org/10.1080/08038740.2014.993423.

Sutherland, Carla, Ben Roberts, Neville Gabriel, Jarè Struwig, and Steven Gordon. 2016. *Progressive Prudes: A Survey of Attitudes towards Homosexuality & Gender Non- conformity in South Africa*. Pretoria: Health Science Research Council.

Theuninck, Jan. 2000. "The Traumatic Impact of Minority Stressors on Males Self-Identified as Homosexual or Bisexual." Unpublished master's dissertation, University of the Witwatersrand.

Victor, Cornelius, and Juan Nel. 2016. Lesbian, Gay, and Bisexual Clients' Experience with Counselling and Psychotherapy in South Africa: Implications for Affirmative Practice." *South African Journal of Psychology* 46 (3): 351–63. https: //10.1177/0081246315620774.

Victor, Cornelius, Juan Nel, Ingrid Lynch, and Khonzi Mbatha. 2014. "The Psychological Society of South Africa Sexual and Gender Diversity Position Statement: Contributing Towards a Just Society." *South African Journal of Psychology* 44 (3): 292–302. https://10.1177/0081246314533635.

Wells, Gary. 2006. "Homophobic Victimisation and Suicide Ideation Among Gay and Lesbian People in Gauteng." Unpublished master's dissertation, University of South Africa.

Woulfe, Julie, and Lisa Goodman. 2018. "Identity Abuse as a Tactic of Violence in LGBTQ Communities: Initial Validation of the Identity Abuse Measure." *Journal of Interpersonal Violence* 36 (5-6): 2656–76. https://doi.org/10.1177 /0886260518760018.

Chapter 6

The Quest for a First-Born

Boys' Reproductive Desires and the
Un/intentionality of Teenage Pregnancy

Busisiwe Nkala-Dlamini and Thobeka Nkomo

Pregnancy in the teenage years has received much attention and has been presented unequivocally as problematic. When examining pregnancy among young people, the literature often uses terms such as "unintended," "unplanned," "mistimed," and even "unwanted" (Mchunu et al 2012; Raushen and Raushen 2017). These terms are often used interchangeably to mean that it is either socially unacceptable or "normal" for young people to be pregnant or parent, much less *by desire or intention*. This literature overlooks the fact that teenage pregnancy occurs in a social context, alongside biological changes, where pregnancy, childbearing, and child-rearing have significant personal, cultural, and social value, including for young people. Moreover, within this work, girls[1] are often blamed for failing to prevent pregnancy, while the experiences of teenage boys and their understandings of and desires in relation to pregnancy and fatherhood are frequently overlooked (Swartz and Bhana 2009).

Despite advances in the management of pregnancy, delivery, and infant management, the problematisation of teenage pregnancy persists and reveals that people's right to decide when to have a child normatively excludes teenagers, particularly males. Cook and Fathalla (1996) argue that it is the right of everyone to have access to information and services that will support their right to have children, space pregnancies, and have the best chance of having a healthy infant. A Reproductive Justice approach recognises the history of controlling the reproduction of people of colour, those who are poor, or otherwise deemed "unfit parents" (Ross 2017), including young people. Indeed, while the problematisation of early or teenage pregnancy is based on the assumption that teenage pregnancy is inherently problematic, the normative focus tends to be on Black working-class teenagers' reproduction (Hans and White 2019). Research frequently understands unintended pregnancy among Black teenagers in relation to socio-economic deficit, whereas White teenagers' unintended pregnancy is given a psychological explanation (Macleod and Durrheim 2002). Extending Cook and Fathalla's (1996) argument, a Reproductive Justice perspective highlights the experiences of people who are marginalised in the reproductive sphere and acknowledges that reproductive choices are shaped by intersecting factors such as race, class, gender, and age (Smith 2006). This is true for Black teenagers living in under-resourced settings whose reproductive choices are constrained by various intersecting relations of power.

In line with the problematisation of young people's sexuality and reproduction, society tends to focus on what *behaviours* young people engage in, at what age, and what gender, but overlooks the nature of their relationships (e.g., social-sexual relations) and pays little attention to what such sexual relationships *mean* to young people themselves. Addressing this oversight, in this chapter we present extracts from young people's narratives about intimate relationships and prevention of unintended pregnancies.

We pay special attention to teenage cisgender boys' desires and intentions regarding childbearing and fatherhood, given the lack of research including them in mainstream research as well as Reproductive Justice scholarship. Studies taking a Reproductive Justice perspective have (of necessity) focussed on women in disadvantaged circumstances (Morison and Macleod 2015). Our findings highlight that this is insufficient. As Morison and Macleod (2015, 165) argue, "it is important to recognise men as reproductive beings who are invested in particular understandings of sexualities, reproduction and parenting, who form an integral part of the gendered matrix that coheres around reproduction." Accordingly, we explore boys' intentions and desires in relation to constructions of masculinities, the meaning of pregnancy, what it means to parent, and motivations for impregnating a partner. We consider the interface between boys' perspectives of childbearing and patriarchal ideals. Our analysis is underpinned by a "creative sexual developmental framework" (explained in more detail further below) that encourages researchers to approach young people as active agents in their socio-sexual context rather than passive observers or victims and, in line with a Reproductive Justice perspective, emphasises the importance of considering young people's understandings and practices within these contextual constraints.

THE STUDY

This chapter reports on data drawn from a larger study conducted by the first author, Busisiwe. The study aimed to explore the responsiveness of youth-friendly services to unintended teenage pregnancy and was conducted in a highly urbanised township (areas that were designed for exclusive occupation by people not White, that is Blacks, Indians, and Coloureds in South Africa) (Donaldson 2014) near Johannesburg in South Africa. To do so, the objective was to reach cisgender young people, girls and boys, who have been pregnant, are most likely to fall pregnant, and/or have impregnated a partner in the context of sexual relationships. Three datasets were collected and analysed, namely: (1) a survey of opinions of 233 teenagers, (2) 6 focus group discussions with teenagers in 2 age cohorts, namely, 3 with 13- to 15-year-olds (female only, male only, and mixed gender) and 3 with 16- to 19-year-olds (female only, male only, and mixed gender), and (3) 15 in-depth narrative interviews conducted with pregnant or previously pregnant teenagers. The young people interviewed by the first author identified themselves as heterosexual or described their engagement in heterosexual relationships.

In this chapter, we present data collected from focus group discussions (FGDs) and in-depth narrative interviews. The research instruments were in English pitched at grade six level. While participants in the FGDs were given an option of using any language that they were comfortable with, three languages (i.e., English, IsiZulu, and SeSotho) were used interchangeably, with English being the main language spoken during the discussions.

For data analysis we used the "creative sexual development framework" adopted from Suleiman et al.'s (2017) work that interrogates adolescent childbearing and parenting, understanding it as shaped by the demands of adolescents' social contexts. The authors therefore challenge researchers to look at the knowledge that enables teenagers to take on social roles such as those within romantic and sexual relationships. Similarly, Harden (2014) understands adolescents as having the capacity to navigate early romantic and sexual experiences safely but as also needing necessary support in this. Here, we use the framework to understand how young people's narratives around sex and un/intended pregnancy may be shaped by culture, beliefs, patriarchal gender norms, and young people's lived experiences.

The analysis generated data in three different domains: (1) dating, sexual activity, and teenage pregnancy; (2) perceptions, use, and expectations of youth-friendly services; and (3) meaningful impact of teenager relationships in teenage pregnancy prevention. The themes presented in this chapter are derived from the first area, "dating, sexual activity, and teenage pregnancy" as it relates to teenage parenting taking into consideration boys' and girls' sexual and reproductive health rights.

The study protocol was reviewed by the University of the Witwatersrand's Human Research Ethics Committee (HREC) and ethical approval was granted. Participants aged 18 years or older provided consent for participating in the study. All participants younger than 18 years provided assent and their parents provided consent, as per the South African Children's Bill, which defines the age of majority as 18 years (South African Government 2005).

FINDINGS

In this chapter, we present focus group and interview data extracts in which young people speak about their engagement in sex, which we interpret drawing on the creative sexual development framework discussed above. Overall, our analysis of the participants' talk showed that young people, including girls, are active sexual agents and contrary to the common view of young people's sexual engagement as a problem, FGD participants' perceptions were that young people do have sex and that this is natural and enjoyable, as evident in the following comments from male participants: "we all know that with sex two people must enjoy" (Participant #5, FGD, boys 16–19); "I was taught that sex is not a bad thing, which means it is something that is there that is natural" (Participant #4, FGD, boys 16–19). The girls' narratives indicate that they too are not passive participants but creative and resourceful in creating spaces to have fun and sex. For instance, a girl described misleading her parents into allowing them to go out to meet boys: "My friend and I will write letters to our parents stating that there is a function like Valentine's ball or something at school" (Narrative Participant #6, A girl who experienced "unintended" pregnancy). In these accounts, girls demonstrate agency and resourcefulness so that they can meet their needs and their relational and sexual desires, challenging dominant stereotypes and gendered expectations of women and girls as mere passive victims in heterosexual activity (Jewkes, Morrell, and Christofides 2009).

These findings, read through a creative sexual development lens, suggest that young people are sexual beings, without the need for sanctioning by society (Schalet 2004; Suleiman et al. 2017) and add to an evidence base showing that young people largely engage in intimate relationships willingly and may practice sexual relations in different ways (Bhana and Pattman 2011; Mchunu et al. 2012; Morrell, Bhana, and Shefer 2012; O'Sullivan et al. 2006).

Importantly, our data show how participants' sexual and reproductive decision-making is "influenced by local ideas of how to be and act" (Mkhwanazi 2006) during the process of exploring how they fit into social structures (Jones 2009). In the remainder of this section, we focus on boys' thoughts about and desires around pregnancy and parenthood, presenting two themes drawn from male participants' accounts, namely, (1) provider masculinity and acceptable masculinity and (2) boys' quest for a first-born child.

Theme 1: Provider Masculinity and Acceptable Masculinity

The boys' accounts and the behaviour they described appear to be associated with traditional notions of heterosexual masculinity, such as having a family and providing financially or materially for girls, which Bhana and Pattman (2011) refer to as "provider masculinity." Male participants in this study were self-assured about their ability to fulfil a girl's material needs and quest for attention. The older male participants (16- to 19-years-old) reported that in relationships they give attention to girls and assume provider roles giving girls money, purchasing needed items, or gifts. For example:

Extract 1, Participant #Boy (FGD, mixed, 16–19)
That is what lead me into wanting a 13-year-old girl while I am 16, because I know that no, I will just buy her snack, and tell her that I will do for you anything you want. (laughter).

Extract 2, Participant #5 (FGD, boys 16–19)
I have already spotted her needs, I am able to satisfy her, I will compromise my needs for her. It is a goal that everyone can achieve but because you as a boy.

The speaker in extract 2 describes his preference for young girls who will accept "being provided for" and implicitly are easier to attract than older girls. Likewise in extract 1, the speaker takes up the role of provider within the constraints of economic resources. These two quotes demonstrate how boys adhered to a heterosexual script which places men as providers who "propose love" and initiate the first move in intimate relationships (Morison, Macleod, and Lynch 2021; Bhana and Pattman 2011). Boys are expected to be experienced with sex (Mantell, Smit, and Stein 2009) and to actively seek heterosexual sex to prove their manhood (Allen 2003). Such ideas about "normal" heterosexuality, including the perception of men as active and women as passive in their sexuality, were a dominant discourse within the participants' talk. These ideas were considered normal by participants. Research suggests that such assumptions about feminine and masculine identities show that the roles prescribed by society for boys and girls motivate young people to engage in sexual activity (Buga, Amoko, and Ncayiyana 1996).

The quotes above suggest that romantic and sexual relationships are important to the boys in the study, most often because of the status it grants them among their male peers. We observe that romantic relationships and especially "sexual activity provided an arena for the performance of self, for the demonstration of . . . [socially valued] masculine identity" (van der Riet et al. 2019). The link between sexual relationships and social reputation is also shown in several other South African studies (e.g., Morison, Macleod, and Lynch 2021; van der Riet et al. 2019). For instance, echoing our findings, a recent study in a township in Cape Town shows that boys "persuaded" girls to have sex through gift giving, flattery, and other means to gain social status among male peers and avoid being labelled as *isishumane* (impotent or sexually inactive) (Morison, Macleod, and Lynch 2021). Likewise, in our study boys' motivation to engage in romantic and sexual relationships was to some extent motivated by their male peer relationships. Male peer relationships appeared to fulfil an immediate need for affirmation and at the same time encourage adherence to a traditional heterosexual script.

Theme 2: Boys' Quest to Father a First-born Child

In our study, the older boys viewed pregnancy and parenthood as an important aspect of their socio-sexual relationships, with an urgent quest to have a child of their own soon. This quest was described as driven by the fear that they may not have an opportunity to father their own first-born child if they delay sex and fatherhood. The expression "first-born" appeared to be widely known by participants in the FGDs. Along with the boys, some female participants also spoke about how boys are pressured to father babies by the age of 18, although in the girls' discussion it was not clear who had placed this pressure on the boys. Male participants' accounts suggest that the pressure was associated with traditional male gender roles and status associated with getting married and becoming a father, as shown in the following quote.

> *Extract 3*, *Participant #Boy* (FGD, mixed, 16–19)
> If you can look you will see that girls aged 15 have children? Now we think of the future, say you want to marry that very girl and that has a child already. So when we say the first-born are getting finished we mean just that, so that at least if you have a child let that child be mine so it is going to be easy for me to take you and marry you. Because if you have another man's child, no, it means I don't have first-born anymore. (laughter)

Such accounts of how boys seek to fulfil culturally assigned roles may be related to the perception of masculine "success" given by adopting the role of provider and father. As the above extract shows, the boys in the FGD described this pressure as emanating from the notion that the "first-born children are getting finished," meaning that because girls are having babies at an earlier age, it is more likely that the woman they marry will already have had her first child. They would therefore only be the stepfather to the first-born child, depriving them of the opportunity of fathering their own first-borns. It, therefore, appears to be important to boys' manhood to be able to claim that they had fathered a first-born child, which may distinguish them from other boys who might not be able to claim that.

This shines a spotlight on the role that gendered cultural norms play in (un/intended) pregnancy among young people. The boys' wish to father a first-born child suggests a conscious intention to impregnate a partner, irrespective of what her reproductive wishes and plans might be. There was evidence to suggest that while boys have their own agenda, girls may not always have the same intentions to become pregnant and parent, largely because the weight of any negative consequences will be borne by them. For example, one female participant said, "I think after giving birth to a child, you still have a problem of taking care of that child, and that you have to feed [the child], you will need money" (Participant #7, FGD, girls, 13–15). Such statements may highlight gendered differences in the meanings and consequences that pregnancy may have.

Indeed, participants in our study related how community members labelled girls who had been pregnant "midwives" and called their school a "birth centre," a comment implying that there are high numbers of pregnancies at the school and that the school is functioning as a place where girls become pregnant. This stigma extended to all female learners who attended the same school, as one girl reported: "they call it [the school] 'birth centre', imagine, when you show up they just say 'here is midwife birth centre'; another person thinks that we also have given birth" (Participant #4, FGD, girls, 13–15). The stigma of teenage pregnancy she describes is notably directed only at girls, who are held responsible for and tainted by teenage pregnancy. Such reactions of course ignore the possibility that pregnancy intentions are not only driven by individual choices but also by social rules and expectations that shape sexual behaviour. Notably, this labelling is made in the absence of any engagement with pregnant girls to determine the un/intentionality or reason behind the pregnancy.

Boys' intentions, and the possibility that girls may not be aware of these, can be explained by gendered inequalities within heterosexual intercourse which constrain girls' ability to make decisions about sex and reproduction (Holland et al. 1990; Wood, Maforah, and Jewkes 1998). Similarly, a Reproductive Justice approach views choices as being enabled and restricted by systems of power (Price 2010). Where girls do not wish to become pregnant, perceived pressure for boys to father babies by the time they turn 18 and boys' belief that their community is accepting of young people's reproduction potentially undermine girls' desire not to become pregnant. None of the male participants disclosed having impregnated a girl; having had participants with this experience could have provided valuable views of the quest for a "first-born."

DISCUSSION

Our study sought to move beyond a sexual risk framework, instead of adopting a "creative sexual developmental framework" (Suleiman et al. 2017) that aligns with Reproductive Justice principles. From this perspective, young people's engagement in sex, their pregnancy, and child-rearing should not be viewed as inherently problematic but understood in relation to their social contexts. Following this approach, we observed that young people are active and creative in negotiating their psycho-sexual lives.

In particular, we showed how participants' sexual and reproductive decision-making is shaped by local gender ideals (Mkhwanazi 2006). We demonstrated how cultural ideals related to manhood, notably enacting provider masculinity and fathering a first-born child, shaped boys' desires and intentions around pregnancy and fatherhood. Following dominant heterosexual scripts (Morison, Macleod, and Lynch 2021) boys described themselves as initiating sexual relationships, with some room for negotiation. Considering our findings, however, this negotiation possibly did not include pregnancy and parenthood intentions and reproductive decision-making.

Davies (1989) notes that dominant discourses of gender sexuality are powerful and legitimise existing power relations by defining what is normal and what is not. Indeed, hetero-patriarchal norms are central to socialisation and young people's identity creation. This is key to understanding our findings around boys' motivations for dating and engaging in sexual relationships and their desires to father a first-born child, irrespective of what their partner's wishes or plans may be. These accounts, particularly around the notion of having their own first-born child, demonstrate boys' enactment and reinforcement of gender power relations already defined by society.

Notably, our participants framed boys' decision-making and reproductive desires within the context of peer pressure. Similarly, the literature understands social relationships as fulfilling teenagers' need to belong, receive attention, and not be left out from their peer group (Korkiamäki 2014; McElhaney, Antonishak, and Allen 2014; Sunwolf and Leets 2004). Furthermore, research demonstrates how gender norms and peer relationships regulate and police young people's sexuality in ways that conform with and reproduce dominant gendered norms and power relations (Morison, Macleod, and Lynch 2021).

Considering boys' desires for pregnancy and fatherhood, the *un*intended nature of teenage pregnancy should not simply be assumed. It is also important to note that their desires might not align with those of their female partners, potentially impacting the negotiation of sex and reproduction in intimate heterosexual relationships. Yet, boys' role in sexual and reproductive decision-making is largely overlooked, and girls are largely portrayed as responsible for becoming pregnant, based on the assumption that they are *able to* prevent this.

Our findings suggest that boys' reproductive desires—based on pressure to attain status by being the father of a first-born child and a provider—may restrict girls' ability and right to choose whether to have children or not and under what conditions, as stipulated by Reproductive Justice advocates (Ross 2017, 290). These traditional gender norms reinforce men's role as decision-maker and potentially encourage boys to disregard and/or overlook a female partner as a decision-maker, potentially placing girls in a vulnerable position as they may often be unaware of the boy's intention to conceive a first-born. Indeed, gendered power relations in heterosexual encounters have been shown to affect female sexual and reproductive health outcomes directly, as these relations restrict a woman's ability to protect herself from unwanted sexual acts and pregnancy (Wood, Maforah, and Jewkes 1998).

Our findings highlight the importance of including young people in Reproductive Justice efforts by addressing how young people think about and measure the outcome of their social-sexual behaviours, without condemning young people's sexuality and reproduction. Current sexual and reproductive messages aimed at teenagers may be inadequate, conflicting, or overwhelming (Kirby, Laris, and Rolleri 2007; Thorogood 2000; Schaalma et al. 2004; Wellings et al. 1995). (See also chapters 3, 10 and 11 in this volume.) Rather, interventions are needed that empower teenagers to evaluate their behaviour and support adolescents to experience their sexual selves safely (Harden 2014). This process may include engaging in discussions that encourage youth to reflect on their motivations and intentions of future parenthood, including whether or not they wish to become parents, the timing of child-bearing in their lives, and various factors involved in child-rearing. As part of this, norms need to be interrogated in young people's discussions about pregnancy intentionality. Doing so may encourage young men to reflect on gendered and parenting roles, and meanings around parenthood, towards challenging gendered norms in heterosexual romantic relationships, including gendered responsibilities in parenting. Doing so may also ensure that in the process of boys' realising their desire to have a first-born child, their female partner's right to have children if/when she desires to do so, is protected. Sexual and reproductive health programmes must encourage boys to value their partner's reproductive desires, including when their partner's desires and plans are not the same as their own. Thus, in line with the Reproductive Justice approach, the reproductive rights and desires of boys can be acknowledged, but not in a way that undermines their partners' reproductive rights not to have children if they do not wish to.

Moving forward, the creative sexual developmental framework could be used to understand how young people's cultures and beliefs shape their understandings, intentions, and motivations related to sex, pregnancy, and future parenthood. Drawing on the creativity and resourcefulness demonstrated by the young people in our study, this framework could be used to encourage them to be equally creative in preventing pregnancy where pregnancy is not desired by one or both partners. It could incorporate apply-ing the knowledge young people may have about pregnancy prevention to a consideration of the timing and outcome of pregnancy, so that parenthood occurs only when both partners desire it and when it aligns with both part-ners' plans.

NOTE

1. We recognise the sex and gender diversity of young pregnant people. Much of the literature, however, focusses on young cis women specifically.

REFERENCES

Allen, Louisa. 2003. "Girls Want Sex, Boys Want Love: Resisting Dominant Discourses of (Hetero) Sexuality." *Sexualities* 6 (2): 215–36. https://doi.org/10.1177/1363460703006002004.

Bhana, Deevia, and Rob Pattman. 2011. "Girls Want Money, Boys Want Virgins: The Materiality of Love Amongst South African Township Youth in The Context of HIV and AIDS." *Culture, Health & Sexuality* 13 (8): 961–72. https://doi.org/10.1080/13691058.2011.576770.

Buga, Geoffrey, Donald Amoko, and Daniel Ncayiyana. 1996. "Sexual Behaviour, Contraceptive Practice and Reproductive Health Among School Adolescents In Rural Transkei." *South African Medical Journal* 86 (5): 523–27. https://pubmed.ncbi.nlm.nih.gov/8711547/.

Cook, Rebecca J., and Mahmoud F. Fathalla. 1996. "Advancing Reproductive Rights Beyond Cairo and Beijing." *International Family Planning Perspectives* 22 (3): 115–21. https://doi.org/10.2307/2950752.

Davies, Bronwyn. 1989. *Frogs, Snails and Feminist Tales: Preschool Children and Gender.* Sydney: Allen and Unwin.

Donaldson, Ronnie. 2014. "South African Township Transformation." In *Encyclopedia of Quality of Life and Well-Being Research*, edited by Alex C. Michalos. Dordrecht: Springer. https://doi.org/10.1007/978-94-007-0753-5 4186.

Hans, Sydney L., and Barbara A. White. 2019. "Teenage Childbearing, Reproductive Justice, and Infant Mental Health." *Infant and Mental Health* 40: 690–709. https://doi.org/10.1002/imhj.21803.

Harden, K. P. 2014. "A Sex-Positive Framework For Research On Adolescent Sexuality." *Perspectives on Psychological Science* 9 (5): 455–69. https://doi.org/10.1177/1745691614535934.

Holland, Janet, Caroline Ramazanoglu, Sue Scott, Sue Sharpe, and Rachel Thomson. 1990. "Sex, Gender And Power: Young Women's Sexuality In The Shadow of AIDS." *Sociology of Health and Illness* 12 (3): 336–50. https://doi.org/10.1111/1467-9566.ep11347264.

Jewkes, Rachel, Robert Morrell, and Nicola Christofides. 2009. "Empowering Teenagers To Prevent Pregnancy: Lessons From South Africa." *Culture, Health & Sexuality* 11 (7): 675–88. https://doi.org/10.1080/13691050902846452.

Jones, Gill. 2009. *Youth (Key Concepts).* Cambridge: Polity Press.

Kirby, Douglas B., B. A. Laris, and Lori A. Rolleri. 2007. "Sex and HIV Education Programs: Their Impact on Sexual Behaviors of Young People Throughout The World." *Journal of Adolescent Health* 40 (3): 206–17. https://doi.org/10.1016/j .jadohealth.2006.11.143.

Korkiamäki, Riikka. 2014. "Rethinking Loneliness — A Qualitative Study About Adolescents' Experiences of Being An Outsider In Peer Group." *Open Journal of Depression* 3 (4): 125–35. https://doi.org/10.4236/ojd.2014.34016.

Macleod, Catriona, and Kevin Durrheim. 2002. "Racializing Teenage Pregnancy: 'Culture' and 'Tradition' in the South African Scientific Literature." *Ethnic and Racial Studies* 25 (5): 778–801. https://doi.org/10.1080/014198702200000268.

Mantell, Joanne E., Jennifer A. Smit, and Zena A. Stein. 2009. "The Right To Choose Parenthood Among HIV Infected Women and Men." *Journal of Public Health Policy* 30 (4): 367–78. https://doi.org/10.1057/jphp.2009.35.

McElhaney, Kathleen B., Jill Antonishak, and Joseph P. Allen. 2014. "'They Like Me, They Like Me Not': Popularity and Adolescents' Perceptions of Acceptance Predicting Social Functioning Over Time." *Child Development* 79 (3): 720–31. https://doi.org/10.1111/j.1467-8624.2008.01153.x.

Mchunu, G., K. Peltzer, B. Tutshana, and L. Seutlwadi. 2012. "Adolescent Pregnancy and Associated Factors in South African Youth." *African Health Sciences* 12 (4): 426–34. https://doi.org/10.4314/ahs.v12i4.5.

Mkhwanazi, Nolwazi. 2006. "Partial Truths: Representation of Teenage Pregnancy in Research." *Anthropology Southern Africa* 29 (3&4): 96–104. https://doi.org/10 .1080/23323256.2006.11499935.

Morison, Tracy, and Catriona Ida Macleod. 2015. *Men's Pathways to Parenthood: Silences and Heterosexual Gender Norms.* Cape Town: HSRC Press.

Morison, Tracy, Catriona Ida Macleod, and Ingrid Lynch. 2021. "'My Friends Would Laugh At Me': Embedding The Dominant Heterosexual Scripts in the Talk of Primary School Students." *Gender and Education.* https://doi.org/10.1080 /09540253.2021.1929856.

Morrell, Robert, Deevia Bhana, and Tamara Shefer. 2012. "Pregnancy And Parenthood In South African Schools." In *Books and babies: Pregnancy and Young Parents in Schools*, edited by Robert Morrell, Deevia Bhana and Tamara Shefer, 1–30. Cape Town: HSRC Press Books.

O'Sullivan, Lucia F., Abigail Harrison, Robert Morrell, Aliza Monroe-Wise, and Muriel Kubeka. 2006. "Gender Dynamics In The Primary Sexual Relationships of Young Rural South African Women and Men." *Culture, Health & Sexuality* 8 (2): 99–113. https://doi.org/10.1080/13691050600665048.

Price, Kimala. 2010. "What is Reproductive Justice?: How Women of Color Activists Are Redefining The Pro-Choice Paradigm." *Meridians Feminism Race Transnationalism* 19 (S1): 42–65. https://doi.org/10.1215/15366936 -8566034.

Raushen, Rajesh, and Mukesh Ravi Raushen. 2017. "Level and Correlates of Unintended Pregnancy Among Currently Pregnant Young Women in India." *Journal of Population and Social Studies* 25 (3): 194–212. https://doi.org/10.25133 /JPSSv25n3.003.

Riet, Mary van der, Sofika Dumisa, Jacqueline Akhurst, and Harry Daniels. 2019. "Young People's Investments in Sexual Relationships: A Different Prioritization of Self in the Negotiation of Safe Sex Practices in South Africa." *Sexualities* 22 (7–8): 1035–52. https://doi.org/10.1177/1363460718780865.

Ross, Loretta J. 2017. "Reproductive Justice as Intersectional Feminist Activism." *Souls: A Critical Journal of Black Politics, Culture, and Society* 19 (3): 286–314. https://doi.org/10.1080/10999949.2017.1389634.

Schaalma, Herman P., Charles Abraham, Mary Rogers Gillmore, and Gerjo Kok. 2004. "Sex Education As Health Promotion: What Does It Take?" *Archives of Sexual Behaviour* 33 (3): 259–69. https://doi.org/10.1023/B:ASEB.0000026625 .65171.1d.

Schalet, Amy. 2004. "Must We Fear Adolescent Sexuality?" *Medscape General Medicine* 6 (4). http://www.ncbi.ncbi.nlm.gov/pmc/articles/PMC148090/.

Smith, Andrea. 2006. "Beyond Pro-Choice Versus Pro-Life: Women of Color and Reproductive Justice." *NWSA Journal* 17 (1): 119–40. https://doi.org/10.2979/ NWS.2005.17.1.119.

South African Government. 2005. *The South African Children's Act As Amended By The Children's Amendment Act (No.41 of 2007).* Government Gazette, 2007, Cape Town: South African Government.

Suleiman, Ahna Ballonoff, Adriana Galván, K. Paige Harden, and Ronald E. Dahl. 2017. "Becoming a Sexual Being: The 'Elephant in The Room' of Adolescent Brain Development." *Developmental Cognitive Neuroscience* 25: 209–20. https:// doi.org/1016/j.dcn.2016.09.004.

Sunwolf, and Laura Leets. 2004. "Being Left Out: Rejecting Outsiders and Communicating Group Boundaries In Childhood and Adolscent Peer Groups." *Journal of Applied Communication Research* 32 (3): 195–233. https://doi.org/10 .1080/0090988042000240149.

Swartz, Sharlene, and Arvin Bhana. 2009. *Teenage Tata: Voices of Young Fathers in South Africa.* Cape Town: HSRC Press.

Thorogood, Nicki. 2000. "Sex Education As Disciplinary Techniques: Policy and Practice in England and Wales." *Sexualities* 3 (4): 425–38. https://doi.org/10.1177 /136346000003004004.

Wellings, K., J. Wadsworth, A. M. Johnson, J. Field, L. Whitaker, and B. Field. 1995. "Provision of Sex Education and Early Sexual Experience: The Relation Examined." *The BMJ* 311 (7002): 417–20. https://doi.org/10.1136/bmj.311.7002 .417.

Wood, Katharine, Fidelia Maforah, and Rachel Jewkes. 1998. "'He Forced Me To Love Him': Putting Violence On Adolescent Sexual Health Agendas." *Social Science & Medicine* 47 (2): 233–42. https://doi.org/10.1016/S0277-9536(98)00057-4.

Chapter 7

Weighing In

Reimagining Fat Reproductive Embodiment through the Lens of Sexual and Reproductive Justice

George Parker

Sexual and Reproductive Justice is both a movement and a framework for reconceptualising questions of reproductive health, rights, and autonomy. With its emphasis on the intersecting structures, dynamics, and interests that can curtail people's reproductive freedom, dignity, and health, Sexual and Reproductive Justice provides an important analytical tool for engaging critically with wide-ranging sexual and reproductive health issues that extend reproductive politics far beyond abortion access and notions of individual choice. The focus of this chapter is to explore the utility of the framework of Sexual and Reproductive Justice to inform a response to the recent problematisation of the fat reproductive body in Western reproductive healthcare settings through the emergence of a dominant medical discourse on maternal obesity (Bombak, McPhail, and Ward 2016; LaMarre 2020; McPhail et al. 2016; Parker 2014; Parker, Pausé, and Le Grice 2019).

Drawing on semi-structured qualitative interviews with self-identified fat pregnant people and midwives in Aotearoa New Zealand, I trace the problematisation of the fat reproductive body and its harmful effects on fat pregnant and birthing people. I argue that, understood through these harmful effects, this process of problematisation constitutes a reproductive oppression that undermines fat people's self-determination over their reproductive destinies and acts as a powerful instrument of social control enacted through fat reproductive bodies. I also demonstrate how fat reproductive oppression intersects with and amplifies other axes of oppression, including race and class, with particularly harmful effects on poor fat pregnant people and fat pregnant people of colour.

Importantly, Sexual and Reproductive Justice is not a framework confined to critique but also opens the possibility for thinking about transformation and social change. Grounded in the framework of Sexual and Reproductive Justice, I trace a counter story about fat reproductive embodiment that proposes a holistic and just view of fatness and reproductive health. Such a counter story would take account of the social, political, and cultural context of health, body weight, and parenting and emphasise collective responsibility for pregnancy health in place of individual blame and sanction. I argue that should this counter narrative come to form the basis of fat pregnant peoples' engagement with reproductive healthcare, the result would likely be a flourishing of possibilities for more peaceful and positive fat birthing and parenting subjectivities and a much more constructive pathway to the health and well-being of fat parents and their children.

WAGING WAR ON "MATERNAL OBESITY"

The problematisation of fat reproductive embodiment is a relatively recent phenomenon in Western reproductive healthcare but has had significant effects. Pregnancy was once considered a time of release from social ideas about ideal feminised slender embodiment, and maternal fatness was viewed as either benign or even a signifier of the maternal (e.g., Earle 2003; Strings 2015; Williams and Potter 1999). However, the emergence and enactment of a medical discourse that has problematised fatness in relation to reproductive health and the resulting moral panic about "maternal obesity" have transformed how the fat reproductive body is conceptualised over the past decade. The fat reproductive body has become a site of medicalised risk and harm, both to the main subjects of pregnancy—the pregnant person and developing foetus—*and* to maternal healthcare providers and systems tasked with "carrying the weight" of maternal fatness (Parker 2014).

The emergence of this medical discourse has been driven by an ever-expanding body of medical and health science literature. Such literature emphasises growing rates of fatness among people of reproductive age and frames fatness as a risk factor for a broad range of reproductive health complications from infertility to newborn intensive care unit requirement (e.g., Avcı et al. 2015; Catalano and Shankar 2017; Poston et al. 2016). Concurrently, in the expanding field of epigenetics, maternal obesity has been extensively associated with a range of long-term health effects for children born to fat people, (e.g., pre-disposition for childhood and later obesity, heart disease, poorer cognitive performance, see Godfrey et al. 2017; Shrestha et al. 2020). Fuelled by sensationalist media reporting on an epidemic of maternal fatness threatening public health systems and future generations, "maternal obesity" has been described as having "profound public health implications" (Godfrey et al. 2017, 10) and as a "global public health priority" (Poston et al. 2016, 1025).

In response to this crisis framing, Western reproductive healthcare systems have mobilised to address and manage fat reproductive bodies, resulting in widespread changes to reproductive healthcare service delivery. System responses have been underpinned by several Western, weight-based assumptions, including that: weight is mostly within individual control; fatness is caused by a simple imbalance between energy intake and usage; weight determines current and future health status; and losing weight will result in better health and can largely be achieved by changes to individual diet and physical activity (O'Hara and Gregg 2006). These assumptions centre the individual as both the cause and solution to the problem of maternal fatness and have been embedded in a range of government and health service enquiries, reviews, and committees aiming to address the maternal obesity "crisis" (Parker 2014).

The resulting policy and service guidelines and programmes have focussed on what can be done to modify lifestyle behaviours before, during, and after pregnancy, and to manage the risks and costs fat people ostensibly pose to themselves, their babies, and public maternity services. A range of healthy eating and activity programmes targeted at pregnant people and new mothers/ parents have consequently been introduced (Ministry of Health 2014, 215), as well as pregnancy weight surveillance programmes, like recording of Body Mass Index when registering for maternity care and routine weighing at reproductive healthcare appointments (Parker 2014). Fat pregnant people are advised to limit weight gain or attempt weight loss during pregnancy, are informed that they have placed their babies at risk because of their weight, and describe humiliating interactions with healthcare providers leading to feelings of guilt, shame, and self-blame (Fahs 2019). Reproductive health services have been reconfigured to manage the risks fat people purportedly pose to their own health, that of their babies, and to perinatal health services. Public fertility services have introduced weight-based criteria to qualify for access to fertility treatment, largely excluding fat people unless they lose weight or can afford the high cost of private care (Farquhar and Gillet 2006).

In Aotearoa New Zealand, the use of weight-based criteria to determine access to publicly funded fertility care has particularly disadvantaged Māori Indigenous and Pacific people, who have a higher mean body mass, compounding racialised inequalities in fertility care access (Farquhar and Gillet 2006). Weight-based criteria have also been introduced in maternity care, for example, restricting fat people's access to primary birthing facilities, the use of water for labour and birth, and choice of caregiver during pregnancy and birth (Parker 2014).

The need to medically manage fat people's pregnancies and births has been accepted as common-sense fact in maternity care, leading to increased medical surveillance. This includes increased ultrasound scans and gestational diabetes screening and referral for planned caesarean sections in the absence of any actual deviation from a physiological pregnancy (Ward and McPhail 2019). This results in higher rates of medically unnecessary interventions and restrictions on fat pregnant people's birth choices and plans (Cook et al. 2019).

System responses have also not been confined to reproductive healthcare but have extended to parenting more generally with documented reports of the exclusion of fat people as adoptive parents (Carter 2009) and the involvement of child protection services in the management of "obese" infants and young children (Friedman 2014). Taken together, the health and social system responses to maternal obesity constitute an oppressive web of surveillance, control, and medicalisation in the reproductive lives of fat people. Undermining fat people's dignity and self-determination in relation to fertility, pregnancy, and birth constitutes a reproductive *injustice*, which is compounded by ethnocentric/racist metrics. In the following section, I describe the key features of the study including participant demographics, data collection, and my analytical approach.

THE STUDY

In this chapter, I draw on one-on-one in-depth semi-structured interviews with 27 self-identified fat, ethnically diverse, cis-gender people who were pregnant, new parents, or were trying to conceive. Participants represented a range of ethnicities (as commonly defined in Aotearoa New Zealand): Māori (5), Pasifika (6), Pākehā/New Zealand European (10), other-European (4), and Asian (2). I also draw on one-on-one interviews and small focus groups with 25 hospital-employed and case-loading community midwives. All interviews were undertaken in Auckland, the largest city in Aotearoa New Zealand with 1.6 million inhabitants. Once the audio recordings of the interviews and discussions were transcribed and anonymised, the transcripts were analysed using a form of critical discourse analysis that incorporates the theoretical and methodological principles of intersectionality that underpin the Sexual and Reproductive Justice framework (Staunaes 2003).

Intersectionality directs attention to how claims about women's experience often produce "hegemonic generalisations" by universalising the experiences and problems of privileged (most often White, Western, middle class, heterosexual) women to all women (Ross 2017). Intersectional analysis complicates feminist analyses by attending to the "interlocking effects of identities, oppressions, and privileges" to understand the range and complexity of women's experiences more fully (Price 2011, 55; see also Collins 1986; Crenshaw 1989). Analytically, a commitment to intersectionality requires a refusal to analyse "gender" in isolation, or "women" as a homogenous group. In critical discourse analysis, this means attending to how the effects of discourse (ways of constituting authoritative knowledge) are differentiated by various axes of social power and by the effects of oppression in its myriad forms: colonisation, racism, heterosexism, cis-centrism, economic marginalisation, ableism, sizeism, and ageism (Ross 2017).

I have incorporated intersectionality in my approach to critical discourse analysis, asking how multiple intersecting categories of difference stratify subject construction within maternal obesity discourses, their regulatory and governing effects, and how these are navigated and resisted. The following section presents some of the study findings that demonstrate the ways in which the problematisation of fat maternal bodies in perinatal healthcare constitutes a reproductive injustice.

NAMING AND ADDRESSING FAT
REPRODUCTIVE *INJUSTICE*

My analysis is presented in three parts. The first part describes the discursive context of intensified fat phobia in maternity care that resulted from escalating concern about maternal obesity and its impact on maternal and infant health, and health service delivery. The following two parts of my analysis explore two of the discursive and subjective effects of this discursive context. The first explores how participants took up this discursive context as a form of pre-emptive biopolitics in pursuit of "healthy" maternal subjectivity. The second describes the resulting constrained agency as pregnant and maternal/parental subjects. I demonstrate how both of these effects are heightened for women/people in marginalised social locations.

A Discursive Context of Intensified Fat Phobia

An intensifying focus on weight as a perinatal health risk was accompanied by an intensification of fat phobia in reproductive health services and a general disregard for fat pregnant people's dignity and rights. Such fat phobia has been well documented as a feature of Western health services contributing to health harms and inequities for fat people (Fahs 2019; Parker 2017; Tomiyama et al. 2018), as illustrated by the following extract.

Extract 1, *Sara* (midwife)
When you think about how empowering a midwife can be, well I think the opposite is true too. And midwives aren't talking about it. We go to study days to achieve the right weight gain for their BMI [Body Mass Index] but we don't have any discussions about the emotional and the psychological care of large women.

Rather, midwives described discussions about maternal obesity in their services and positioned their colleagues including midwives, obstetric, and allied medical staff, such as anaesthetists and paediatricians, as responsible for the escalation of fat phobic attitudes and practices. This manifest as negative commentary about fat people at handovers and directly to fat people during their care, rough and gruff treatment, and a lack of will or commitment to providing size-inclusive facilities and equipment, as seen below.

Extract 2, *Rachelle* (midwife)
It's horrible, it's demoralising, it's insulting, it's belittling, it's unprofessional, "Oh well you're too big for our theatre bed, *you'll break it!*" that's the inference, "our beds just aren't designed to take women your size." Or you get the anaesthetist, and maybe they're not having a good day and struggling to put it [IV line] in, and they get frustrated so they say to the woman, "well how did you sneak in?"

Amia (MW) agreed, observing, "What I see is a lot of judgement and frustration amongst my colleagues." Riley (parent) captured the painful experience of fat phobia from the perspective of fat pregnant people themselves, describing the hurt caused by the intense focus on her weight when she was in the hospital giving birth:

Extract 3, *Riley* (parent)
They told me I shouldn't be eating so much, that my blood pressure was too high, and that was because I was overweight, and that I should have been exercising more. And I was just in tears, I was in here to give birth, and they just weren't treating me right. I felt really bad about myself, and I felt stressed out and anxious. I felt like I had been judged as soon as I had walked in the door without them knowing me.

Zoe (parent) described similar negative attitudes towards her fatness from hospital staff during birth:

Extract 4, *Zoe* (parent)
It definitely changes how they treat you, mainly because those assumptions [about your weight] are always there. It doesn't matter what they say to you,

in the end you're just like "get me out of here," and then you come home and you're like, no, that was my time, those two days with my new baby were taken away from me because I was treated like that, and so the blues kick in.

These findings describe the escalation of fat phobia resulting from a discursive context in which greater emphasis has been placed on weight as a health issue in maternity care with material effects on how care is provided to pregnant people. These effects are consistent with existing evidence that has shown the deleterious effects on fat people's health from exposure to obesity epidemic discourses and the resulting fat phobic attitudes and practices in healthcare (see LeBesco 2011). Material effects have been shown to include reduced access to care for fat people, along with misdiagnosis and mistreatment (Fahs 2019; Parker 2017; Tomiyama et al. 2018). Where public health and medical discourses are implicated in the framing of fatness as a health issue and public health threat, fat phobic attitudes and practices by health providers are legitimised as a reasonable response to the threatening fat body and even as a moral good (Tomiyama et al. 2018).

"I WAS TRYING TO BE REALLY HEALTHY": THE WORK OF PRE-EMPTIVE BIOPOLITICS

In addition to legitimising and driving an escalation of fat phobic attitudes and practices in reproductive healthcare, public health and medical discourses about maternal obesity amplify the construct of individual (maternal) responsibility for the problem and solution of pregnancy fatness (Parker 2014; Parker and Pausé 2018). The focus on the choices and behaviours of individuals without regard to the social, economic, and environmental context of people's lives that determine health and well-being is a typical feature of health discourses under neoliberal political regimes that govern Western societies (LeBesco 2011; Rail 2012).

In the context of pregnancy, maternal obesity discourses that mobilise notions of individual responsibility can be understood as an expression of a Foucauldian "pre-emptive biopolitics" (Parker and Pausé 2018). Within a pre-emptive biopolitics, public health and medical discourses are implicated in the responsibilisation of pregnant people not only with the health of their own baby in the womb but also projected forward to the citizen of the future (Evans 2010). In this way, pre-emptive biopolitics attempts to control the future by precipitating an individual's sense of responsibility for action in the present. Responsibilising the individual for health diminishes state and social responsibility for the conditions of people's lives that produce poor health and health inequities both now and in the future (Lupton 2012; Parker and Pausé 2018). The self-responsible and disciplined citizen is a central subject in neoliberal healthism, laying blame for poor health as the result of poor citizenship and a failure of self-management rather than social and economic inequities and structural violence (Lupton 2012). Combined with a longer-standing gendered tradition of mother-blame in the West for health and social problems (Parker 2014), a pre-emptive biopolitics embedded in maternal obesity discourse positions fat pregnant people and new parents as subjects of blame and sanction for their current and future body weight and reproductive health. This is without attention to the material conditions of their lives that are so determining on body weight and reproductive health (Parker and Pausé 2018).

Participants' accounts of navigating their pregnancies as fat people revealed starkly the ways in which they reiterated the notion that they were failing in their responsibilities as citizens and mothers-to-be because of their fatness. These accounts demonstrate how participants framed their body size as a personal choice. They described an acute awareness that their fatness was harmful to their babies and meant that they were taking up more space and resources than rightfully allocated to them in maternity care. As illustrated in the extract below, limits are set on what a citizen can expect from the public healthcare system, and entitlement to care is construed as established on meeting certain requirements, including slenderness.

Extract 5, Zoe (parent)
It makes you feel guilt, that you're taking away stuff, for me, that you're taking away stuff from the health system that could be used elsewhere, instead, because I have chosen to be a larger lady having a baby it's going to require more resources put into me, and they wouldn't have to do that if I was smaller.

Here Zoe positions herself as personally responsible for her fatness, constructing it as an outcome of her "irresponsible choice." Similarly, in an account of her pregnancy and birth, Lisa (parent) also made sense of her fatness as irresponsible and a personal failure. However, in the following excerpt, she frames this as a failing of maternal responsibility towards her baby. Like Zoe, Lisa (parent) positions herself as less deserving of maternal health care due to her failure to conform to citizenry and maternal requirements.

Extract 6, Lisa (parent)
I was made to feel so bad about it, like I was going to be a bad mother because I was fat, or a bad person because I was pregnant *and fat*. And it's like, well, I don't smoke, or drink, and I don't take drugs, you know? I was doing everything I could. I upped my exercise. I took the supplements. I was trying to be *really* healthy, but they were still going, "Your BMI is too high and you're going to

have to have a caesarean." And it made me feel guilty, that I was inflicting this onto my baby, and I wasn't deserving of care. [. . .] So I just worked harder. You know, I would do another lap of the pool swimming, I don't know what I was trying to do, eat some more salad, yeah just, I tried not to get down too much, I tried to see, like even though I felt really guilty, and I felt really upset, I just tried to make it into a positive thing, like "Ok well I'll go and do some more exercise, I'll go and do some more laps," I really, really tried, you know?

In the above extract, Lisa describes how she drove herself through a range of self-disciplined, pre-emptive actions aimed at offsetting the harms her fatness poses to her child's health. She describes feelings of guilt and failure, demonstrating how maternal responsibilisation for fatness results in a negative affective response whereby parents feel that they have failed before they even hold their babies in their arms (Parker and Pausé 2018).

Pre-emptive biopolitics were not only evident in the accounts of fat pregnant people in my study. Discourses of individual responsibility, in which pregnant fatness is rendered the result of poor self-management and an unacceptable burden on maternity care providers and health systems, were also evident in the accounts of midwives about providing care for fat pregnant people, as described below.

Extract 7, Angela (midwife)
It's frustrating, it's almost like they're not aware that their weight is a problem and they aren't motivated to do anything about it. And I worry for them and I worry for myself. I worry about New Zealand's future. I worry for myself in terms of, am I up to speed when these women are having heart attacks in our unit because I feel like it's going to happen.

Through an intersectional lens, neoliberal discourses of maternal responsibility and blame for reproductive health do not implicate all fat pregnant people and new parents equally. Rather, they are focussed on families who—because of the intersecting oppressions of racism, colonisation, ableism, poverty, heteronormativity, and cis-genderism—have the least resources and capacity to meet the requirements of the responsible and self-managing neoliberal maternal citizen who secures slenderness and health for herself and her family. Consequently, the most marginalised families are placed as the most vulnerable to blame and sanction for poor reproductive health outcomes for themselves and their families and are positioned as less deserving of government resourced reproductive health care.

The additional burden of discourses of self-responsibility and self-blame for pregnancy fatness on participants marginalised along intersecting axes of indigeneity, race, and socio-economic status was stark in my analysis. For example, the following two extracts are the challenges faced by two participants living in areas of high socio-economic deprivation.

Extract 8, Mere (parent, Samoan)
I'd walk out angry at myself sometimes because I hadn't tried hard enough to lose the weight. I just couldn't fit it into my daily life. My work has moved into the city, so it now takes two hours out of my day. I work eight hours, so that's, what, ten hours already gone in a day. I come home and it's time to quickly get my son sorted. My partner leaves at five in the morning and he finishes at 2.30 pm so he can pick up my son. I leave later so I can get my son ready for school. So, we work around the clock, and it's like by the time you get home you're exhausted and there's just no willpower to actually go out and do something, because it's dark by then.

Extract 9, Kahu (parent, Māori)
They tell me I'm heavy and I need to lose the weight, but no one has ever asked me what my job is. You know it's hard to be told you're heavy, and not have any options to do anything else about it. They tell me what I need to eat for my baby, that I can't have McDonalds, but that's the thing, there's just no other options, they haven't suggested any options for me to do anything.

Mere, a Pacific person, juxtaposes self-blame with the impossibility of taking responsibility for getting her weight down in the context of parenting, long hours of shift work, and constrained material resources. Similarly, Kahu, a Māori pregnant person, describes a lack of alternatives in relation to the difficulties of navigating a sense of personal responsibility for weight management during pregnancy with limited resources, limited time, and a job involving heavy labour. These extracts illustrate how fat phobic, individualised discourses of failed self-management and maternal blame constrain dignity and self-determination. Participants described how negative or hostile encounters with maternity providers and within maternity services—along with the affective toll of feeling as though they were bad mothers before they had even given birth—had deleterious effects including guilt, shame, feeling undeserving of their pregnancies, and of good quality care, with some describing the desire to withdraw from or avoid maternity care altogether.

"I'D JUST GIVEN UP": CONSTRAINED AGENCY

For some participants, being treated as a problem to be dealt with resulted in passive positioning in relation to maternity providers. Participants recounted how they abandoned their desires and wishes for how their pregnancy and birth would progress in acquiescence to medical management. As Lisa (parent) described, "I remember my midwife was asking me about my birth plan and I said well, you know, the hospital's got my birth plan, it doesn't matter what I want, I'd just given up." As a result, poor treatment went unchallenged. In addition to the impact on agency in maternity care, participants also described being robbed of the ability to enjoy their pregnancies. As Riley (parent) described:

Extract 10, Riley (parent)
I don't think you enjoy your pregnancy as much, and I don't think, you know it's a beautiful thing to be pregnant, and have this baby, and you should be able to enjoy this beautiful bump that you have, not think "holy crap, I'm fat and I've got this giant baby."

Here Riley constructs pregnancy as something "beautiful" that ought to be enjoyable, but which is undermined by the awareness of not meeting normative expectations. Instead, they described the anticipated joy being replaced with anxiety, concern, and hypervigilance that they were harming their babies and needed to do everything they could to offset this harm. Thus, as discussed above, some participants told how they attempted to pre-emptively manage risk by exercising excessively and dieting. Others' accounts described themselves as passive: they spoke of a loss of self-esteem, declining interest or investment in their own self-care leading to excessive eating, and loss of enjoyment in exercise. As one parent described:

Extract 11, Lisa (parent)
If I wasn't so focused, I think I would have just come home and eat and not bothered exercising and just gone, "oh well," cause they were saying that he was going to be a caesarean because they thought I wasn't allowed to have a natural birth.

Lisa describes her impulse to give up in response to not being "allowed" to give birth how she wished; her wish to do so is rendered contingent on regulating her eating and exercise. Her account points to a scenario of constrained agency in which participants either actively attempt to comply with the restrictions and conditions imposed upon them by healthcare providers or resign themselves to failure and defer to expert opinion.

The constraint was compounded for participants marginalised along multiple axes of race, indigeneity, and class who had to negotiate these effects with and alongside institutional and interpersonal racism, colonised reproductive healthcare, and the health and healthcare access impacts of poverty. As Kahu (parent) reflected:

Extract 12, Kahu (Māori)

I think those in the health care system would like us [Māori and Pacific women] to be like Pākehās[1] like you know, Pākehās and their body shape and everything. Like that's what they think healthy is, but I'd be sick if I was like that. But I try to keep quiet because they told me I'm a danger to my son.

Kahu's comments highlight the racialised standards against which Polynesian women are held and construct these as unrealistic and harmful ("I'd be sick if I was like that"). Yet, her positioning as a risky mother is implied to disqualify her from speaking up against this. Instead, her description of being silenced suggests deference to healthcare providers.

TALKING BACK: IN SEARCH OF FAT REPRODUCTIVE JUSTICE

My analysis highlighted the ways in which the problematisation of pregnancy fatness constitutes a reproductive oppression that acts as a powerful instrument of social control enacted through fat reproductive bodies and undermines fat people's agency over their reproductive destinies. I have demonstrated how this domination intersects with and amplifies other axes of oppression, including race and class, with particularly harmful effects on poor fat pregnant people, and fat pregnant people of colour. In this way the problematisation of pregnancy fatness constitutes a reproductive injustice and my findings speak to the critical importance of the framework of Sexual and Reproductive Justice to wider struggles to secure reproductive rights and self-determination.

The framework of Sexual and Reproductive Justice applied to the problematisation of pregnancy fatness insists that reproductive health can only be secured if the problems (and solutions) to reproductive health challenges are located in a broader social justice context and by securing the dignity and self-determination of pregnant and birthing people. As I have traced in this chapter, the alternative that actively undermines the agency, dignity, and health of pregnant and birthing people will not achieve public health goals and is unjust. The problematisation of pregnancy fatness, as I have intimated, is not only incapable of improving maternal and child health but in fact actively undermines it.

Faced then with the question of what we should do in response to calls for maternal obesity to be addressed as a public health issue, the short answer is when it comes to the complexity of weight, and considering the risk of harm, we should do nothing at all. The long answer is that efforts to improve health outcomes for fat people and their babies may be better spent bringing to light the nature and dynamics of the stigmatisation of fatness in maternity care and its intersections with other processes of marginalisation with and beyond maternity care systems, including institutional and interpersonal racism, classism, ableism, and heteronormativity, and developing strategies to address them.

However, Sexual and Reproductive Justice is not a framework confined to critique but also opens the possibility for thinking about transformation and social change. The challenge then is to ask how we might draw on the framework of Sexual and Reproductive Justice to facilitate a much more complex, holistic, and just set of meanings about body weight and reproductive health. To fulfil the challenge of Sexual and Reproductive Justice we need stories and knowledges about reproductive health that affirm and secure the safety, dignity, and self-determination of fat people, and that protect and honour their right to have children and to parent those children in a safe and healthy environment. Such stories are, as hooks (1986) proposed, an opportunity to pursue liberation from oppressive influences in our lives by "talking back."

A counter story of pregnancy fatness informed by Sexual and Reproductive Justice could begin by outright rejecting the idea that fat pregnant people and new parents should be held entirely responsible for the outcome of their pregnancies, the health of their children, and the future health of Western societies. Further, it would challenge the assumptions that the derogation of fat pregnant people's dignity, safety, and well-being could ever be in their own interests or in the interests of public health. Revealing neoliberal healthism in the context of pregnancy as a health fallacy would connect a Sexual and Reproductive Justice approach to pregnancy fatness with wider political struggles and scholarly agendas. This connection would assist in reclaiming the meanings of health from neoliberalism and re-socialising health instead (Rail 2012). By re-socialising health, I mean global and inter-disciplinary scholarly and activist movements to recover a model of health and healthcare that is holistic and open to a plurality of meanings of health and embodiment; recognises the determining force of politics, social structures, environmental health, and human relationships on peoples' ability to be healthy; and centres kindness, compassion, and care as core values in health systems and interactions (e.g., Lee 2012).

In the place of neoliberal healthism, a counter story of pregnancy fatness informed by the framework of Sexual and Reproductive Justice could draw on a holistic and arguably non-Western epistemological view of pregnancy health that takes account of the social, political, and cultural context of health, body weight, and parenting. It could draw on the knowledges afforded by a mātauranga Māori epistemology of reproduction and other Indigenous and cultural frameworks of reproduction (Le Grice 2014; Le Grice and Braun 2016; Parker, Pausé, and Le Grice 2019) to emphasise the significance of the social, spiritual, and ecological, alongside the biological, in the life-giving forces of human reproduction. From this perspective, pregnancy health could never be achieved by undermining the dignity of pregnant people, and healthy pregnancy would be understood in the context of a complex web of relationships and factors that include cultural differences in patterns of fertility and reproductive norms, socio-economic disparities, food and housing security, diverse family realities and challenges, access to education and healthcare, and safe and sustainable communities.

Through the framework of Sexual and Reproductive Justice, pregnant people in all their diversity would be treated with dignity and respect and celebrated for their life-giving potential. Fat pregnant peoples' motivation for healthy pregnancy and birth would be valued as a resource to be harnessed rather than dismantled. This would be achieved through the extension of unmitigated support, care, and resources to ensure pregnant people would be able to achieve health and well-being on their own terms and in the context of their own circumstances. Fat pregnant people's diverse cultural and Indigenous epistemologies of reproduction would help shape and be centred in reproductive health knowledges, as would fat people's own stories of pregnancy and birthing as they "talk back" to the oppressive discourses about their bodies and generate new possibilities for being (Parker and Pausé 2018).

Should this counter story come to form the basis of fat people's engagement with reproductive healthcare, I suggest that the result would likely be a flourishing of possibilities for more peaceful and positive fat parental subjectivities and a much more constructive pathway to the health and well-being of fat people and their children. This was of course the stated goal of public health interventions motivated by maternal obesity discourse anyway, so what are we waiting for?

NOTE

1. People from Aotearoa New Zealand who are not indigenous and primarily from European descent.

REFERENCES

Avcı, Muhittin Eftal, Fatih Şanlıkan, Mehmet Celik, Anıl Avcı, Mustafa Kocaer, and Ahmet Göçmen. 2015. "Effects of Maternal Obesity on Antenatal, Perinatal and Neonatal Outcomes." *The Journal of Maternal-Fetal & Neonatal Medicine* 28 (17): 2080–83. https://doi.org/10.3109/14767058.2014.978279.

Bombak, Andrea E., Deborah McPhail, and Pamela Ward. 2016. "Reproducing Stigma: Interpreting "Overweight" and "Obese" Women's Experiences of Weight-Based Discrimination in Reproductive Healthcare." *Social Science & Medicine* 166: 94–101. https://doi.org/10.1016/j.socscimed.2016.08.015.

Carter, Helen. 2009 "Too Fat to Adopt- the Married, Teetotal Couple Rejected by Council Because of Man's Weight." *The Guardian.* January 13. https://www.the-guardian.com/society/2009/jan/13/adoption-rejected-couple.

Catalano, Patrick M., and Kartik Shankar. 2017. "Obesity and Pregnancy: Mechanisms of Short Term and Long Term Adverse Consequences for Mother and Child." *BMJ* 356. https://doi.org/10.1136/bmj.j1.

Collins, Patricia Hill. 1986. "Learning from the Outsider Within: The Sociological Significance of Black Feminist Thought." *Social Problems* 33 (6): s14–s32.

Cook, Katie M., Andrea LaMarre, Carla Rice, and May Friedman. 2019. ""This Isn't a High-risk Body": Reframing Risk and Reducing Weight Stigma in Midwifery Practice." *Canadian Journal of Midwifery Research and Practice* 18 (1): 26–34. http://hdl.handle.net/10214/17830.

Crenshaw, Kimberlé. 1989. "Demarginalizing the Intersection of Race and Sex: A Black Feminist Critique of Antidiscrimination Doctrine, Feminist Theory and Antiracist Politics." *University of Chicago Legal Forum* 140 (1): 139–67.

Earle, Sarah. 2003. ""Bumps and Boobs": Fatness and Women's Experiences of Pregnancy." In *Women's Studies International Forum,* 26 (3): 245–52.

Evans, Bethan. 2010. "Anticipating Fatness: Childhood, Affect and the Pre-Emptive 'War on Obesity'." *Transactions of the Institute of British Geographers* 35 (1): 21–38. https://doi:10.1111/ j.1475-5661.2009.00363.x.

Fahs, Breanne. 2019. "Fat and Furious: Interrogating Fat Phobia and Nurturing Resistance in Medical Framings of Fat Bodies." *Women's Reproductive Health* 6 (4): 245–51. https://doi.org/10.1080/23293691.2019.1653577.

Farquhar, C. M., and W. R. Gillett. 2006. "Prioritising for Fertility Treatments—Should a High BMI Exclude Treatment?." *BJOG: An International Journal of Obstetrics & Gynaecology* 113 (10): 1107–09. https://doi.org/10.1111/j.1471-0528.2006.00994.x.

Friedman, May. 2014. "Reproducing Fat-phobia: Reproductive Technologies and Fat Women's Right to Mother." *Journal of the Motherhood Initiative for Research and Community Involvement* 5 (2): 27–41. https://jarm.journals.yorku.ca/index.php /jarm/article/view/39755.

Godfrey, Keith M., Rebecca M. Reynolds, Susan L. Prescott, Moffat Nyirenda, Vincent W. V. Jaddoe, Johan G. Eriksson, and Birit F. P. Broekman. 2017. "Influence of Maternal Obesity on the Long-term Health of Offspring." *The Lancet Diabetes & Endocrinology* 5 (1): 53–64. https://doi.org/10.1016/S2213-8587(16)30107-3.

hooks, bell. 1986. "Talking Back." *Discourse* 8: 123–28.

LaMarre, Andrea, Carla Rice, Katie Cook, and May Friedman. 2020. "Fat Reproductive Justice: Navigating the Boundaries of Reproductive Health Care." *Journal of Social Issues* 76 (12): 338-62. https://doi.org/10.1111/josi.12371.

LeBesco, Kathleen. 2011. "Neoliberalism, Public Health, and the Moral Perils of Fatness." *Critical Public Health* 21 (2): 153–64. https://doi.org/10.1080/09581596 .2010.529422.

Lee, Wenshu. 2012. "For the Love of Love: Neoliberal Governmentality, Neoliberal Melancholy, Critical Intersectionality, and the Advent of Solidarity with the Other Mormons." *Journal of Homosexuality* 59 (7): 912–37. https://doi.org/10.1080/00918369.2012.699830.

Le Grice, Jade. 2014. "Māori and Reproduction, Sexuality Education, Maternity, and Abortion." PhD diss., University of Auckland. https://researchspace.auckland.ac.nz/bitstream/handle/2292/23730/whole.pdf?sequence=2.

Le Grice, Jade, and Virginia Braun. 2016. "Mātauranga Māori and Reproduction: Inscribing Connections Between the Natural Environment, Kin and the Body." *AlterNative: An International Journal of Indigenous Peoples* 12 (2): 151–64. https://doi.org/10.20507/AlterNative.2016.12.2.4.

Lupton, Deborah. 2012. "'Precious cargo': Foetal Subjects, Risk and Reproductive Citizenship." *Critical Public Health* 22 (3): 329–40. https://doi.org/10.1080/09581596.2012.657612.

McPhail, Deborah, Andrea Bombak, Pamela Ward, and Jill Allison. 2016. "Wombs at Risk, Wombs as Risk: Fat Women's Experiences of Reproductive Care." *Fat Studies* 5 (2): 98–115. https://doi.org/10.1080/21604851.2016.1143754.

Ministry of Health. 2014. *Guidance for Healthy Weight Gain in Pregnancy.* Wellington: Ministry of Health. https://www.health.govt.nz/your-health/healthy-living/food-activity-and-sleep/healthy-weight/healthy-weight-gain-during-pregnancy.

O'Hara, Lily, and Jane Gregg. 2006. "The War on Obesity: A Social Determinant of Health." *Health Promotion Journal of Australia* 17 (3): 260–63. https://doi.org/10.1071/HE06260.

Parker, George. 2014. "Mothers at Large: Responsibilizing the Pregnant Self for the 'Obesity Epidemic'." *Fat Studies* 3 (2): 101–18. https://doi.org/10.1080/21604851.2014.889491.

———. 2017. "Shamed into Health? Fat Pregnant Women's Views on Obesity Management Strategies in Maternity Care." *Women's Studies Journal* 31 (1): 22–33. http://www.wsanz.org.nz/journal/docs/WSJNZ311Parker22-33.pdf.

Parker, George, and Cat Pausé. 2018. "'I'm Just a Woman Having a Baby': Negotiating and Resisting the Problematization of Pregnancy Fatness." *Frontiers in Sociology* 3 (5): 1–10. https://doi.org/10.3389/fsoc.2018.00005.

———. 2018. "Pregnant with Possibility: Negotiating Fat Maternal Subjectivity in the 'War on Obesity'." *Fat Studies* 7 (2): 124–34. https://doi.org/10.1080/21604851.2017.1372990.

Parker, George, Cat Pausé, and Jade Le Grice. 2019. "You're Just Another Friggin' Number to Add to the Problem": Constructing the Racialised (M)other in Contemporary Discourses of Pregnancy Fatness. In *Thickening Fat: Fat Bodies, Intersectionality and Social Justice*, edited by May Friedman, Carla Rice, and Jen Rinaldi, 97–109. New York: Routledge.

Poston, Lucilla, Rishi Caleyachetty, Sven Cnattingius, Camila Corvalán, Ricardo Uauy, Sharron Herring, and Matthew W. Gillman. 2016. "Preconceptional and Maternal Obesity: Epidemiology and Health Consequences." *The Lancet Diabetes & Endocrinology* 4 (12): 1025–36. https://doi.org/10.1016/S2213-8587(16)30217-0.

Price, Kimala. 2011. "It's Not Just About Abortion: Incorporating Intersectionality in Research about Women of Color and Reproduction." *Women's Health Issues* 21 (3): S55–S57. https://doi.org/10.1016/j.whi.2011.02.003.

Rail, Geneviève. 2012. "The Birth of the Obesity Clinic: Confessions of the Flesh, Biopedagogies and Physical Culture." *Sociology of Sport Journal* 29 (2): 227–53. https://doi.org/10.1123/ssj.29.2.227.

Shrestha, Nirajan, Henry C. Ezechukwu, Olivia J. Holland, and Deanne H. Hryciw. 2020. "Developmental Programming of Peripheral Diseases in Offspring Exposed to Maternal Obesity During Pregnancy." *American Journal of Physiology-Regulatory, Integrative and Comparative Physiology* 319 (5): R507–16. https://doi.org/10.1152/ajpregu.00214.2020.

Staunæs, Dorthe. 2003. "Where Have All the Subjects Gone? Bringing Together the Concepts of Intersectionality and Subjectification." *NORA: Nordic Journal of Women's Studies* 11 (2): 101–10. https://doi.org/10.1080/08038740310002950.

Strings, Sabrina. 2015. "Obese Black Women as 'Social Dead Weight': Reinventing the 'Diseased Black Woman.'" *Signs: Journal of Women in Culture and Society* 41 (1): 107–30. https://doi.org/10.1086/681773.

Tomiyama, A. Janet, Deborah Carr, Ellen M. Granberg, Brenda Major, Eric Robinson, Angelina R. Sutin, and Alexandra Brewis. 2018. "How and Why Weight Stigma Drives the Obesity 'Epidemic' and Harms Health." *BMC Medicine* 16 (123): 1–6. https://doi.org/10.1186/s12916-018-1116-5.

Ward, Pamela, and Deborah McPhail. 2019. "A Shared Vision for Reducing Fat Shame and Blame in Reproductive Care." *Women's Reproductive Health* 6 (4): 265–70. https://doi.org/10.1080/23293691.2019.1653582.

Williams, Lauren, and Jane Potter. 1999. "'It's Like They Want You to Get Fat': Social Reconstruction of Women's Bodies During Pregnancy." In *A Sociology of Food and Nutrition: The Social Appetite*, edited by John Germov and Lauren Williams, 228–41. Melbourne, Australia: Oxford University Press.

Chapter 8

The Possibilities and Limitations of Midwives Practicing Compassionate Care in Maternity Care

Jessica Dutton and Lucia Knight

Maternal health facilities play a fundamental role in shaping experiences of pregnancy and childbirth. Maternity clinics and wards are systemically and structurally regulated by the state, and their everyday practices therefore reflect the local and global bio-political landscape in which they are located. In South Africa, pronounced socio-economic inequalities and institutionalised racism structure access to quality healthcare (Fried et al. 2013). Everyday practices in the clinic are often governed by state order as much as they are by the implementation of clinical guidelines and formalised codes of behaviour. Reproductive injustice is undoubtedly produced and reproduced within the clinic as an institutional setting. Yet, it can also be a place of compassion and resistance as healthcare providers and patients go against the grain of systemic violence in everyday practices of being together.

In the context of a poorly resourced public health system, where are midwives and nurses situated within the politics of Reproductive Justice? What possibilities for Reproductive Justice can midwives and nurses assemble and what are the limitations? Much of the current writing on obstetric violence, a major barrier to achieving Reproductive Justice, positions midwives within the rigid language of either perpetrator or victim. In this chapter, we take the position that the role of the public healthcare worker, as state employee, is equivocal: to provide healthcare and, simultaneously, to police the population they serve. In the South African public health system, as in other countries, policing is achieved through acts of shaming, scolding, neglecting, and refusing to recognise the autonomy of their patients (Lappeman and Swartz 2019). Policing reproduction is also carried out through systemic violence, as particularly evident in many of the country's severely under-resourced clinics (Chadwick 2017).

The position of midwives and nurses is therefore more complicated than the uncompromising language of victim or perpetrator allows for. The midwife's position to in/justice is always relational to the health system and never static. In this we follow Bhakuni's (2021) thinking on Reproductive Justice as requiring non-domination in our reproductive lives. Bhakuni (2021, 5) states:

> The notion of freedom as non-domination is therefore useful for reproductive justice because it places emphasis on the circumstances that make separate instances of oppression possible rather than on the individual and her choices. Non-domination focuses on the ways in which human beings are systematically situated in relation to the structures that limit (or empower) us. Similar to non-interference, non-domination comes in degrees, meaning that a person is not either free or unfree, but *relatively* free depending on the extent of non-domination the person enjoys. (Emphasis in original)

We think about the circumstances and conditions of the maternal health clinic and how forms of structural and gender-based violence shape midwifery care. What are nurses' and midwives' relationship to freedom and what does this mean for the possibilities of compassionate care?

In this chapter we explore the ways in which midwives and nurses care for their patients, drawing on empirical data generated at three government maternity facilities in low-resource settings in Cape Town (South Africa) through site observations and qualitative interviews conducted with midwives working there. We demonstrate how the act of offering compassionate care while working under difficult and distressing conditions is a form of resistance to reproductive injustices as a form of mundane and systematised violence in under-resourced public maternity care settings. Through compassionate care, midwives and nurses imagine and create possibilities the health system does not currently provide for. However, due to limitations imposed by inequality and violence, such as resource shortages in economically disadvantaged locations, possibilities for structural changes are always already compromised. This chapter offers narratives of compassion told by midwives that expose both the possibilities for and limitations of Reproductive Justice available to those seeking maternity care[1] in the public sector in South Africa, predominantly accessed by poorer, Black women.

OBSTETRIC VIOLENCE IN SOUTH AFRICA

Obstetric violence is an expression of violence during the provision of healthcare that ranges from neglect and absence of informed consent to physical harm. It most commonly involves dehumanising, disrespectful, aggressive, and humiliating treatment of labouring and birthing patients, most of whom are women, in social contexts that foster uneven power relationships between patients and healthcare providers (Lappeman and Swartz 2019). The body of work exploring obstetric violence in economically disadvantaged communities, where under-resourced health facilities are the norm, has grown over the past decade or so (Chadwick 2018; Rucell 2017). South African research has shown that acts of disrespect and abusive treatment by healthcare providers towards their patients are not a simple result of individual wrongdoings (Jewkes, Abrahams, and Mvo 1998), but forms of systemic violence (Chadwick 2017), a particular form of gender-based violence (Rucell 2017). Drawing on these findings, we regard obstetric violence as structural violence, acknowledging that the problems and hardships in South Africa's health system are shaped by historical and contemporary injustice (Rucell 2017).

We apply the term gender-based violence to capture "violence that occurs as a result of the normative role expectations associated with each gender, along with the unequal power relationships between the two genders" (Sabri 2016, 2). In South Africa, like the rest of the world, women are more likely to be victims of gender-based violence; however, South Africa's rates of violence against women are much higher than the global average (Chadwick 2018). Gender-based violence is pervasive and touches on all aspects of South African society, public and private spaces alike (Kim and Motsei 2002; Rucell 2017). Obstetric violence is the form gender-based violence takes in the maternity ward, across the continuum of maternity care.

South Africa's healthcare is divided into public and private sectors, with 84% of the population using public health services (de Villiers 2021). The private sector, accessed by those who can afford the costs of medical aid, is still compensated by government expenditure and offers high-quality care to patients. In contrast, public health services are characterised by a lack of resources and high numbers of patients. To give an idea of the severe imbalance between the two sectors, only 30% of doctors in South Africa work in the public system, the sector that serves the majority of the public (de Villiers 2021). Severe economic and racial segregation in South Africa means that the vast majority of Black people cannot access private healthcare. Though obstetric violence may occur in private healthcare settings, it may take particular forms in these settings. Moreover, some patterns of obstetric violence may be more pervasive in government maternal health services where the majority of patients are poor, Black women. In this context, obstetric violence functions to shame and punish those who live in poverty for being pregnant and becoming mothers; a clear instantiation of reproductive injustice in which the rights to motherhood and good healthcare are denied to poor, Black women. The normative (White, middle class) role expectations attached to

who *ought* to be a mother, or *will* be a "good mother," are violent constructions that penalise those outside the narrow definition of "good mother"
(Chadwick 2017). When such normative role expectations are institutionalised in public healthcare, obstetric violence, as a form of gender-, race-,
and class-based violence, can be committed with impunity. Discipline in the
clinic, accordingly, manifests in acts such as refusing care and neglect.

   Much of the research being conducted on obstetric violence in Africa—
often referred to as disrespect and abuse towards women during pregnancy—has focussed on defining, categorising, measuring, and developing
interventions (Bohren et al. 2015; Bowser and Hill 2010).[2] Understanding
the issue as something definite with concrete boundaries may be useful for
developing interventions, such as workshops and human rights training,
but this approach does not adequately address the complexity of obstetric
violence as a systemic form of violence. Nor does it effectively consider the
roots of the issue, especially the contemporary and historical context in which
the maternity clinic is located. Such research often relies on maternal health
standards of care developed in the West, far from low-resource settings, leading to impossible expectations being placed on healthcare providers (Arnold
et al. 2019).

   When discussing the role of nurses and midwives in situations where
obstetric violence has been reported, the discourse often oscillates between
two positions—nurses as perpetrators *or* as victims (Arnold et al. 2019).
When nurses and midwives are seen simply as *perpetrators*, the problem is
often individualised and reduced to an issue of human behaviour to be cor-
rected through training or education. Yet, portraying staff only as victims
of under-resourced health systems misses the ways in which they negotiate and make decisions in their work environment and profession. Neither
extreme provides a complex understanding of the ways healthcare providers
are implicated in, and act within, the healthcare system. The call to rethink
obstetric violence requires tools of analysis that go beyond understanding
obstetric violence as strictly an (interpersonal) incident between a caregiver
and patient. We therefore work towards broadening the scope of our understanding about these relationships and what repair and justice can look like
in maternal healthcare, especially in contexts where gender-based violence
against women is extreme.

MATERIALITY OF CARE

The challenges of working in an under-resourced health facility have
received attention in the literature on obstetric violence (Bohren et al. 2015).
Recognising that under-resourced clinics functioning without basic supplies

and equipment is itself a form of undignified care and constitutes obstetric violence, much of the literature on obstetric violence acknowledges the impact materiality of care has on providers and patients (Bradley et al. 2019). There have been a number of studies highlighting the stress caused by having to offer midwifery care in a clinic without the basic equipment and supplies (Freedman and Kruk 2014; Freedman et al. 2018). However, a common perception is that this issue can be overcome or is expected to be prevailed over, in order to prioritise the quality of care in the facility (Tantchou 2018). Similar treatment of the issue can be found in South African maternal health policy documents and guidelines (South Africa DOH 2016). These documents maintain that no matter how poor the working conditions are, respectful maternity care should be a guarantee.

Tantchou's (2018) notion of "materiality of care" provides a framework to think about this, particularly the extent to which the material aspects of the clinic impact relationships in it. Tantchou (2018) defines materiality of care as encompassing

> Infrastructures, spatial organization, equipment and supplies, income, and the ways professional status is managed–all of which are determined by history, broad economic and political forces, a specific position in medicoscapes, and thus the "visibility" and "invisibility" of a specific place. (272)

She explains that the requirements for constant tinkering with broken equipment, working with missing supplies, limited space for privacy, low salaries, and societal beliefs towards care work and midwifery play an undeniable role in the tensions that grow between clinic staff and their patients and patient's families. What enriches Tantchou's (2018) standpoint is that she not only understands material constraints as frustrating and stressful but also connects these to historical and contemporary politics that explain how such adverse conditions have come to exist.

In this view, structural violence plays out through visible means—such as the lack of supplies and broken equipment—as well as forms of invisible violence, such as diminishing respect for care work and reproductive injustices that affect the clinic daily. Considering both the visible and invisible forms of violence, "materiality of care" is greatly influential in nursing and midwifery professional practice and where the clear connection between the materiality of care and the quality of care is made. In the following section we document some of the findings of our study, demonstrating how the materiality of care in the clinic setting and the impact of uncertainty shape possibilities for compassionate care. We offer a perspective of neglect as an institutionalised form of violence that plays a role in structuring the patient–provider relationship. Providing evidence of obstetric violence, our intention is to give some context to the clinic space we are discussing and further the conversation on possibilities for Reproductive Justice for those it has been often refused.

OUR STUDY

This study was conducted in three midwifery obstetric units (MOUs) situated in community health centres in Cape Town (South Africa). Community health centres serve the majority in South Africa and serve primary healthcare. MOUs are midwifery-run health facilities staffed by nurses and midwives and comprise an antenatal clinic, labour ward, and post-partum care. They are accessible and provide free-of-charge care for low-risk pregnancies and the postpartum period. Midwives are trained to provide care across the continuum of maternity care, as well as to detect pregnancy-related complications and transfer the care to a doctor and local referral hospital when necessary.

The MOUs visited in this study operate with two midwives and one or two auxiliary nurses in the labour ward. From auxiliary nurses to advanced midwives,[3] nurses from all levels of qualifications were included in this study.

Ethics approval was given from the University of Western Cape Bio-Medical Research Ethics Council and the Western Cape Department of Health and informed consent was sought from all participants prior to data collection. The first author undertook observations of at least 24 hours at each MOU and conducted 24 semi-structured, in-depth qualitative interviews with nurses and midwives working there. All participants were South African nurses or midwives aged between 24 and 60 years, residing in the cape flats area of Cape Town, and identifying as Black or Coloured women. Further characteristics are summarised in table 8.1.

The interviews aimed to generate personal narratives of experiences working in the MOU. The transcripts were coded and analysed using grounded theory followed by a combination of feminist theory, including Reproductive Justice theory, for interpretation. We discuss three themes that speak to the question of midwives' situation and role in the politics of Reproductive Justice, namely, (i) neglect as the norm in the MOU, (ii) working with constant uncertainty, and (iii) the limitations and possibilities for realising compassionate care.

Neglect as a Norm in the MOU

After spending close to a year interviewing nurses and midwives as well as observing each MOU, our interpretation of the relationship between the midwives and those seeking maternity care was that it seemed to be largely

Table 8.1 Participant Characteristics

	N (24 total)
Role	6
Advanced midwife	6
Auxiliary nurse	12
Professional nurse	
First/home language	3
Afrikaans	2
English	18
Xhosa	1
Zulu	
Religion	22
Christian	2
None	
Reproductive status	
No children	2
Has children	22
Relationship status	10
Single	14
Partnered (Married)	

structured by the confines of the healthcare facilities as under-resourced. For the most part, healthcare providers were working with what they had available, which was never enough. The staff were repeatedly having to make do with lack, whether it be equipment, supplies, or time. Obstetric violence, we observed, did not commonly take the form of direct mistreatment (such as verbal or physical assault) but a more subtle and pervasive practice of neglect and an accompanying normalised lack of communication. This observation aligns with another study conducted in a nearby hospital maternity ward (Lappeman and Swartz 2019).

The observed neglect seemed to involve different levels of intent on the part of healthcare providers. Incidences of neglect ranged from pregnant in a crowded and short-staffed antenatal clinic waiting excessively long times to be seen by a nurse to what appeared to be a more intentional refusal to provide care during and immediately after childbirth. While these forms of neglect varied in terms of the severity of the implications, and also the perceived callous or uncaring nature of the treatment, they came across as fairly ritualised and normalised. Instances of neglect did not seem to be regarded as poor treatment by staff and seemed to be commonplace.

Nurses and midwives rarely spoke directly about neglect but did speak candidly about the ways in which those attending the antenatal care clinic, labour ward, and postpartum care would have to wait for a considerable amount of time before being seen. Waiting would take place on a wooden bench alongside the hallways or a plastic chair in one of the designated wait areas. Tension would build throughout the day in the antenatal clinic waiting area. In the morning, the patients and the nurses and midwives seemed reasonably pleasant and relaxed, the waiting room was lively and often full of conversation. As the day passed, restlessness and discomfort set in and the mood shifted, both staff and patients displayed impatience ranging from mild frustration to anger. Those arriving at the MOU and present in labour would not necessarily be attended to immediately and, depending on how busy the MOU was at that time, might spend the duration of the second stage of labour (when experiencing strong contractions) without the support of a birth companion. The maternity ward offers limited privacy and therefore the company of a family member or spouse is not always possible. The combination of waiting for care while in labour and labouring without a companion has been identified in similar studies and seems to be characteristic of government maternal health facilities in South Africa (Lambert et al. 2018; Rucell 2017).

Our efforts to rethink obstetric violence in the context of low- and under-resourced maternal health facilities in South Africa require a particular engagement with neglect, and how and why it is so commonplace. Although the concept of materiality of care does not explicitly include the temporal constraints on healthcare providers, it does allow for a reflection on the status of care work (Tantchou 2018). There are several ways in which neglect speaks to the status of the midwifery and nursing profession, and the lack of value placed on maternal healthcare more broadly in South Africa (and beyond). If quality of care is to exist in the MOU, then it is the midwife who must deliver it. When the ratio of patients to midwives/nurses at ante- or post-natal care becomes unmanageable, and there is limited time to give during childbirth, one outcome is neglect and escalated tensions. Although there is evidence that patients' perceptions of nurses and midwives are changing, the belief that nurses are rude and gratuitously punitive still remains and for good reason; disrespect and abuse are still carried out by healthcare providers (Lappeman and Swartz 2019). Disrespectful behaviour, including but not limited to, neglect by midwives and nurses may be direct responses to their working conditions. Linking acts of neglect to the disregard for quality maternal healthcare by the state does not condone the act of neglecting a patient but allows for the nurses' and midwives' actions to be understood as part of a broader pattern of systemic violence (Solnes Miltenburg et al. 2018).

During one clinic visit, shortly before the day-staff were handing over to the staff on night shift, the antenatal care clinic (ANC) was closed and the clinic was relatively quiet. There were two patients and their newborns in the post-natal section of the labour ward and one in labour in a room off the nurses' station referred to as the consultation room. The woman in labour was alone and, from the intensity of her moans, seemed to be experiencing strong contractions. In the nurses' station, which separated the consultation room from the labour ward, two senior midwives sat at a table with two nurses and a student nurse. One midwife was reviewing patient charts while the other went briefly into the consultation room to examine the woman in labour. The midwife returned to the nurses' station and was followed shortly thereafter by the labouring woman, who entered the nurses' station alone, breathing intensely and holding onto the wall for balance. She slowly made her way through the room without assistance, stopping when a contraction came on, passing the table where the nurses sat, to the labour ward and got herself onto a bed. Approximately ten minutes later, the same midwife who had examined her, along with the student, entered the labour ward and assisted in the birth of the baby. The midwife and student remained in the labour room with the patient and her baby to, presumably, continue with newborn and postpartum care.

One may not consider the event discernibly violent but there seemed to be something cold and unfeeling in the treatment towards the woman who was labouring alone without support. That not one of the four members of staff assisted her from the consultation room to the labour ward shortly before giving birth appeared to lack compassion. Observing, it seemed that the labouring woman was struggling to walk unassisted, and a wheelchair would have been helpful and safer for her. The unresponsiveness displayed by nursing staff can be understood as a collaborative effort to refuse care. Of course, one can make an individual choice to neglect a patient in labour, but that not one member of staff responded to a patient clearly needing assistance is a demonstration of a shared attitude.

Overall, the ritualisation of neglect appears to sum up much of the mistreatment observed in the MOUs. Midwives speak of their inability to be as attentive as they would like to be when the antenatal care clinic and labour ward are busy and unmanageable; however, neglectful treatment continues, even when the clinic is quiet and few patients require care.

Working with Constant Uncertainty

Midwives at all three clinics spoke frequently about shortages of supplies, broken equipment, and the restrictions they feel due to the MOU's spatial limitations. Having to provide care without some of the most basic of midwifery supplies was considered to be part of the daily routine. Supplies including speculums, auto-hooks, catheters, urine bags, sterile gloves, bed linen, and bed-linen savers may be missing from the labour ward on any given day. Making do without these essentials or finding ways to minimise their use in the effort not to run out, such as limiting bed-linen savers, were discussed as part of working at the clinics.

Working at a maternal health facility that functions in a constant state of uncertainty is something midwives are tasked with daily. This uncertainty comes in many forms—from unreliable emergency transportation services and lack of basic supplies, such as linen and sterile gloves, to caring for people in labour who have received no antenatal care and managing a patient/ staff ratio that is unsafe for those seeking care. Midwives and nurses spoke about this uncertainty with great familiarity and frustration. In the last year, one of the clinics had undergone a change in management and a new midwife was brought in as sister in charge.[4] Nurses and midwives spoke positively of this and how much change the new sister in charge was bringing to the clinic. They felt that the clinic was more organised and better care was being offered to the patients due to the new sister. However, when the issue of supplies was discussed, old frustrations remained, as one nurse explained in a conversation about the supply chain:

Extract 1 (Advanced Midwife, Age 50)
Yeah, yeah that is the bad part of it. It is, I don't think they [people working in the supply chain] follow up and if one person says, "Ag[5] man," the next person just says, "Ag man, I am not going to do it now. I will just pass the blame onto the next person." It's terrible, even linen! There was a time when people [patients] had to sleep on thin papers because there were no sheets and it is uncomfortable, and they are bleeding. Even when you order, you must follow up on your order. You must phone and find out, and according to them [supply chain], they say there is no stock. It's terrible.

Improvements in one area of the clinic may therefore not translate to improvements in other areas. Limitations imposed by the health system, such as an unreliable supply chain, hinder the clinic staff's professional potential to offer quality care. Staff at this specific clinic were not alone in stressing discontent with the lack of necessary supplies. In the following quote, a midwife from another of the MOUs stresses the difficulty of having to work without enough sterile gloves, a basic requirement for offering safe midwifery care.

Extract 2 (Professional Midwife, Age 38)
Even with the gloves we are using, like when you do a PV [per vagina examination] to a patient, you are supposed to use the very sterile glove, but because we are saving, you use only one of the gloves and you cannot use the other one. When you do a PV on another client, you need to twist that other side of the glove, so you see how difficult that is?

Similar descriptions were commonplace in several midwives' stories. Supply shortages and faulty equipment featured frequently in the narratives and were often normalised as just the way in which the clinic functioned. Another area of tension regarding supplies is that patients often arrive without the personal essentials (such as newborn nappies, maternity pads, or food) required for childbirth and these are not provided by the facility. Familiar with their communities, midwives were sympathetic, but the dilemma was still theirs to deal with and try to solve. As one midwife explains:

Extract 3 (Professional Midwife, Age 42)
Sometimes even the plastic aprons are getting finished, even the pads. . . . We are telling them (patient) to bring their own pads but now if the person doesn't have the pads, what must we do? Because you know that person is bleeding already and let's say she is here and has never received a visitor, how do you expect her to get the pads? Also, the nappies for the babies; people are really suffering.

Giving birth without necessary supplies such as pads and newborn nappies is an affront to the right to a dignified childbirth enshrined as an international human right (Lokugamage and Pathberiya 2017). The responsibility to make pads and nappies available to those who cannot afford to buy their own falls on the state. There is something particularly dehumanising about requiring maternity pads and not having access to them—particularly considering that women are routinely shamed when their bodies bleed and "make a mess." This was not a finding in our study, but there are South African findings of disrespectful and punitive treatment of women during childbirth, such as patients having to clean the floors after childbirth as a punishment for "making a mess" (Odhiambo and Mthathi 2011).

In the interviews, nurses and midwives were sympathetic to the conditions of poverty that patients live in such that they cannot access basic supplies needed for childbirth. However, they also raised the issue as creating stress in the clinic. The absence of basic material necessities affects both patients and the staff, influencing the relationship between them and refusing possibilities for reproductive freedoms to be assembled within the clinic space. This refusal is not new. For example, a long history of denying Black women dignity in childbirth has existed in racist, anti-poor nation-states (Rucell 2017).

The Limitations and Possibilities for Realising Compassionate Care

Nurses' and midwives' position towards in/justice, as stated previously, is dynamic and always in relation to the health system. Throughout this research we have asked what possibilities for Reproductive Justice midwives can assemble and what the limitations are. This question has allowed us to consider why compassionate care seems so hard to maintain as common practice. As we have stated in an article looking at the possibilities of compassionate care:

Both the patient and midwife are entangled within an inherently violent system that treats women's labour and bodies as if they are disposable. When we understand that there is a violence to working under conditions of constant resource shortages and uncertainties then neglect becomes predictable and a constitutive aspect of public maternal healthcare. Without a radical deconstruction and transformation of a system that perpetually devalues or makes invisible social reproduction we can expect to produce the same outcome which in this case is substandard care despite a high degree of clinical skill. (Dutton and Knight 2020, 8)

When considering materiality of care, time constraints characterise much of the clinics' operations and staff interaction with patients. Compassionate care is time consuming; it requires nurses and midwives to slow down and attend to patients in an attentive and personable manner. Midwives expressed feeling that their workload was unmanageable, that time did not allow for all that was expected of them and they felt generally underappreciated in the health system. The healthcare worker's time—the aspect that often seems to pit the midwife and patient against one other—is required by patients attending the clinic but also protected by midwives and nurses who feel the demands are too high. In one instance, nurses and midwives scramble to manage increasing amounts of paperwork, high patient volume, and tinkering with broken equipment, while compensating for staff shortages. Meanwhile, patience dwindles as the patients await care. The ways in which midwives guard their time, and how such practice becomes normalised in the clinic, could help us understand why nurses and midwives neglect patients, even when their time is available.

After talking to the nurses and midwives in the clinic and listening to their ongoing struggle to manage their workload, and also witnessing the ways neglect is leveraged against patients, it seems that in some ways, how time is managed is a way to hold onto and exercise power. For one not to give their time to someone else, even by neglecting someone in labour, is also to preserve what is valued. The hierarchical nature of health systems that places patients at the bottom creates conditions where nurses and those receiving care are set against each other. Freedman et al. (2018), a public health writer who has written extensively on the mistreatment of women during childbirth, calls for an examination of "the ways in which hierarchies of power that permeate health systems and the marginalizing demeaning practices that go with those hierarchies are internalized, naturalized and/or normalized" (108). On one hand, through the ongoing devaluing of social reproduction, nurses and midwives feel their time is deprecated and on the other, their time is what patients require. Neglecting a patient who requires care can be understood as one such marginalising and demeaning practice that is naturalised into the health system hierarchy. The devaluing of midwifery work due to its affiliation with care and caring labour (and therefore feminine) is bound up in the ways reproductive labour is erased and negated. Reproductive labour is either not recognised or is poorly recognised in the formal system of exchange; it is often done without the exchange of money (Andaiye 2020). Dignified maternity care not only requires caring labour but also requires that caring labour be valued and even prioritised. Through denying the right to a dignified birth, healthcare workers participate in the devaluing of reproductive labour; they are not outside the very system that devalues their care.

Compassionate care is not a formalised characteristic of care in the clinic; it is not built into everyday practices nor does the organisation of the clinic support it. This is not to say compassion was absent. The primary researcher witnessed nurses staying past their shift to attend to all patients in the ANC queue and there was often an exchange of food and laughter. On the same evening that she observed a patient in labour being neglected, one of the nurses involved had earlier shared in an interview that she had given an undisclosed amount of her own money to a woman returning for postpartum care. She had told the nurse in private that she had not eaten. Midwives shared stories of counselling women who had experienced gender-based and sexual violence. Some patients were dealing with drug and alcohol addiction and there were occasions where they were under the influence while in labour. Unemployment was extremely common, and many pregnant women did not have a secure place of residence. Midwives spoke frequently of the effects of violence in the communities being served by the MOUs, which included poverty and the lack of employment, on them and the women in their care. The tone of these conversations was rarely of blame or condemnation but more of a deep understanding of the realities of poverty and motherhood under these conditions.

The compassion observed seemed to take the form of individual acts of kindness rather than part of the standard delivery of maternal healthcare. Those seeking maternity care could therefore not expect compassionate treatment across the continuum of the care received. To practise compassionate care also requires a level of freedom, freedom in the sense that Bhakuni (2021) refers to: that one is not systemically dominated by oppressive hierarchies and other forms of structural violence. Working under constant uncertainty and duress interferes with midwives' relationship to their own freedom and, as Bhakuni (2021) points out, people are only "*relatively* free depending on the extent of non-domination the person enjoys" (5). When midwives act compassionately, they do so amid circumstances not designed for such interactions to flourish.

Individual acts of compassion are in no way solutions to a health system that must be reimagined and transformed. However, in a system predicated on inequality, acts of kindness go against the grain and disrupt the healthcare provider's role in maintaining this dehumanising system. Healthcare providers recognise the humanity in their patients and resist the devaluing of their own reproductive labour by finding ways of sharing under conditions of duress. Even in considering the limitations of the clinic as a place for compassionate care, when it occurs, it is worth taking the time to explore. Healthcare providers' acts of compassion demonstrate resistance from inside the very systems that devalue the work they do and those they care for.

CONCLUDING COMMENTS

In South Africa, obstetric violence is rarely the outcome of policy or guidelines but rather how past and present classed, raced, and gendered hierarchies shape healthcare services. It would be inaccurate to think of nurses and midwives as simply vessels of classist, racist, and patriarchal beliefs, but they are at the interface between discriminatory systems and those multiply affected by systematic violence, including poor, Black women. The clinic is one place where reproductive injustice plays out (Dutton and Knight 2020). This injustice harms those seeking maternal healthcare, including through the material conditions of the clinic. Nurses and midwives are not exempt from this, they too are part of the population that is systematically discriminated against (Jewkes and Penn-Kekana 2015; Kim and Motsei 2002). Their status as midwives gives them power in the healthcare provider–patient relationship but does not protect them from a system built on racism and patriarchy.

Childbirth demands compassionate, humanising care; that this is denied because of economic and social status is a clear mark of injustice. Maternal health facilities in low-resource settings are places where compassion is practised piecemeal but is extremely difficult to sustain, given the ways inequality dominates the health system at present. When compassionate care is practised in the maternity clinic, it is a demonstration of the possibilities for a Reproductive Justice that resists systematic domination. That compassionate care is not sustained as a model of care in the clinic requires an examination of the conditions that maternal healthcare exists in, as suggested by Bhakuni (2021), with her notion of non-domination in Reproductive Justice. Neglectful acts such as guarding time, withholding care, and shaming are forms of obstetric violence and are inexcusable. They may also be demonstrable forms of surviving a system that constrains and attacks social reproduction in multiple ways (Frederici 2013).

It is in acts of compassion that the knowledge needed to imagine improving the quality of maternity care offered in low-resource clinics is produced and reproduced. Such knowledge production, if we are to learn from it, needs to be free from any romanticised analysis or understanding of what is being assembled and violently unassembled. The possibility of reproductive freedom, which is assembled partially through acts of compassion, also reimagines the value given to social reproduction and caring labour. The relative freedom one experiences in an MOU, both care provider and patient, is regulated, in part, by a lack of recognition that care is essential to life (Andaiye 2020). Without this recognition, freedom within an MOU is always already severely constrained. One of the possibilities for Reproductive Justice lives is through compassionate acts that work against a system of domination that structures much of the South African health system.

NOTES

1. In this chapter, we use gender-inclusive terms (e.g., "patients," "pregnant people," "those seeking maternity care," etc.) as far as possible to recognise the sex and gender diversity of pregnant people, those seeking maternity care, and those therefore subjected to obstetric violence in healthcare settings.

2. The focus here, and in much of the scholarship on obstetric violence elsewhere, is on cisgender women.

3. South Africa has no direct-entry midwifery programme; midwifery is a component of the nursing degree, with the option for an additional one-year training in midwifery. Auxiliary nursing training involves a two-year diploma.

4. A sister in charge is a senior midwife who manages the MOU. Her office is within the MOU and their duties are expansive.

5. A filler word used to express irritation or resignation

REFERENCES

Andaiye. 2020. *The Point Is to Change the World*, edited by Alissa Trotz. London: Pluto Press.

Arnold, Rachel, Edwin van Teijlingen, Kath Ryan, and Immy Holloway. 2019. "Villains or Victims? An Ethnography of Afghan Maternity Staff and the Challenge of High Quality Respectful Care." *BMC Pregnancy and Childbirth* 19 (307): 1–12. https://doi.org/10.1186/s12884-019-2420-6.

Bhakuni, Himani. 2021. "Reproductive Justice: Non-Interference or Non-Domination?" *Developing World Bioethics* April: 1–6. https://doi.org/10.1111/dewb.12317.

Bohren, Meghan A., Joshua P. Vogel, Erin C. Hunter, Olha Lutsiv, Suprita K. Makh, João Paulo Souza, Carolina Aguiar, et al. 2015. "The Mistreatment of Women during Childbirth in Health Facilities Globally: A Mixed-Methods Systematic Review." *PLoS Medicine* 12 (6): 1–32. https://doi.org/10.1371/journal.pmed.1001847.

Bowser, Diana, and Kathleen Hill. 2010. "Exploring Evidence for Disrespect and Abuse in Facility-Based Childbirth Report of a Landscape Analysis USAID-TRAction Project." http://www.tractionproject.org/sites/default/files/Respectful _Care_at_Birth_9-20-101_Final.pdf.

Bradley, Susan, Christine McCourt, Juliet Rayment, and Divya Parmar. 2019. "Midwives' Perspectives on (Dis)Respectful Intrapartum Care during Facility-Based Delivery in Sub-Saharan Africa: A Qualitative Systematic Review and Meta-Synthesis." *Reproductive Health* 16 (116): 1–16. https://doi.org/10.1186/ s12978-019-0773-y.

Chadwick, Rachelle. 2017. "Ambiguous Subjects: Obstetric Violence, Assemblage and South African Birth Narratives." *Feminism & Psychology* 27 (4): 489–509. https://doi.org/10.1177/0959353517692607.

———. 2018. *Bodies That Birth: Vitalizing Birth Politics.* Oxfordshire: Routledge. https://doi.org/10.4324/9781315648910.

Department of Health South Africa. 2016. *Guidelines for Maternity Care in South Africa: A Manual for Clinics, Community Health Centres and District Hospitals*, 4th ed. https://www.knowledgehub.org.za/system/files/elibdownloads/2020-08/ CompleteMaternalBook.pdf.

Dutton, Jessica, and Lucia Knight. 2020. "Reproducing Neglect in the Place of Care: Normalised Violence within Cape Town Midwifery Obstetric Units." *Agenda* 34 (1): 14–22. https://doi.org/10.1080/10130950.2019.1704481.

Freedman, Lynn P., and Margaret E. Kruk. 2014. "Disrespect and Abuse of Women in Childbirth: Challenging the Global Quality and Accountability Agendas." *The Lancet* 384 (9948): e42–e44. https://doi.org/10.1016/S0140-6736(14)60859-X.

Freedman, Lynn P., Stephanie A. Kujawski, Selemani Mbuyita, August Kuwawenaruwa, Margaret E. Kruk, Kate Ramsey, and Godfrey Mbaruku. 2018. "Eye of the Beholder? Observation versus Self-Report in the Measurement of Disrespect and Abuse during Facility-Based Childbirth." *Reproductive Health Matters* 26 (53): 1–16. https://doi.org/10.1080/09688080.2018.1502024.

Frederici, Silvia. 2013. *Women, Reproduction, and the Construction of the Commons.* Presented at the Reproducing Values Series, Museum of Arts and Design, New York.

Fried, Jana, Alia Sunderji, Steve Birch, and John Eyles. 2013. "The Reason That I Did Not Go – Determinants of the Use of Antenatal Care Services in South Africa, Two Decades after the End of Apartheid." *Canadian Journal of African Studies/ La Revue Canadienne Des études Africaines* 47 (1): 27–50. https://doi.org/10.1080 /00083968.2013.770340.

Jewkes, Rachel, and Loveday Penn-Kekana. 2015. "Mistreatment of Women in Childbirth: Time for Action on This Important Dimension of Violence against Women." *PLoS Medicine* 12 (6): e1001849. https://doi.org/10.1371/journal.pmed .1001849.

Jewkes, Rachel, Naeemah Abrahams, and Zodumo Mvo. 1998. "Why Do Nurses Abuse Patients? Reflections from South African Obstetric Services." *Social Science & Medicine* 47 (11): 1781–95. https://doi.org/10.1016/S0277 -9536(98)00240-8.

Kim, Julia, and Mmatshilo Motsei. 2002. "'Women Enjoy Punishment': Attitudes and Experiences of Gender-Based Violence among PHC Nurses in Rural South Africa." *Social Science & Medicine* 54 (8): 1243–54. https://doi.org/10.1016/S0277-9536(01)00093-4.

Lambert, Jaki, Elsie Etsane, Anne Marie Bergh, Robert Pattinson, and Nynke van den Broek. 2018. "'I Thought They Were Going to Handle Me like a Queen but They Didn't': A Qualitative Study Exploring the Quality of Care Provided to Women at the Time of Birth." *Midwifery* 62 (July): 256–63. https://doi.org/10.1016/j.midw.2018.04.007.

Lappeman, Maura, and Leslie Swartz. 2019. "Rethinking Obstetric Violence and the 'Neglect of Neglect': The Silence of a Labour Ward Milieu in a South African District Hospital." *BMC International Health and Human Rights* 19 (30): 1–11. https://doi.org/10.1186/s12914-019-0218-2.

Lokugamage, Amali U., and S. D. C. Pathberiya. 2017. "Human Rights in Childbirth, Narratives and Restorative Justice: A Review." *Reproductive Health* 14 (17): 1–8. https://doi.org/10.1186/s12978-016-0264-3.

Odhiambo, Agnes, and Siphokazi Mthathi. 2011. *Stop Making Excuses: Accountability for Maternal Health Care in South Africa*. Johannesburg: Human Rights Watch. https://www.hrw.org/sites/default/files/reports/sawrd0811webwcover.pdf.

Rucell, Jessica Zerucelli. 2017. "Obstetric Violence & Colonial Conditioning in South Africa's Reproductive Health System." PhD Diss., University of Leeds.

Sabri, Bushra, and Douglas A. Granger. 2016. "Gender-Based Violence and Trauma in Marginalized Populations of Women: Role of Biological Embedding and Toxic Stress." *Physiology & Behavior* 39 (9): 1–16. https://doi.org/10.1080/07399332.2018.1491046.Gender-based.

Solnes Miltenburg, Andrea, Sandra van Pelt, Tarek Meguid, and Johanne Sundby. 2018. "Disrespect and Abuse in Maternity Care: Individual Consequences of Structural Violence." *Reproductive Health Matters* 26 (53): 88–106. https://doi.org/10.1080/09688080.2018.1502023.

Tantchou, Josiane Carine. 2018. "The Materiality of Care and Nurses' 'Attitude Problem.'" *Science, Technology, & Human Values* 43 (2): 270–301. https://doi.org/10.1177/0162243917714868.

Villiers, Katusha de. 2021. "Bridging the Health Inequality Gap: An Examination of South Africa's Social Innovation in Health Landscape." *Infectious Diseases of Poverty* 10: 1–7. https://doi.org/10.1186/s40249-021-00804-9.

Chapter 9

Doing the Work of the State?

Class Inequalities and Motherhood in Neoliberal Times

Kristina Saunders

In the context of neoliberalism, reproductive decisions are imbued with notions of individual responsibility, free choice, self-investment, and are deeply connected to class inequalities and perceptions of value (Saunders 2020). These judgements are based upon, and reinforce, an idealised (White) middle-class reproductive trajectory, suggesting the "right" time and conditions under which to have children and constructing an appropriate citizen/ mother. Despite being understood as freely chosen, reproductive trajectories and constructions of motherhood are, of course, inseparable from intersecting systems of ableism, colonialism, heteropatriarchy, nationalism, and racism. Using empirical data from in-depth interviews with women in Scotland, in this chapter I draw on Bourdieusian theory to explore the stigma directed towards working-class mothers, resulting from an unjust neoliberal state agenda that shapes and is reproduced and upheld through mothering practices.

The perspectives of both working and middle-class mothers demonstrate how it is possible that political discourses seep into everyday life to reproduce and sustain class inequalities. As Angela Davis suggests, "we often do the work of the state in and through our interior lives" (2016, 142). Participants' accounts therefore reflect constructions of neoliberal motherhood that intersect with middle-class values to position some women as more or less desirable mothers based on notions of individual responsibility, self-investment, and access to appropriate economic, social, and cultural resources.

The findings presented in this chapter speak to one of the key demands of Reproductive Justice—the right to parent in safe and healthy environments, and the right to do so without coercion (Price 2010)—considered here in a novel way through an exploration of how neoliberal and classed notions of parenting are engaged with, reproduced, and resisted in everyday life. In what follows, I show how this process of reproduction and resistance occurs, as participants negotiate neoliberal ideals of "good" motherhood in their accounts of parenting practices in such a way that upholds the political status quo and deepens classed inequalities.

NEOLIBERAL MOTHERHOOD

The free-market ideology at the core of neoliberalism supports a lack of state intervention in the lives of citizens (Harvey 2005). An emphasis on individual responsibility, independence, and consumer choice underpins neoliberal politics and economies and is transposed from the macro to the micro as citizens are constructed as avid consumers and held responsible for making "good" or "bad" choices in all aspects of their lives. This hierarchy of choice further legitimises state withdrawal, depicting the welfare state as burdensome and associated with dependency (Hall 2011) and those who require its support as moral failures (Tyler 2008). Consequently, understandings of "good" parenting, particularly motherhood, come to be characterised by self-sufficiency and intense (maternal) investment in families' futures so that the state does not have to (Allen and Taylor 2012; Sollinger 2013).

Motherhood is therefore framed in an individualised way, as a job that has economic value through the raising of children as citizens who are also self-investing and individually responsible (Allen and Taylor 2012; Tabatabai 2020). Neoliberal motherhood involves what Lowe (2017) refers to as maternal sacrifice: the expectation that mothers will take responsibility to minimise risks not only when raising children but before and during pregnancy. Women must therefore adopt a future-oriented approach to (potential) motherhood (Skeggs 2011). The individualising of reproductive risk, for example, is evident in the UK's health policies related to pregnancy that construe diet, alcohol consumption, and stress as risks to unborn children and an economic cost to society (Lowe 2017). This individual-level focus ignores the structural, social, and biological factors that shape pregnancy and motherhood.

Similar ideas support the ideology of "intensive mothering" (Hays 1996), which goes beyond essential care and requires an increasing amount of additional, expert-informed work and responsibility to ensure children's optimal development and safeguard them from risk (Hays 1996). Lareau (2003) refers to such practice as "concerted cultivation": the intense investment of time, energy, and financial resources primarily by the middle classes to enhance children's development, for example, paying for extra-curricular activities to expand children's skillsets. For Phipps (2014), these parenting approaches— underpinned by the neoliberal values of responsibility, productivity, and self-sufficiency—ultimately uphold a classed agenda as they work to construe marginalised mothers with differential access to resources as irresponsible and requiring education.

Some authors have also pointed to the contemporary expectation that women must "do it all" by combining intensive mothering and paid employment (McRobbie 2013, 130). This balancing act reflects the demands of neoliberalism as "good" mothers are called upon to be "labourers/consumers and mothers/carers, shifting responsibility away from the welfare state and towards individuals" (Orgad and De Benedictis 2015, 3), reinforcing its ideals of self-reliance and productivity. This idealised form of motherhood stands in contrast to the figure of the British "chav[1] mum," held contemptuously in the public imagination as embodying "failed" femininity due to her economic dependency and thus evoking disgust (Tyler 2008).

Idealised, neoliberal motherhood, as described in this chapter, is not universal and is bound up with varying geopolitical, cultural, and religious norms (Al-deen 2019). However, scholars have noted the transnational reach of neoliberalism in shaping experiences, including motherhood, beyond the Global North (Vandenbeld Giles 2014; Dosekun 2015).

REPRODUCTIVE JUSTICE AND PARENTING

A Reproductive Justice perspective, with its attention to the social, political, and historical contexts of marginalisation, compels the critical examination of how neoliberal discourses and constructions impinge upon the experiences and practices of raising children (Ross 2017). The appropriateness of reproduction has historically been decided by those holding power and seeking to restrict and reduce the number of births to those deemed socially "undesirable" (Davis 1983). Reproductive freedom and decision-making are therefore deeply connected to social and public policies that "immediately and urgently touch upon race and class" (Solinger 2013, 50). This is evident when considering neoliberal welfare responses that demonise poor families (particularly mothers) and locate social and structural issues of poverty and marginalisation within families themselves (Roberts 1993; Sollinger 2013).

While mainstream, Western feminist movements have focussed their energies on how reproductive rights could be realised through the state, Reproductive Justice scholars and activists highlighted the need to consider the surveillance and interference exerted by the state over the lives of Black women, Women of Colour, and working-class White women. Reproductive justice therefore highlights the structural and political barriers to having and raising children that many marginalised women face (Luna and Luker 2013; Ross 2017). In particular, family life and parenting practices are experienced by these women as more intensely governed by the state and its actors (i.e., social workers, the care system, child protection services) (Roberts 1993; Price 2010). Reproductive Justice scholarship crucially draws our attention to these top-down mechanisms of the state that discipline motherhood. My aim in this chapter is to add to this body of literature by using a Bourdieusian lens to show the subtle and insidious ways that neoliberal and class-based ideals of motherhood are re/produced, and resisted, in everyday practices.

THE PROBLEMATISING OF POOR PARENTS IN BRITISH SOCIAL POLICY

Despite an ideological commitment to providing a post-WW2 safety net for all, successive UK governments and their agencies have continued to discipline and demonise poor families and those requiring welfare culminating in more recent times as "antiwelfare commonsense" (Jensen and Tyler 2015, 470). Such a consensus has taken hold and is exacerbated by the individualising and responsibilising logics of neoliberalism, and the political project of austerity following the 2008 Great Recession (Lupton et al. 2016). In the United Kingdom, depressed wage levels and cuts to public spending and state benefits have accompanied (and partly justified) an intensified stigmatising narrative that construes welfare and poverty as the result of people's "bad" choices—especially parents. Poverty and welfare assistance are posited as the *causes* of inequalities and social problems, rather than the effects (Jensen and Tyler 2015).

Somewhat contradictorily (or perhaps conveniently), while the state withdraws from family life, its surveillance of and governance in this sphere intensifies. The policy focus of the last 20 years has been on parenting as the answer to alleviating social and structural issues and creating future economic potential (Jensen and Tyler 2015; Vincent 2017). For example, as Gillies (2013) points out, the UK New Labour Government's (1997–2010) provision of parenting classes took on a regulatory role, as predominantly mothers from poor families were threatened with fines and imprisonment for non-attendance at classes. During this time, Gillies (2013, 95) argues, "the family was hailed as the formative site through which 'competent personhood' is cultivated." Such rhetoric absolves the state of its duties, firmly placing responsibility onto (largely) mothers for children's educational, emotional, and physical development (Vincent 2017).

In Scotland, where I conducted my research, it is widely held that the Scottish National Party, in power since 2007, is more progressive than the UK government (Mooney 2016). However, the Scottish Government's Early Years Framework (2009) displays an interventionist approach to ensure that parents "maximise life chances" (9) and ultimately generate "positive economic returns" (8) for the nation. The policy establishes the time prior to birth and home learning as crucial to improving child development outcomes thereby expecting families to adopt a future-oriented approach to mitigate possible developmental risks. This policy focus on early intervention and parental responsibility are largely directed towards poor mothers, effectively shifting attention from the need for more progressive strategies to reduce inequalities (Horsley, Edwards, and Gillies 2017;[2] McKendrick 2016). Instead, the blame for social problems is seen to lie with poor parenting or, *poor parents* (Allen and Taylor 2012), who are ultimately held responsible for socio-structural issues and their own experiences of inequality.

This section has provided a snapshot of the neoliberal policy context in the United Kingdom and the inequalities it produces. This background provides context for the rest of the chapter, which focusses on how these neoliberal discourses of motherhood and good citizenship underpin policies that shaped the everyday experiences and decision-making of research participants in such a way as to reinforce the classed hierarchisation of motherhood.

THE PRESENT STUDY

For my doctoral research exploring reproductive decision-making, I conducted 22 in-depth interviews with women aged 21- to 60-years-old, and with service providers working in Scottish reproductive and sexual health and maternal services.[3] I was interested in a wide range of reproductive topics including abortion, contraception, pregnancy, and raising children; therefore, recruitment was open to mothers and women without children, and this chapter includes the experiences of both groups. The women who participated in the study were all cis-gender, heterosexual, and from either a middle- or working-class background. Most of the participants were White (three participants identified as mixed race) and non-disabled (two participants discussed experiencing ongoing mental distress).

To make sense of participants' class positions, I followed the approach taken by Gillies (2006) when doing research with working-class mothers, which is based on their access to Bourdieu's (1990) capitals: economic, cultural, and social. A Bourdieusian approach allows for a symbolic and cultural view of class that is useful when focussing on inequalities in everyday practices and interactions, as connections and boundaries are drawn between social actors due to the transmission and possession of capitals. To briefly outline the capitals, economic capital refers to money and property; cultural capital describes the possession of formal knowledge (e.g., obtained through school or university education) and informal or more general knowledge (e.g., manners and way of speaking); and social capital refers to connections forged through relationships. Power is drawn from specifically middle-class forms of cultural capital that are afforded higher status and legitimated to produce symbolic capital that allows for processes of distinction to occur between and within classes. As I will show, capitals were evidenced during my research when middle-class participants expressed a desire to avoid budget supermarkets due to the perceived low quality of food or highlighted a preference for having an au pair to culturally enrich children's lives; whereas, one working-class participant discussed having "no money" and felt a need to justify her spending to me.

Bourdieu (1990) focusses on the distinctions created through interactions and displays of capitals, creating a picture of discreet, roughly standardised groups. However, the Black feminist roots of Reproductive Justice would ask us to attend to the difference within groups, and Vincent (2017) rightly reminds us that middle- and working-class are not homogenous groupings, despite frequently being presented as such within research. Understandings of parenting practices are also complicated by the intersecting experiences of class and racism. For instance, research from the United Kingdom points to the intensive educational investment made by Black mothers when attempting to counter racist stereotypes regarding their children's intelligence, and to their deliberate self-presentation when meeting White teachers to challenge potential negative views of their parenting (Vincent et al. 2012). These intersections and fractions (Vincent 2017) are crucial to attend to in analyses of parenting and interlocking inequalities.

In the next section, I will present findings from the research that are grounded in participants' accounts and demonstrate the pervasive power of neoliberal ideology and its classed construction of motherhood.

FINDINGS AND DISCUSSION

Participants' accounts reflected and sometimes challenged dominant neoliberal constructions of motherhood. In what follows, I first analyse the accounts of middle-class women, demonstrating how middle-class mothers maintain unequal class relations and do the work of the state as they prioritise individual responsibility for and investment in their children, transferring privilege to their children while at the same time demonising those with less resources for their apparent irresponsibility and dependency. I then turn to their working-class counterparts, showing how these women's present-focussed accounts differed from those of their middle-class counterparts as they emphasised trying to do the best for their children in the here-and-now, while apparently aware of the stigmatisation of their mothering practices. I highlight instances in which the described parenting practices break with the neoliberal norm, suggesting agency and presenting alternative mothering possibilities.

Middle-Class Women's Perspectives on Raising Children

Middle-class participants were able to use material resources, social connections, and legitimated cultural capital to plan for the future and facilitate their role as responsible parents. For instance, discussing what they considered to be appropriate ways of raising children, two participants who did not have children expressed the importance of investing in children's education. However, in their accounts "education is not just school it's also from the people you talk to, and places you go to travel" (Diana, mc, 33, no children, council supervisor), and also might involve "having an au pair in the house. It would be good for children to learn about different cultures and learn a different language" (Chiara, mc, 26, no children, student). Diana and Chiara's comments illustrate how middle-class women placed value on education which is construed as including knowledge and experiences that go beyond formal education. Such views reflect how middle-class parents often seek to accrue value from investing cultural and social capital in their children, transferring and maintaining privilege while differentiating themselves from working-class families (Lareau 2003; Gillies 2005).

The view of ideal childrearing as going beyond essential care also arose when Diana outlined further aspects of parenting she considered important, including "not living in a deprived or a rough environment" and providing "good quality food rather than from *Iceland* [a budget supermarket chain]." Diana considers the location where children are raised to be an important part of parenting, which necessitates taking responsibility to avoid living in areas of deprivation. It is not simply being able to meet basic needs (food) that are described as important, what Diana suggests goes beyond basics ("*good quality* food"). In her account, class is signified by devaluing the consumption practices of those who purchase (implicitly poorer quality) food from cheaper supermarkets, thus creating a mark of distinction by "increasing positions of otherness" (Wills et al. 2011, 73). This example shows how the middle-class can utilise economic and valued cultural capital to shape children's tastes, thereby maintaining a position of privilege through cultural distinction.

Participants with children also framed parenting as involving individual investment and requiring advanced planning. For Isabel, this began at the early stages of her children's lives by making use of private childcare. This is shown below in her response to my question about whether she had always wanted to send her children to a private nursery.

Isabel (mc, 46, 3 children, university administrator)
Emm . . . that was always the outset. We visited the council nursery and it was like, oh wow! There's like . . . 50 children in here! (*laughs*). No doubt they get good care but . . . what also played a role was, when the first child went to the

nursery there were lots of other families who had their first child there and we sort of made friends with those families. And our children made friends, and it was like . . . "Oh, your child is friends with mine, could we maybe nurture that friendship?"

Isabel emphasises the need to invest in education from a young age through paying for marketised private childcare, a decision made prior to having children. In her account, a distinction is made between the care delivered at a private nursery and a council-run, state-funded nursery. Her intimation that state-funded care is less desirable distinguishes between those able to pay more for childcare and those who are not. Isabel also emphasises the value of establishing social networks with families whose children attend the private nursery. This too can be viewed as a form of investment: accruing social capital through fostering friendships with other middle-class families (Gillies 2008). Like Isabel, Julie also adopted a future-oriented perspective when discussing the importance of being involved in her three-year-old daughter's future education:

Julie (mc, 37, one child, council manager)
I'm quite focused on that (daughter's education), and for her to have a good education and do well in life and get a good career. I'm not forcing her, but I want her to do a degree with an outcome like a doctor, solicitor, engineer. I know a lot of people that went to uni [university] and are now working in *Tesco* [supermarket], and you think, "It hasn't got you anything!"

Interviewer:
So, do you see yourself as being quite involved when it comes to her education in the future?

Julie:
Yeah, I do. I hope to help her and guide her in the right direction . . . I do hope to be involved.

Julie is already contemplating the involvement she will have in her daughter's education, with university attendance presented as an expectation and a means to upward social mobility (despite her recognition that this is not a guaranteed route to a good career). Julie's and Isabel's orientation towards the future reflects the middle-class alignment with the "individualised subject of value, who is always accruing through exchange and investment in order to enhance futures" (Skeggs 2011, 502), with the hope that taking the responsibility to invest in and transfer potential to children will ensure productive and "valued" futures (Allen and Taylor 2012; Gillies 2013). The valued futures (of high-status professional employment) are distinguished from those deemed less valuable (waged labour) and serve as evidence of making the "wrong" choices. The emphasis on individual choices also obscures the role of structural inequalities in shaping educational options and outcomes (Reay et al. 2001). Julie went on to describe other aspects of parenting she considered important:

Julie:
I want her to have the best and that's why we moved, so we could get her to a better school than she would have went to. I want her to grow up into a well-adjusted adult that's going out to work and has a good job, and I think it's a huge responsibility on parents to do that from the start. I mean, where I lived was lovely, but you went out on the main street and there was a chemist there and they were all waiting on their methadone, and people with amputated legs through drugs . . . It's not normal for kids to be going to school with people whose parents are addicts; I didn't want her to see that. So, I think it's a huge responsibility for parents to try and protect children from all that.

Interviewer:
And before she was born, were you thinking about these things?

Julie:
I thought about it all beforehand . . . just hoping that she would grow up into a decent person.

Julie's account echoes the view of parenting contained in the previously discussed neoliberal early intervention policies: taking responsibility for an individualised investment project, beginning before children's birth or soon after, to ensure children will grow into "well-adjusted adults" and therefore "decent" members of society. Julie's reference to a neighbourhood with a "better school" also reflects the Western middle-class discourse of intensive motherhood and emphasis on childhood innocence (Gutman 2013), through which mothers are held responsible for individually protecting children from structural inequalities. Julie's access to the resources to move home to "protect" her child from perceived risks and exposure to "undesirable elements" ("people whose parents are addicts") upholds dominant neoliberal norms of responsibility and early intervention. In this way, Julie secures the position of responsible mother who plans in advance to secure a better life for her daughter.

Perceptions of individualised responsibility are also featured in the accounts of participants without children, evident in the excerpt below where Pam articulates the view that some parents are not responsible enough for their children, which she raised in relation to the rise of school breakfast clubs.[4]

Pam (mc, 41, no children, social worker)
I was watching TV and they were talking about—and it's horrendous that we have to do this—but you send in your mobile phone and that goes towards

buying food for breakfast clubs. The parenting responsibilities are going over to the school! The school is now responsible for feeding them. The school is now responsible for—I saw, recently that teachers are now responsible for teaching them how to brush their teeth! There has to be something that puts the onus back on the parents to parent their children, because the nanny state is churning out parents who don't know what they're doing, or are on drugs, or are too young.

The way poverty impacts parenting is again framed here as an individual and moral failing of families whose irresponsibility is attributed to a seemingly overprotective "nanny" state. Those with adequate resources (and who are old "enough" and not using substances) are therefore classified as taking responsibility to invest in their families and are aligned with an idealised middle-class trajectory, while those with fewer resources are responsibilised as welfare is withdrawn (Gillies 2013). With regard to breakfast clubs, Holloway and Wilson (2016) found that affluent parents paid for this service as an extension of childcare to facilitate their labour market productivity, whereas in lower-income areas, breakfast clubs were subsidised to ensure children had eaten before classes and to improve school attendance. This demonstrates the class-based use of this service and the anti-welfare commonsense (Jensen and Tyler 2015) expressed by Pam, for whom working-class parents' use of breakfast clubs signifies irresponsibility, due to "dependency" on the state and its institutions.

Working-Class Women's Perspectives on Raising Children

In comparison to middle-class participants, those from the working class appeared to be less focussed on accruing neoliberal forms of value for the future. In the excerpt below, Stephanie's feelings of shame and disappointment arise from the concern that her three children may be unlikely to attend university, and she is afraid this reflects negatively on her as a mother.

> *Stephanie* (wc, 36, 3 children, not in paid work)
> I feel . . . like I've lost out a wee bit—it's a bad thing to say—but I kinda get envious of people whose kids are going to university. I want them to do well, but I've got to be realistic and be like, right well, they're never gonna go to university because that's not within their capabilities so why push them? (*sighs*). I mean, ma kids aren't workshy. My youngest is *really* tryin' to get a job— delivering leaflets, anything he can do. He got two jobs but as soon as they knew he was 13 he didn't get them. But they're no' workshy. It's hard not to be envious of people who've got kids that are gonna be like really successful and everything, but at the same time, I'm confident that they will be successful in what they do as long as they're happy. But you know, a lot of people are kinda judgemental, are people gonna think bad upon me and upon ma kids?

Stephanie is aware of the neoliberal construction of parenting as an educational project, so that not having one's children achieve highly in education is equated with bad parenting and a devalued trajectory (Gillies 2008). She also emphasises that she wants her children "to do *well*" (in contrast to Julie's desire for her daughter to have the *best*) but believes this will not be in the realm of education. Research has shown that for some working-class parents, their children's education is "contained by resignation and realism" (Gillies 2006, 287) due to possessing less capital to invest in educational goals. At the same time, traditional working-class trajectories involving labour market entry straight from school are now politically constructed as indicative of low aspirations (Roberts and Evans 2013).

Stephanie's account also implies a sense of shame, resonating with Lawler's (1999) argument that the pathologisation of working-class life can lead to feelings of failure or lack due to perceived or actual judgements from middle-class others. This potential judgement of laziness (being "workshy") is evident as Stephanie emphasises that her children are not afraid of hard work. Her claims demonstrate how working-class parents may emphasise non-academic qualities but also highlight engagement with neoliberal discourses that prioritise productivity. Here, Stephanie attempts to negotiate the neoliberal terrain to classify herself and her children as productive and therefore valuable and respectable citizens (Skeggs 1997), as well as to distinguish them from others within her class who may be deemed politically and socially "unproductive."

Stephanie expressed further feelings of lack and shame when reflecting on her experience as a mother to three autistic children, and their frequent interactions with agents of the state (i.e., teachers, social workers, psychologists) stating, "These people are pedigrees and I'm like a mongrel. I'm just like . . . this . . . wee mum who hasn't got a great intelligence, so I just feel kinda inferior to them." In contrast to this expression of inferiority, research indicates that middle-class parents are often confident to negotiate with and command respect from professionals (Gillies 2008). The way in which class inequality is felt can be seen through Stephanie's self-deprecating use of the word "mongrel" associated with the notions of dirt and impurity that working-class women and their children are thought to embody (Skeggs 2005). The feelings Stephanie expresses highlight the pervasiveness of neoliberal perceptions of "good" motherhood in the political and economic sphere that shape marginalised women's relationship with state actors and their sense of themselves.

Like Stephanie, other working-class participants also expressed a sense of inferiority. Holly (wc, 27, 1 child, not in paid work) indicated a feeling of being out of place at a more individual level when expressing anxiety about living close to middle-class families from affluent neighbourhoods. She worried this proximity may negatively impact her son's sense of self due to their different class position. Kirsten expressed similar views when describing her interactions with middle-class mothers:

> *Kirsten* (wc, 36, 2 children, receptionist)
> I have a *WhatsApp* group with some mums from school, and most of them are alright, but there's a couple who are like, "I'm super mum"—really stuck up. [. . .] It's just like, gymnastics at 9 o'clock on a Saturday, swimming at 10 o'clock, church every Sunday. And the mums are never at the school because they're workin', so they're not there first thing, and not there last thing at night. And quite a few of us will say "The kids are strugglin' with the reading homework" or whatever. Some people will tell you how it really is, but others won't tell you these things because they see that as a failure and want you to think their kids are the best at everythin'.

Kirsten is critical of middle-class mothers' "concerted cultivation" (Lareau 2003) and engagement with paid work, rendering this as secondary to being there for their children. This portrayal is akin to what Skeggs (2011, 503) refers to as a "moral value reversal" whereby the socially valued decisions of middle-class women to return to full-time paid work are viewed negatively by working-class mothers. In this way they defend their lack of paid work by assigning greater worth to the attention and time spent with their children. Criticism is also directed towards how these mothers talk about their children, emphasising children's academic performance and concealing difficulties. Similar themes were discussed by Gillies (2005) who found that middle-class parents demonstrated pride when talking about children's academic performance, emphasising their "brightness." Kirsten's sense of support from sharing children's struggles at school with other mothers is depicted as compromised by the more individualistic and competitive approach taken by "stuck up" mothers, who refuse to share struggles but differentiate their children by presenting them as exceptional. This resonates with Skeggs' (2011) research on the *Mumsnet* parenting website, which found working-class mothers to be critical of middle-class mothers' displays of competition and entitlement, portraying this to be self-centred and pretentious. The connection or camaraderie between mothers that Kirsten describes suggests a more supportive network and differs from middle-class participants' accounts of individually accruing social capital as a process of investment for future success and maintaining privilege.

The moral value reversal described above was also evident in other working-class participants' accounts, as they emphasised mothering practices deviating from the neoliberal norm. The excerpt below from my interview with Stephanie provides a good illustration of this.

Stephanie (wc, 36, 3 children, not in paid work)
I don't have a lot of money. I don't go out. I don't smoke. I drink in the house, like, a bottle of wine—£4 a bottle. Any disposable income goes on holidays. And I like that because I want to make the nicest, most perfect memories because our life is really hard . . . It's just really, really hard going day-to-day life, so just having that break to look forward to. And we don't have money at all—any we do have goes on holidays—but ma kids have so many memories. I like to give them quality time, and the most time I can give them is when we're away from everything and you can't put a price on that . . . But I think a lot of people will judge me and think, "Oh she's goin' on all these holidays how can she afford that?"

Here Stephanie depicts "quality time" as priceless and important for children's well-being. This resonates with Gillies' (2006) finding that working-class parents valued quality time over academic and economic success. Unlike middle-class parents' use of financial resources to invest in tutors, private education, or moving to affluent neighbourhoods for school catchment areas, working-class mothers described saving money for holidays to be an important part of parenting. Accordingly, Stephanie expresses a sense of pride in being able to ease the difficulties of her children's lives through "quality time" and time "away from everything," in a similar way to the meanings Kirsten attached to her mothering practices (above). Money is not viewed as a means of investing in children as part of a process of self-accumulation for the future but as an emotional investment in the *present* and a form of escape for her children from the difficulties of their "hard going day-to-day life" and to show them how much they are valued, as they may often feel devalued in everyday life.

In a similar way to her previous account of marking herself and her children as respectable, Stephanie anticipates—and attempts to mitigate—judgement for going on holiday when she does not undertake paid work. This again can be viewed as an attempt to differentiate herself from those of a similar class background who may be viewed as engaging in the "wrong" consumption practices such as smoking or drinking alcohol. When these practices are undertaken by working-class women, they are pathologised and associated with excess and irresponsibility (Skeggs 2005).

Holly also presented an alternative to the neoliberal values of middle-class mothers when considering the importance of fostering relationships for her son. This involved "socialising and seeing people that are important in my life like my family and best friends." These relationships are not, however, presented as an investment in social capital, as discussed previously. Rather, the priority placed on relationship building reflects research findings indicating the value of immediate support and care from social networks for working-class families (Skeggs 2011). Neoliberal norms may therefore be negotiated through valuing alternative practices such as prioritising attention, time, and emotional support for children in the present, which also demonstrates a form of resistance to neoliberal and middle-class motherhood, in a struggle over the meaning of value and worth (Skeggs 2011).

CONCLUSION

In this chapter, I have traced how neoliberal policy rhetoric is reproduced through the actions and views of citizens who thereby come to do the work of the state in everyday life. I demonstrated how the stigmatisation of working-class motherhood, and the middle-classes enactment of parenting as an intensive educational project, operates at the macro and micro political levels as a form of governance, entrenching an individualised and entrepreneurial approach to parenting as common sense. Neoliberal political and economic ideology therefore shapes reproductive lives and experiences of parenting by inscribing relations of value/lack and judgement/shame, which simultaneously upholds its political dominance by moulding citizens in its image.

The findings show how neoliberalism is engaged with and classed inequalities upheld through everyday accounts of raising children and parenting practices. Middle-class participants demonstrated their embodiment and reproduction of the neoliberal state agenda through the desire and ability to distinguish themselves from "other" working-class mothers, who were viewed as irresponsible as they fail to adhere to ideals of productivity or "correctly" use educational, economic, and cultural resources. Working-class mothers often experienced or were aware of their "difference," but at times also engaged with neoliberal ideology by marking their children as "productive" or otherwise valuable in neoliberal terms. These findings add to Reproductive Justice scholarship by demonstrating how wider systems of oppression and inequality play out in the views and everyday parenting practices of those attempting to navigate dominant neoliberal conceptions of "good" motherhood, with an ever-present classed gaze at the micro and macro levels overseeing decisions about how children are raised.

I also showed how working-class mothers referred to parenting practices that deviated from and resisted the neoliberal norm. They were thus able to carve out agency in the face of the classed inequalities shaping their motherhood experiences, thereby creating their own supportive conditions for raising children. These demonstrations of resistance, no matter how small, remind us that alternative ways of parenting are possible and allow us to think beyond taken-for-granted ideals, which have wider applicability for the parenting practices and experiences of many others who experience marginalisation. In order to move closer to a world where parenting practices and decisions are supported, as envisaged by the Reproductive Justice framework, considerable work is required to challenge and radically rethink the neoliberal common-sense contained in policy and wider society that shapes the everyday experiences and rights of parents.

NOTES

1. A British pejorative for the working-class underpinned by constructions of an "undeserving poor" and social "underclass," and who are placed beyond working-class respectability.

2. Horsley, Edwards, and Gillies (2017) also point to the pervasive influence of brain science over UK policy, with mothers held responsible for babies' brain development during pregnancy which is said to determine social and economic inequalities.

3. Findings from service provider interviews are not discussed here.

4. The Scottish Government (2012) defines breakfast clubs as fulfilling "a range of functions for children who attend them and parents who use them" by offering a nutritious breakfast and fulfilling an element of childcare. In 2012, the Scottish Government reported that children tended to use breakfast clubs multiple days each week, and over one-fifth of parents surveyed reported that breakfast clubs were required for children to have access to a meal. Children whose parents were unemployed were more likely to attend a breakfast club than children from households where parents were employed.

REFERENCES

Al-deen, Taghreed J. 2019. *Motherhood, Education and Migration: Delving into Migrant Mothers' Involvement in Children's Education.* Singapore: Palgrave Macmillan.

Allen, Kim, and Yvette Taylor. 2012. "Placed Parenting, Locating Unrest: Failed Femininities, Troubled Mothers and Rioting Subjects." *Studies in the Maternal* 4 (2): 1–25. https://doi.org/10.16995/sim.39.

Bourdieu, Pierre. 1990. *The Logic of Practice.* Stanford: Stanford University Press.

Davis, Angela. 1983. *Women, Race and Class.* New York: Vintage Books.

———. 2016. *Freedom Is a Constant Struggle: Ferguson, Palestine, and the Foundations of a Movement.* Chicago: Haymarket Books.

Dosekun, Simidele. 2015. "For Western Girls Only? Post-feminism as Transnational Culture." *Feminist Media Studies* 15 (6): 960–75. https://doi.org/10.1080/14680777.2015.1062991.

Gillies, Val. 2005. "Raising the 'Meritocracy': Parenting and the Individualization of Social Class." *Sociology* 39 (5): 835–53. https://doi.org/10.1177%2F0038038505058368.

———. 2006. "Working Class Mothers and School Life: Exploring the Role of Emotional Capital." *Gender and Education* 18 (3): 281–93. https://doi.org/10.1080/09540250600667876.

———. 2008. "Childrearing, Class and the New Politics of Parenting." *Sociology Compass* 2 (3): 1079–95. https://doi.org/10.1111/j.1751-9020.2008.00114.x.

———. 2013. "Personalizing Poverty: Parental Determinism and the Big Society Agenda." In *Class Inequality in Austerity Britain*, edited by Will Atkinson, Steven Roberts, and Mike Savage. London: Palgrave Macmillan.

Gutman, Marta. 2013. "The Physical Spaces of Childhood." In *The Routledge History of Childhood in the Western World,* edited by Paula S. Fass. London: Routledge.

Hall, Stuart. 2011. "The Neoliberal Revolution." *Cultural Studies* 25 (6): 705–28. https://doi.org/10.1080/09502386.2011.619886.

Harvey, David. 2005. *A Brief History of Neoliberalism.* Oxford: Oxford University Press.

Hays, Sharon. 1996. *The Cultural Contradictions of Motherhood.* New Haven: Yale University Press.

Holloway, Sarah L., and Helena Pimlott-Wilson. 2016. "New Economy, Neoliberal State and Professionalised Parenting: Mothers' Labour Market Engagement and State Support for Social Reproduction in Class-Differentiated Britain." *Transactions* 41 (4): 376–88. https://doi.org/10.1111/tran.12130.

Horsley, Nicola., Rosalind Edwards, and Val Gillies. 2017. *Challenging the Politics of Early Intervention: Who's 'saving' Children and Why.* Bristol: Policy Press.

Jensen, Tracey, and Imogen Tyler. 2015. "'Benefits broods': The Cultural and Political Crafting of Anti-Welfare Commonsense'." *Critical Social Policy* 35 (4): 470–91. https://doi.org/10.1177%2F0261018315600835.

Lareau, Annette. 2003. *Unequal Childhoods.* Berkley: University of California Press.

Lawler, Steph. 1999. "'Getting Out and Getting Away': Women's Narratives of Class Mobility." *Feminist Review* 63 (1): 3–24. https://doi.org/10.1080%2F014177899339036.

Lowe, Pam. 2017. *Reproductive Health and Maternal Sacrifice: Women, Choice and Responsibility.* London: Palgrave Macmillan.

Luna, Zakiya, and Kristen Luker. 2013. "Reproductive Justice." *Annual Review of Law and Social Science* 9 (1): 327–52. https://doi.org/10.1146/annurev-lawsocsci-102612-134037.

Lupton, Ruth, Tania Burchardt, John Hills, Kitty Stewart and Polly Vizard, eds. 2016. *Social Policy in a Cold Climate: Policies and Their Consequences Since the Crisis.* Bristol: Policy Press.

McKendrick, John H. 2016. "Poverty in Scotland: The Evidence." In *Poverty in Scotland 2016: Tools for Transformation,* edited by John H. McKendrick, Gerry Mooney, Gill Scott, John Dickie, and Fiona McHardy. London: Child Poverty Action Group.

McRobbie, Angela. 2013. "Feminism, The Family and the New 'Mediated' Maternalism." *New Formations* 80–81: 119–37. https://doi.org/10.3898/newF.80/81.07.2013.

Mooney, Gerry. 2016. "Poverty in Scotland 2016: Beyond 'Austerity'?" In *Poverty in Scotland 2016: Tools for Transformation,* edited by John H. McKendrick, Gerry Mooney, Gill Scott, John Dickie, and Fiona McHardy. London: Child Poverty Action Group.

Orgad, Shani, and Sara De Benedictis. 2015. "The 'Stay-at-Home' Mother, Postfeminism and Neoliberalism: Content Analysis of UK News Coverage." *European Journal of Communication* 30 (4): 418–36. https://doi.org/10.1177%2F0267323115586724.

Phipps, Alison. 2014. *The Politics of the Body: Gender in a Neoliberal and Neoconservative Age.* London: Polity.

Price, Kimala. 2010. "What is Reproductive Justice? How Women of Color are Redefining the Pro-choice Paradigm." *Meridians* 10 (2): 42–65. https://doi:10.2979/meridians.2010.10.2.42.

Reay, Diane, Jacqueline Davies, Miriam David, and Stephen Ball. 2001. "Choices of Degree or Degrees of Choice? Class, `Race' and the Higher Education Choice Process." *Sociology* 35 (4): 855–74. https://doi.org/10.1177%2F0038038501035004004.

Roberts, Dorothy. 1993. "Racism and Patriarchy in the Meaning of Motherhood.*" Journal of Gender and Law* 1–38.

Roberts, Steven, and Sarah Evans. 2013. "'Aspirations' and Imagined Futures: The Im/possibilities for Britain's Young Working Class." In *Class Inequality in Austerity Britain*, edited by Will Atkinson, Steven Roberts, and Mike Savage. London: Palgrave Macmillan.

Ross, Loretta J. 2017. "Reproductive Justice as Intersectional Feminist Activism." *Souls: A Critical Journal of Black Politics, Culture, and Society* 19 (3): 286–341. https://doi.org/10.1080/10999949.2017.1389634.

Saunders, Kristina. 2020. "'I Think I Stick Out a Bit': The Classification of Reproductive Decision-Making." *Sociological Research Online* 26 (1): 75–91. https://doi.org/10.1177%2F1360780420909139.

Scottish Government. 2009. *The Early Years Framework.* https://www.gov.scot/Resource/Doc/257007/0076309.pdf.

———. 2012. *Growing up in Scotland: Early Experiences of Primary School.* Scotland: Scottish Government. https://www.gov.scot/binaries/content/documents/govscot/publications/research-and-analysis/2012/05/growing-up-scotland-early-experiences-primary-school/documents/00392709-pdf/00392709-pdf/govscot%3Adocument/00392709.pdf.

Skeggs, Beverley. 1997. *Formations of Class and Gender: Becoming Respectable.* London: Sage.

———. 2005. "The Making of Class and Gender through Visualizing Moral Subject Formation." *Sociology* 39 (5): 965–82. https://journals.sagepub.com/doi/10.1177/0038038505058381.

———. 2011. "Imagining Personhood Differently: Person Value and Autonomist Working-class Value Practices." *The Sociological Review* 59 (3): 496–513. https://doi.org/10.1111%2Fj.1467-954X.2011.02018.x.

Sollinger, Rickie. 2013. *Reproductive Politics: What Everyone Needs to Know.* New York: Oxford University Press.

Tabatabai, Ahoo. 2020. "Mother of a Person: Neoliberalism and Narratives of Parenting Children with Disabilities." *Disability & Society* 35 (1): 111–31. https://doi.org/10.1080/09687599.2019.1621739.

Tyler, Imogen. 2008. "Chav Mum Chav Scum: Class Disgust in Contemporary Britain." *Feminist Media Studies* 8 (1): 17–34. https://doi.org/10.1080/14680770701824779.

Vandenbeld Giles, Melinda. 2014. *Mothering in the age of Neoliberalism*. Toronto: Demeter Press.

Vincent, Carol. 2017. "'The Children Have Only Got One Education and You Have to Make Sure it's a Good One': Parenting and Parent–School Relations in a Neoliberal Age." *Gender and Education* 2 (5): 541–57. https://doi.org/10.1080/09540253.2016.1274387.

Vincent, Carol, Nicola Rollock, Stephen Ball, and David Gillborn. 2012. "Intersectional Work and Precarious Positionings: Black Middle-class Parents and Their Encounters with Schools in England." *International Studies in Sociology of Education* 22 (3): 259–76. https://doi.org/10.1080/09620214.2012.744214.

Wills, Wendy J., Kathryn Backett-Milburn, Mei-Li Roberts, and Julia Lawton. 2011. "The Framing of Social Class Distinctions through Family Food and Eating Practices." *The Sociological Review* 59 (4): 725–40. https://doi.org/10.1111/j.1467-954X.2011.02.

Chapter 10

Vroeg Ryp, Vroeg Vrot (Early to Ripen, Early to Rot)

Stigma and Young Coloured Women's Negotiation of Heterosex and Motherhood

Andrea Alexander

Teen pregnancy continues to be a great concern in the South African context, as it is in many other countries across the world (Bhana et al. 2010). The moral panic associated with early childbearing and parenting in South Africa is not only linked to fearmongering about HIV/AIDS but, similar to international discourse, also raises concerns about national economic development and declining morality (Mkhwanazi 2012; Salo and Moolman 2013; Sniekers 2017). Teenage mothers are frequently characterised as "deviant" and "immoral" in public discourse, linked to poverty, social assistance, poor academic achievement and being school dropouts, and having inadequate mothering abilities. Many social ills—such as poverty or poor child outcomes—are attributed to young mothers rather than inadequate social structures and support systems. As a result, young mothers face negative social judgement and are frequently socially marginalised in their schools and communities (Cohan and Langa 2011).

In this chapter, I move beyond such negative characterisations of young motherhood and examine young mothers' experiences from their own perspectives, drawing on the findings of my qualitative study with coloured young women in South Africa who have been pregnant and had children as teenagers. The research has shown that age plays a big factor in stigma and stereotypes on mothering at a young age. This chapter will make a distinction between "young mother" and "older mother" as it speaks to how their experience was shaped, but also it is useful when distinguishing between the participants and their mothers. With this said, this chapter affirms that age does not determine the quality of the type of mothering but is identified merely to highlight the impacts that age has on stigma as it relates to mothering.

My research is based on the view that the issue needs to be contextualised and understood from the perspectives of young mothers themselves as agents negotiating their own sexual and reproductive choices within their community and the institutions of the home, school, and religion. Investigating young mothers' experiences from their own perspectives is critical to opposing common representations of them as wholly passive and vulnerable, and potentially seeing how their agency manifests within the constraints of their circumstances (Sniekers 2018).

I use feminist standpoint theory to investigate how the young women themselves negotiate and make meaning about sex, sexuality, and (non) motherhood in a community that holds largely conservative and often stigmatising notions about young women's sexuality—encapsulated by the widely repeated Kaaps saying "*vroeg ryp, vroeg vrot*"/early to ripen, early to rot. In this chapter I show how young women's narratives are shaped by the push and pull of respectability politics and desire, notions of stigma and respectability, and infused by raced, classed, and gendered norms, and are made and re-made, with alterations, over time. This approach aligns with the Sexual and Reproductive Justice approach that seeks to centre the experiences of Women of Colour and recognises that supporting young people's sexual agency requires destigmatising teenage parenthood and ensuring adequate support for teenaged and young parents (Hans and White 2019; Ross 2017).

DOMINANT DISCOURSES OF TEEN SEX AND PARENTHOOD IN SOUTH AFRICA

The South African context, which forms the broad backdrop against which various communities form their ideals, values, and norms about sex and reproduction, is largely a conservative one when it comes to young people's sexuality (Mkhwanazi 2012). South African studies about youth sexuality and pregnancy indicate that for the most part teenage sexuality and reproduction are normatively understood and framed in terms of danger and disease (Macleod, Moodley, and Saville Young 2015). Public discussion about youth sexuality frequently focusses on the risks in terms of HIV and (unintended) teen pregnancy. This dominant discourse of danger and disease also permeates formal sexuality education (Francis 2010; Jewkes and Morrell 2012; Shefer and Ngabaza 2015), where the dominant approach hinges on a "framework of protection, regulation and discipline" (Shefer and Ngabaza 2015, 64). Within this framework, abstinence is prescribed as the best outcome of sexual negotiation, and young people who want to know about sex are frequently stigmatised (Ngabaza and Shefer, this volume).

Thus, instead of empowering youth the dominant approach in South Africa, as in many contexts, to young people's sexuality and reproduction remains conservative. This conservative approach in formal sex education often results in an emphasis on abstinence, supported by educators' conservative value systems and discomfort related to teaching about sex and associated topics (Bhana et al. 2010; Cense and Ganzevoort 2019; Snieker 2017). The restrictive abstinence-focussed approach is echoed in religious institutions where sexual exploration is stipulated as needing to be reserved for the sanctity of marriage.

Together these dominant institutional messages serve to problematise teen sexual exploration, pregnancy, and parenthood. Moreover, numerous studies show that institutional responses to teenage sexuality are gendered: those shamed for engaging in sex are young women (Macleod, Moodley, and Saville Young 2015; Bhana et al. 2010; Nkani and Bhana 2011). Young women are thus singled out to suffer the consequences of engaging in "deviant" sex. For example, despite provisions in the South African Schools Act of 2006, principals often prevent pregnant learners from attending school (Nkani and Bhana 2010).

Such responses emerge in relation to the common view of teen pregnancy as a threat to the social order, resulting in the moral degradation not only of the pregnant young woman but her entire community as well (Macleod 2011). This gendered problematisation of teenage pregnancy demonstrates Gqola's (2015) assertion that it is the marginalised in a society who bears its shame.

In contrast to society's blaming and shaming of individual young women, research that takes a critical and/or Reproductive Justice perspective points to the contextual factors that shape teenagers' sexual and reproductive decision-making (Macleod, Moodley, and Saville Young 2015). For example, decision-making can be impeded by poor relationships between healthcare workers and youth at public health clinics, inadequate sexual knowledge, changing attitudes towards sex, and peer pressure (Mushwana et al. 2015). Sexual violence may also impede young people's ability to make sexual and reproductive decisions in line with their desires.

COLOURED IDENTITIES AND
RESPECTABLE WOMANHOOD

The young women who contributed to my study are at the crossroads of multiple intersecting marginalised identities. Not only are they racialised as coloured, but they are also young mothers aged between 16 and 24 years old, living on the outskirts of the Cape Flats,[1] many of whom did not complete secondary education or enter tertiary education. Following feminist standpoint theory and a Reproductive Justice approach, which centres on Women of Colour and marginalised groups (Collins 2009), my research focusses on "race" as a key identity marker for my participants, alongside other intersecting marginalised identities (gender, age, reproductive status). In South Africa, the racial term "coloured" differs from international usage (i.e., Black people/people of colour) but refers to those descended largely from indigenous Africans, those enslaved in the Cape, and others of African and Asian descent who were part of the Cape colonial populace (Adhikari 2006). The designation was granted social and political significance by the racial hierarchy instituted by the Apartheid government (Adhikari 2009; Erasmus 2001, 2017).

South African scholars have explored the meanings of coloured identity in terms of its location within the racial hierarchy as occupying indeterminate status as "less than white, but better than black" (Erasmus 2001, 13), as well as its intersections with gender and class (Erasmus 2001). Although, as Erasmus (2001) explains, there is no monolithic "Coloured experience," there is among coloured communities a shared history of slavery, dispossession, and creolisation. As an ethnic minority group that has always held indeterminate status, coloured people continue to be impacted by historically entrenched power relation and racist stereotypes of coloured identity: immorality or sexual promiscuity, illegitimacy or impurity, and untrustworthiness. In response to this stigma, shame, decency, and respectability are key defining terms of coloured experience and class aspirations, reinforced by religious institutions that police acceptable conduct, particularly with respect to sexuality (Adhikari 2006; Erasmus 2001).

Relevant to my research are the pervasive communal values related to sex, sexuality, and sexual exploration in post-apartheid coloured communities. Among these is the common ideal of coloured young woman as "chaste, virginal and not with child" (Erasmus 2001, 1). This sentiment is encapsulated by the title to this chapter, "*vroeg ryp, vroeg vrot*" which translates as "early to ripen, early to rot," meaning that sexually "precocious" girls/young women soon lose value or worth. This Kaapse[2] idiom encapsulates the veil of shame cast on young, coloured women who contravene dominant cultural understandings of what it means to be an "*ordentlike*" (decent) coloured woman (Erasmus 2001; Salo 2002). It serves as a warning regarding "premature" sexual interest or activity that regulates young, coloured women's sexuality through the construction of young motherhood as problematic and shameful and the associated surveillance of young women's sexual conduct.

Meanings about adolescent sexuality relate to historical and gendered constructions of respectable personhood within local contexts, as shown in Salo's (2002) work on the Cape Flats where my research was also conducted.

The notion of respectability, as I shall show, is central to the ways in which gendered, racialised, and age-related norms about sex position the coloured young mothers in my study as "deviant" or "other" owing to their departure from communal and national norms regarding teenage sex and respectable womanhood. This positioning is reinforced by religious ideas, which also shape communal values regarding sex and young people's sexual exploration. Erasmus (2001) contends that coloured people cling to their religious identities as a result of the dispossession and erasure of Creole heritage. Thus, being a Christian or Muslim may often be more important than racial or ethnic identity markers. With this said, the research also shows how the idea of a respectable coloured womanhood is challenged in that we see the idiom *"vroeg ryp, vroep vrot"* morphs into sayings such as *"kinnes is maar ook 'n blessing"* (children are a blessing).

METHODOLOGY

Due to the stigma that surrounds the notion of teenage sex and teenage pregnancy, I made use of purposive sampling and snowball sampling. To be included in the study participants needed to be teen mothers between the ages of 16 and 24, identify as coloured, and live in the Westlake community before, during, and after pregnancy. Being a resident of the Westlake community made recruitment easier; there had been rapport established between myself and the participants as many of them were known to me before I approached them. Participants were approached via social media, which allowed participants to decline participation without having to feel the pressure of an in-person invitation.

Data were collected by means of one-on-one, semi-structured, in-depth interviews, conducted by me in English and *Kaaps*. Participants were given the opportunity to decide where the interviews would take place. All the participants requested that the interviews take place at my home to avoid the possibility of being overheard or interrupted while discussing a highly stigmatised topic in the coloured community. Considering this stigma and potential harm, confidentiality and anonymity of the participants' identity have been safeguarded using pseudonyms. Participants' ages ranged from 16 to 25 at the time of the interview, but all had their first child before the age of 18. For one out of the five participants who were under the legal consenting age, consent was sought from both the participant and their legal guardian.

I used thematic analysis to analyse the data (Page 2014) and draw on feminist standpoint theory to interpret the themes I generated. Feminist standpoint theory is derived from intersectionality theory (Crenshaw 1991) and enables an even more nuanced understanding of the factors influencing identity-making, power, and life experiences. This theoretical framework emphasises the complexities of people's identities beyond definitions of good or bad, right or wrong, recognising the possibility of occupying both positions simultaneously. It tasks the researcher with looking at the interplay of micro and macro social systems in a particular moment of a person's life (Collins 2009).

FINDINGS

From their narratives, it was clear that the young women demonstrate agency within the constraints imposed by their communities: they negotiate their own sexual exploration, in some instances choose motherhood, and take up the responsibility of raising their children. I identified three themes, which I named: (1) negotiating choice(s), (2) silencing the shame, and (3) becoming worthy mothers. Through these themes one can see how the idiom, "*vroeg ryp, vroeg vrot*" (early to ripen, early to rot) shapes young women's narratives, regulating how they approach sex, sexuality, sexual exploration, and motherhood.

Theme 1: Negotiating Choice(s)

Negotiating choice(s) around sex is a complex push and pull for participants who must contend with home and communal values and institutional teachings (e.g., school, religious institutions) about sex that confine the practice to be enjoyed by married older adults. Young women who are known to be engaging in sex are met with derogatory comments and slurs. For example, Chantel reported that the community would say, "*Jy's ougat*, you're keeping you big." The loose translation of this is "you're promiscuous" or "you desire sexual exploration (with a negative connotation)." Importantly "*ougat*" and "keeping you big" indicates the transgression of normative age restrictions related to sex. In contrast to girls, boys are given space to experiment with (hetero)sexual desire, whereas girls are restricted by communal values and messages that cast girls into roles of virginity and purity. For instance, Chantel stated, "Now he tells us about his [sexual] experience and we listen and laugh because we are also not any wiser. Because we [the girls] don't really know about these things."

Echoing the pervasive sexual double standard, young women are expected to defend themselves against young men's sexual advances to maintain their virginal status or, at least, to preserve the appearance of chastity by ensuring that they do not become pregnant. For instance, Simone recounted how this responsibility was recounted to young women in sex talks at home:

Simone
They say you're a big girl, you mustn't let boys touch you. And when you have sex you use a condom.

Four of the five participants similarly reported receiving messages about their responsibility to prevent pregnancy and, specifically, making use of a condom.

Based on the common view of young women as sexual gatekeepers and as responsible for preventing pregnancy, it is young women who are blamed if pregnancy does occur when they are considered "too young," unable to financially provide, and/or are unmarried. Popular discourse surrounding teen pregnancy assumes that the pregnancy is a result of young women's irresponsibility or ignorance. Possibilities beyond individual control, like contraceptive failure or sexual coercion, are generally not considered (Collumbien, Gerressu, and Cleland 2004). Rather, it is assumed that young women have made poor choices.

The young mothers in this study resisted this assumption of irresponsibility by highlighting circumstances beyond their control. They explained that they do use contraception, but that these are not always effective. Indeed, some of the young mothers described becoming pregnant while using contraceptives. For example, Simone told about her experience of contraceptive failure and how after giving birth she struggled to find contraceptives that worked for her.

Simone
I'm not stupid, when I started doing intercourse I was on the injection and then I fell pregnant. [. . .] Then, I mean like, I went on the three-month injection, the two-month injection, I saw I was still getting my period, which means you might get pregnant again. I was confused because my first time and then I went on the three-month injection. After that when I fell pregnant, I was like "this is just stupid. What is this?" So, I started the three-year one. My friends also fell pregnant like this. So, I'm like, abstaining.

Here Simone explains that even before first sex, she made use of contraception, but due to the ineffectiveness of the contraception she became pregnant. Describing this as a common experience, she highlights the unreliability of contraception so that abstaining from sex is her only certain option to avoid unintended pregnancy. In telling her story, Simone suggests that she is making a responsible choice and in doing so she challenges stereotypes of young coloured women as reckless and irresponsible and the assumption that she is to blame for the unintended pregnancy.

Similarly, other participants reject the assumption of "irresponsibility" and of having made "poor choices" by explaining that they were unable to use contraceptives. For instance, Mishka was afraid to access contraceptives because of the shame of people knowing that she is sexually active. Mishka's narrative shows how, despite the clinic in this community being within walking distance from participants' homes, stigma creates a barrier to access. This is also shown in the extract below where Jessica recounts an unpleasant experience she had at the clinic. Jessica accompanied her friend, Ayesha, to the clinic to assist her as her daughter needed to be inoculated. Jessica then recalls a nurse saying to her:

Jessica
"God, do you have more children?" I looked at the aunty and said, "Aunty [name] are you talking to me?" "Yes, I am talking to you. Can't you close your legs? When the desire comes, you must sit it in cold water." Then I said, "Hello aunty, this is not my child, this is her child." Then I felt very bad, now she comes to our house all the time to apologise, but I don't open the door for her. It was too terrible.

While not all participants had such experiences, with some even reporting positive experiences at clinics, stories such as Simone's suggest that there is still a need to destigmatise young women's use of contraceptives. This includes challenging the gendered double standards related to young women's sexuality that are embedded in cultural ideals of respectable femininity.

For some participants, pregnancy was planned and was therefore a choice made by them. For example, Simone explains:

Simone
When I first got pregnant, I was so disappointed, I was sad, I was really, really sad. I felt, disobedient. I felt bad in every kind of way you can explain it. But the second one, we actually planned on that one . . . ja, we're gonna have a baby.

The above excerpt shows how the veil of shame so badly affects the perception of self. With this said, young women do still choose to have children, which is illustrated in the above comment. Young women's intentional pregnancies and the ways in which they negotiate sex, and in turn take up the responsibility of mothering their children, can be understood from a Reproductive Justice perspective that emphasises the right to have children and raise them in supportive conditions (Ross 2017).

Importantly, this right includes support for parenting. Thus, participants explained that when young women are unable to fulfil some of the roles of mothering, their mothers take up the task. If the participant or her mother are both unable to fulfil the role of mothering, the task is transferred to older women in the community who fill the care gap. For example, Mishka was conceived at the age of 15 and was unable to financially support her child. Her mother, grandmother, and women in the community supported her financially and provided her with other resources to assist her journey of mothering.

Theme 2: Silencing the Shame

Shame pervades participants' narratives of teenage pregnancy and motherhood. Sometimes shame is related to their deviation from the norm of female sexuality among coloured communities in which young women must remain "chaste, virginal and without a child" (Erasmus 2001, 1) until marriage. This theme shows a concerted effort to silence shame. This is done by literally preventing young women from exploring their sexuality resulting in, some instances, an abortion being forced on a participant so that a cloud of shame would not hang over the participant and her mother because of teen pregnancy. Mishka and Jessica reported that community members did not expect them to get pregnant because they were perceived as "innocent" and "shy" girls.

Shame surfaced in many ways, but most significantly it is rooted in the fact that these young women have not engaged in respectable sex, defined through communal values as an act shared by married adults. The stigma of becoming pregnant as a teenager was evident in Jessica's account of her mother's attempt to compel her to have an abortion. Similarly, while Nikita expressed joy at the fact that she was expecting a baby, this emotion soon morphed into shame: "I was excited. I couldn't wait to tell my mother, but then in that moment I was also afraid to tell my mother because I was seventeen years old [and unmarried]." Nikita's shame is associated with becoming pregnant while young and unmarried, considered the "wrong" conditions for pregnancy and motherhood. Such assumptions about appropriate ages for childbearing are evident in the common reference to young women who have children as "*kinnes met kinnes*" (children with children).

The moments of revealing pregnancy also expose the gendered nature of shame and the subsequent stigma attached to it. Upon reflecting on the moment of revealing the pregnancy, Mishka said that the news of her pregnancy was met with shock and anger. Reflecting on her partner's experience, Mishka mentions that, unlike her mother and grandmother, her partner's parents did not get angry, "they were fine . . . obviously because he is a man." Similarly, reflecting on their experiences in the classroom, negotiating sex and sexual expression, participants told how (heterosexual) boys are able to explore sex and sexual expression without punishment and/or shame. This resonates with Eriksson et al.'s (2013) research that was conducted with young people on pre-marital sex that boys' sexual desires are generally seen to be more acceptable. The weight of the shame is therefore exclusively shouldered by these young women and their mothers, who have had to negotiate their motherhood and sexuality in value systems that do not recognise them as active agents or "real" mothers (Mkhwanazi 2012).

Like other participants, for Chantel, revealing that she was pregnant brought up feelings of shame as well as fear. The shame of being an unmarried pregnant 16 year old was amplified by the fact that she had been sexually assaulted. Sexual violence is usually even more stigmatised and shameful than teenage pregnancy in the community, and blame is undeservedly placed on the victim and not the rapist. Chantel explained, saying, "my first child . . . I can't say it was an accident, the child was not an accident . . . but what happened [rape] should not have happened." To cope with the shame and stigma related to the pregnancy and the context in which conception happened, Chantel tried to hide the pregnancy as much as possible. She said, "No one knew. No one knew because I would stay indoors. It was a shame."

Upon telling her mother that she had become pregnant after being raped, an argument ensued. Her mother responded by slamming the door and Chantel recounts, "she says to me that she is not going to raise that child. That I must have an abortion because we don't want those children [born of rape]." After the child was born, Chantel physically distanced herself from her daughter by sending her to live with Chantel's grandmother. Chantel's and her mother's responses can be understood as attempts to silence shame and stigma.

Theme 3: Becoming Worthy Mothers

Overall, the shame described by participants is a manifestation of the highly stigmatised domain of teenage sex and reproduction. In the following theme, I show how participants enact agency and negotiate shame, redeeming themselves by enacting respectable femininity through being a good or "worthy" mother.

The idea of "becoming a worthy mother" constantly arises in participants' accounts of their experiences. This theme focusses on the emphasis placed on worthiness and links to the notion of coloured respectability that prescribes what it means to be a "respectable mother" (Salo 2018). For the young mothers, this may involve taking up the responsibility of parenting their children themselves, instead of "shifting" the responsibility to their own mothers or other older women in the family or the community. In this way, shame can be mitigated by becoming a "good mother."

Chantel's narrative illustrates the value accorded to becoming a worthy mother. After enduring shame from her first pregnancy that resulted from rape (discussed above), she tells how she and her partner decided to have a child. Commenting on the choice to have a baby she said, "I wanted to show that I can care for my child." Caring for her own child allowed her to regain social status as a mother. In her community, young women who fail to do so are seen as undeserving of motherhood, and "shifting" responsibility of motherhood is often one of the ways through which teen mothers are perceived as recklessly "falling" pregnant. This view is founded upon communal values regarding what constitutes "respectable" mothering (Salo et al. 2010).

As discussed in the previous theme, young women bear shame for becoming pregnant at an early age and when unmarried, but their mothers also bear shame for failing to fulfil *their* responsibility as mothers, that is, for failing to produce "a worthy daughter." According to Salo et al. (2010, 304), in order to maintain values of respectability and mothering held by the community, "coloured women police the respectable status of their households." Thus, in the context of Westlake, good mothering is closely connected to surveillance of daughters to ensure that young girls remain chaste and virginal. For instance, pregnant young women were asked, "Didn't your mother teach you about using condoms?" Thus, mothers are expected to provide their daughters with sex education focussed on re/producing a respectable femininity rooted in heterosexuality and chastity and regulated by communal values of shame and respectability.

Consequently, when young women become pregnant, they are commonly seen as bringing shame upon their mothers. For example, Nikita remarked that people would say, "This child is so young and she's pregnant. Does she have no shame? How must her mother feel?" Community responses are generally less sympathetic towards the mother than this, however. For instance, Simone told about her friend's experiences of public shaming when she became pregnant. She recounted, "the comments that she got . . . it was very rude. They even went to her mommy to say that she must keep her child on a leash." Mothers, therefore, are viewed as having failed in their task of surveillance and keeping a daughter from early/unwed pregnancy and are thus shamed and socially chastised.

On the other hand, being able to keep daughters from early/unwed pregnancy elevates a mother's social status. The community views them as worthy mothers for not "allowing" their daughters to "fall" pregnant. This role of safeguarding young women's social respectability is not limited to mothers only. Participants' accounts indicate that any older female figure in the home and community can enact a maternal role and take on this responsibility. For example, Nikita related how she is now tasked by her mother with giving her younger sister the "sex talk," because of her own experiences of teenage pregnancy. She explained:

Nikita
She [her mother] says that I must do it, because she can't handle stuff like that anymore . . . I am now there to speak. I must drill her, you know. My mother already spoke about that [sexual violence] . . . [pause] I must just . . . talk about the sex stuff.

In this way, worthiness can be regained by mothers and older women after they or their daughters become teen mothers.

Although maternal surveillance is a key element in creating worthy daughters and therefore good mothering within the coloured community (Salo et al. 2010; Erasmus 2001), participants did recount instances in which coloured mothers were more forgiving, for instance stating that teenage pregnancy can happen to anyone and that it is part of life. For example, Mishka told of how her grandmother's initial disappointment turned into a less punitive response: "it is life and it is fine." Thereafter, mother, grandmother, and older women in the community supported her financially and provided her with other resources to care for her child. In this way, shame can be averted to some extent as the women, including Mishka, are able to enact respectable femininity through worthy mothering and taking up motherly roles.

Similarly, some participants recounted how after they become mothers, the dominant narrative of shame related to teenage pregnancy turned into a more positive one in which "children are a blessing." Thus, while the communal values remain punitive and filled with different layers of surveillance, participants' narratives illustrate a shift in ideology where the home values have shown to be more flexible and open to changing its tone to be more supportive. In this way, and as Erasmus (2001) highlights, coloured identities are not fixed but make and re-make themselves; this includes the ways in which parenthood, femininity, and respectability are re-imagined.

CONCLUDING DISCUSSION

Teenage pregnancy is a complex phenomenon that needs to be contextualised and understood from the perspectives of teenage mothers themselves. This study explored how participants' experiences of pregnancy and motherhood are shaped by the terms and conditions of respectable womanhood for young, coloured women. Following the idiom, *"vroeg ryp, vroeg vrot"* young women are instructed to remain chaste in order to be seen as respectable (*"ordentlike"*) young women and community members. This means that they are positioned as gatekeepers who must manage young men's sexual advances. If they fail in this, they are instructed to at least uphold the appearance of respectability by refraining from becoming pregnant. Teenage pregnancy belies the appearance of chastity, announces that these young women have engaged in sex, brings shame on the young women (and her mother) albeit that pregnancy "takes two to tango" and the male sexual partner does not have to shoulder the shame, and that pregnancy can also be a result of sexual violence. Young, coloured women's sexuality and reproduction are therefore devalued; young, coloured mothers are seen as bringing decay to themselves, but potentially also the wider community, as highlighted in the idiom, "*vroeg vrot*" (early to rot). This stigma disproportionately disadvantages women—both the young women and their mothers—who must shoulder the shame.

Ironically, while shaming is meant to deter young women from becoming pregnant, the stigma it reproduces potentially constrains their ability to negotiate sex and make reproductive choices. For instance, I showed that although contraception is available to the young women in the study, the stigma attached to young/unmarried women's sexuality is so amplified that they sometimes do not access contraceptives out of shame.

It is important, therefore, to acknowledge that negotiating and navigating sex, "early" reproduction, and young motherhood are part of a complex web of power relations cutting along lines of gender, race, class, and place (Snieker 2017). It is not enough simply to make contraception available and to teach young women to say "no" to sexual advances or to make "good choices" (Shefer and Ngabaza 2015)—as the institutions of home, school, and religion frequently do. Sex education and policy on sexual and reproductive health and rights need to take into consideration how young women's ability to choose and sexual expression is restricted by stigma and community norms of gendered respectability.

Moving beyond the confines of shame and stigmatisation, however, participants' extracts demonstrate that regardless of the limitations put on sexual expression, the young women in this study negotiate sex in complex ways and demonstrate conditional agency (See chapter 13 for a discussion of agency). Contrary to dominant stereotypes of recklessness and promiscuousness placed on young, coloured mothers, many use contraceptives and in some cases, conception occurred while on contraception. Others' pregnancies had been *planned* and *desired*.

Coloured young women need to be recognised as agents with sexual rights and must be afforded full sexual citizenship, including the right to decide if and when to have sex, and the right to pleasure (Garcia and Parker 2007). The findings presented in this chapter highlight that it is important for young women to be included in these efforts. Doing so will require that young women's sexual agency and reproductive rights need to be acknowledged and supported through policy and, just as importantly, within the communities of which they are part. A Sexual and Reproductive Justice approach highlights the conditions necessary to achieve Sexual and Reproductive Justice for all. Thus, following Hans and White (2019), there needs to be a stronger call to "emphasize the rights of women of colour to have children, to decide the conditions under which they give birth, and to parent their children with support, safety and dignity" (Hans and White 2019, 690).

NOTES

1. "Housing projects [in South Africa] that were constructed in the 1960s and '70s for those classified as coloured, who were forcibly removed from areas proclaimed white by the Group Areas Act" (Salo 2009, 13).

2. A language spoken largely within coloured communities in the Western Cape, originat in settler colonial South Africa. As a form of revolt, indigenous Africans and those enslaved by the Dutch (including Malays, West Africans, and Madagascans) refused to speak the colonisers' language, instead creating a new creole to communicate among themselves. This language is the precursor on the now more widely spoken Afrikaans (Haupt 2021).

REFERENCES

Adhikari, Mohamed. 2006. "Hope, Fear, Shame, Frustration: Continuity and Change in the Expression of Coloured Identity in White Supremacist South Africa, 1910-1994." *Journal of Southern African Studies* 32 (3): 467–87.

———. 2009. "From Narratives of Miscengenation to Post-Modernist Denied by Race." In *Burdened by Race Coloured Identities in Southern Afri*ca, edited by Mohamed Adikari, 1–22. Cape Town: UCT Press.

Bhana, Deevia, Robert Morell, Tamara Shefer, and Sisa Ngabaza. 2010. "South African Teachers' Responses to Teenage Pregnancy and Teenage Mothers in Schools." *Culture, Health & Sexuality* 12 (8): 871–83. https://doi.org/10.1080/13691058.2010.500398.

Cense, Marianne, and R. Ruard Ganzevoort. 2019. "The Storyscapes of Teenage Pregnancy. On Morality, Embodiment, and Narrative Agency." *Journal of Youth Studies* 22 (4): 568–83, https://doi.org/10.1080/13676261.2018.1526373.

Cohan, Zarina, and Malose Langa. 2011. "Teenage Mothers Talk About Their Experience of Teenage Motherhood." *Agenda* 25 (3): 87–95. https://doi.org/10.1080/10130950.2011.610993.

Collins, Patricia Hill. 2009. *Black Feminist Thought.* New York: Routledge.

Collumbien, Martine, Makeda Gerressu, and John Cleland. 2004. "Non-Use and Use of Ineffective Methods of Contraception." In *Comparative Quantification of Health Risks: Global and Regional Burden of Disease Attributable to Selected Major Risk Factors,* edited by Majid Ezzati, Anthony D. Lopez, and Christopher J. L. Murray, 1255–1320. Geneva: WHO. https://core.ac.uk/download/pdf/13110877.pdf.

Crenshaw, Kimberlé. 1991. "Mapping the Margins: Intersectionality, Identity Politics, and Violence against Women of Colour." *Stanford Law Review* 43 (6): 1241–99. https://doi.org/10.2307/1229039.

Erasmus, Zimitri. 2001. "Introduction: Re-Imagining Coloured Identity in Post-Apartheid South Africa." In *Coloured by History, Shaped by Place: New Perspectives on Coloured Identities in Cape Town,* edited by Zimitri Erasmus, 1–29. Cape Town: Kwela Books.

———. 2017. *Race Otherwise: Forging a New Humanism for South Africa.* Johannesburg: Wits University Press.

Eriksson, Elisabet, Gunilla Lindmark, Pia Axemo, Beverley Haddad, and Beth M. Ahlberg. 2013. "Faith, Premarital Sex and Relationships: Are Church Messages in Accordance with the Perceived Realities of the Youth? A Qualitative Study in KwaZulu-Natal, South Africa." *Journal of Religion and Health* 52: 454–66. https://doi.org/10.1007/s10943-011-9491-7.

Francis, Dennis A. 2010. "Sexuality Education in South Africa: Three Essential Questions." *International Journal of Education Development* 30 (3): 314–19. https://doi.org/10.1016/j.ijedudev.2009.12.003.

Garcia, Jonathan, and Richard Parker. 2007. "From Global Discourse to Local Action: The Makings of a Sexual Rights Movement?" *Horizontes Antropológicos* 3 (se): 13–41. https://doi.org/10.1590/S0104-71832006000200002.

Gqola, Pumla Dineo. 2015. *Rape: A South African Nightmare.* Auckland Park, South Africa: MF Books.

Hans, Sydney L., and Barbara A. White. 2019. "Teenage Childbearing, Reproductive Justice, and Infant Mental Health." *Infant Mental Health Journal* 40 (5): 690–709. https://doi.org/10.1002/imhj.21803.

Haupt, Adam. 2021. "The First-Ever Dictionary of South Africa's Kaaps Language Has Launched – Why it Matters." *The Conversation* (August), https://theconversation.com/the-first-ever-dictionary-of-south-africas-kaaps-language-has-launched-why-it-matters-165485.

Jewkes, Rachel, and Robert Morrell. 2012. "Sexuality and the Limits of Agency Among South African Teenage Women: Theorising Femininities and their Connections to HIV Risk Practices." *Social Science and Medicine* 74 (11): 1729–37. https://doi.org/10.1016/j.socscimed.2011.05.020.

Macleod, Catriona. 2011. *'Adolescence', Pregnancy and Abortion: Constructing a Threat of Denigration.* London: Routledge.

Macleod, Catriona, Dale Moodley, and Lisa Saville Young. 2015. "Sexual Socialisation in Life Orientation Manuals Versus Popular Music: Responsibilities Versus Pleasure, Tension and Complexity." *Perspectives in Education* 33 (2): 90–107. https://journals.ufs.ac.za/index.php/pie/article/view/1908.

Mkhwanazi, Nolwazi. 2012. "A Tough Love Approach Indeed: Demonising Early Childbearing in the Zuma Era." *Agenda*, 26 (4): 73–84. https://doi.org/10.1080/10130950.2012.759440.

Mushwana, Lenny, Lydia Monareng, Solina Richter, and Helene Muller. 2015. "Factors Influencing the Adolescent Pregnancy Rate in Greater Giyani Municipality, Limpopo Province – South Africa." *International Journal of Africa Nursing Sciences* 2: 10–18. https://doi.org/10.1016/j.ijans.2015.01.001.

Nkani, Nomvuyo, and Deevia Bhana. 2011. "When African Teenagers Become Fathers: Culture, Materiality and Masculinity." *Culture, Health & Sexuality* 16 (4): 337–50. https://doi.org/10.1080/13691058.2014.887780.

Page, Jools Meryl. 2014. "Childcare Choices and Voices: Using Interpreted Narratives and Thematic Meaning-Making to Analyse Mothers' Life Histories." *International Journal of Qualitative Studies in Education* 27 (7): 850–76. https://doi.org/10.1080/09518398.2013.805850.

Ross, Loretta. 2017. "Conceptualising Reproductive Justice Theory: A Manifesto for Activism." In *Radical Reproductive Justice: Foundation, Theory, Practice, Critique*, edited by Loretta Ross, Erika Derkas, Whitney Peoples, Dorothy Roberts, and Pamela Bridgewater Toure, 170–232. New York: Feminist Press at CUNY.

Salo, Elaine. 2002. "Condoms Are for Spares, Not for Besties: Negotiating Adolescent Sexuality in Post-Apartheid Manenberg." *Society in Transition* 33 (3): 403–19. https://doi.org/10.1080/21528586.2002.10419073.

———. 2009. "Coconuts Do Not Live in Townships: Cosmopolitanism and its Failures in the Urban Peripheries of Cape Town." *Feminist Africa* 13: 11–21. http://hdl.handle.net/2263/14465.

———. 2018. *Respectable Mothers, Tough Men and Good Daughters: Producing Persons in Manenberg Township South Africa*. Baltimore, MD: Project Muse.

Salo, Elaine, and Benita Moolman. 2013. "Biology, Bodies and Human Rights." *Agenda* 24 (4): 3–9. https://doi.org/10.1080/10130950.2013.872894.

Salo, Elaine, Mario Ribas, Pedro Lopes, and Márcio Zamboni. 2010. "Living Our Lives on the Edge: Power, Space and Sexual Orientation in the Cape Town Townships, South Africa." *Sexuality Research and Social Policy* 7 (4): 298–309. https://doi.org/10.1007/s13178-010-0028-8.

Shefer, Tamara, and Sisa Ngabaza. 2015. "'And I Have Been Told That There is Nothing Fun about Having Sex While You are Still in High School': Dominant Discourses on Women's Sexual Practices and Desires in Life Orientation Programmes at School." *Perspectives in Education* 33 (2): 63–76. https://journals.ufs.ac.za/index.php/pie/article/view/1906.

Sniekers, Marijke. 2018. "Defining Dreams: Young Mothers' Agency in Constructions of Space." *Social & Cultural Geography* 19 (8): 1073–96. https://doi.org/10.1080/14649365.2017.1344872.

Chapter 11

Sexuality Education for Sexual and Reproductive Justice?

Deconstructing the Dominant Response to Young People's Sexualities in Contemporary Schooling Contexts in South Africa

Sisa Ngabaza and Tamara Shefer

Global concerns related to young people's sexual and reproductive health (SRH) and rights—particularly with respect to unwanted pregnancies, STIs/ HIV, and gender-based violence (GBV)—have been implemented in mainstream school sexuality education or out of school curricula and public health programmes. Sexuality education at school has been regarded as a key platform for gender and sexual justice by equipping young people with appropriate skills and knowledge for reproductive health and sexual agency, freedom, and safety. Despite these good intentions, the sexuality education curriculum has come under increased scrutiny across the globe, including in South Africa. This includes concerns about the relevance of the curriculum to young people (Allen 2007, 2008), parents' lack of understanding of and resistance to sexuality education (Sham et al. 2020), critical questions about the curriculum content and its political intentions and underpinnings (Fine 1988; Francis 2010), and challenges around curriculum delivery (Helleve et al. 2011; Shefer and Ngabaza 2015; Kirby 2008).[1]

The South African "Life Orientation" (LO) curriculum, a prescribed subject directed at providing life skills for young people, has been seen as a key platform for sexuality education. The primary emphasis of LO has been to provide life skills, while also generating awareness of and investment in responsible citizenship and social justice, including gender equality. This is evident in the Department of Basic Education's (DBE's) National Curriculum Statements (NCS) (Grade R-12), also flagged in the primary four LO

Curriculum Assessment Policy Statements (CAPS), directed at "equipping learners irrespective of their socio-economic background . . . with knowledge, skills and values necessary for self-fulfilment and meaningful participation as citizens of a free country" (DBE 2011, 4). In 2017, the DBE developed the National Policy on HIV, STIs, and TB for stakeholders in all primary and secondary schools as a way of enhancing response strategies. Through this policy, the DBE is expected to provide curriculum-based sexuality education and access to SRH services to prevent new HIV infection and STIs, early unintended pregnancies, and school-related GBV, and to retain learners and support their success in schools.

Mturi and Bechuke (2019, 135) show that SRH education in South Africa is generally disseminated through "clinics and health centres, mass media, peers and friends, parent child communication and school-based curriculum." The school is the only source of this knowledge that is regulated and can be evaluated. Curriculum-based sexuality and sexual reproductive health education is crucial in South African schools, given the continued high rates of HIV and STIs, early and often unintended pregnancy at school, GBV, and a general inadequacy of information on sexual health and rights education (DBE 2012).

Implementing sexuality education in schools has the potential to support young people's agency to overcome the numerous barriers that compromise their sexual health and rights (Frohlich et al. 2014; Zulu et al. 2019). Although South Africa boasts numerous public policy documents to enable young people to access SRH services (Strode et al. 2017), many young women, in particular, still lack adequate knowledge and information to make informed decisions about their sexual health and rights (Mturi and Bechuke 2019). Current statistics show that young women still carry the load of HIV in South Africa, with four times as many women as men of their age being infected. Further, 37% of all new infections in South Africa are among young women aged 15–24, while one-third of the country's young women become pregnant before the age of 20 (SANAC 2017). Along with this, South Africa faces unacceptably high rates of violence against women, evident in the normativity of coercive and violent sexual practices in many young women's experiences (Stern et al. 2016) and linked with the gendered dynamics of reproductive health challenges for young South Africans.

Globally (UNESCO 2009) and locally, schools have been viewed as well-positioned to provide sexuality education for young people (Francis 2011). School-based provision of knowledge and skills potentially equips young people with appropriate knowledge and the agency to make responsible choices in their social and sexual reproductive and health matters. However, it is not only knowledge about reproduction and reproductive health that has been valued by critical and feminist scholars and practitioners but also the stated emphasis on human rights, reproductive rights, and sexual and gender justice (DBE 2011, 1.3(c)). The LO curriculum has been understood as having the potential to engage with a larger social and gender justice project, to challenge sexual and gender inequalities, gender binarisms, and heteronormativity. Further, statistics related to the challenges of HIV and STIs that reveal the gendered nature of these, together with the high rates of GBV, add further weight to the imperative to work with gender equality as key for SRH.

Some research on LO at schools has documented positive impacts of sexuality education (Makina et al. 2017; Haberland 2015; Bainame et al. 2016), highlighting how the LO teacher emerges as a primary source of information for young people. However, proliferating research on sexuality education in South African schools has flagged a wide range of problematic effects and challenges with the curricula and the way in which sexuality education is taught (Bhana et al. 2019; Macleod 2009; Ngabaza et al. 2016). Notwithstanding its good intentions, researchers have argued that this classroom is frequently deployed as a regulatory space, directed at controlling young people's sexuality and underpinned by a particular set of moralities about young people, sexuality, relationships, and family. The expectation that sexuality education will provide valuable resources and information for SRH and well-being, and serve as a space for a constructive dialogue for young people in developing their agency to practise safer, equitable, and pleasurable sexuality, seems very far from the reality emerging in research findings. Rather than taking forward the gender justice goal to stimulate critical thinking about gender and sexuality, such spaces seem to reproduce and rationalise rigid binary gender norms and stereotyped practices and identities.

Our argument in this chapter emerges out of a critical and feminist lens to view sexuality education, both the textual curricula and reported experiences of young people and teachers in school settings. While we acknowledge the possible value of sexuality education, it is imperative to also understand and work with its current challenges and limitations in South Africa. In sum, we argue that current efforts at sexuality education in this local context, seen in both the text-based curriculum (Potgieter and Reygan 2012; Wilmot and Naidoo 2014) and in young people's and teachers' reported experiences (Mturi and Bechake 2019), reflect and reinstate a range of practices and narratives that undermine gender, SRH, and justice for young people. In the chapter, we explore and attempt to illustrate these critical concerns within four key themes: (1) sexuality education as directed towards controlling young people's sexual practices through a discourse of damage, danger, and disease; (2) the reproduction of rigid binaries of gender and sexuality and the "othering" of gender and sexual non-conforming people and practices; (3) the assumption and legitimation of global northern values about family and sexuality; and (4) dominant practices of adult authority over young people which assume the adult as expert and the young person as in a state of development requiring discipline and direction. Drawing on a growing body of qualitative research on sexuality and SRH education at secondary school, we unpack these discourses and argue for a re-thinking and re-articulation of sexuality education in ways that enable alternative practices and principles, in particular those that centralise young people's voices for gender and Sexual and Reproductive Justice.

DISCIPLINING YOUNG PEOPLE'S SEXUALITY

It remains important to make appropriate, accurate, and current knowledge about and resources towards SRH available and accessible for young people (UNESCO 2018). This means engaging with and accepting their sexual agency and activity to facilitate safe and equitable practices and well-being, rather than denying or disciplining such practices. In this respect, it is concerning that a well-documented finding in much current South African research is the way in which sexuality education is taught through a lens of negativity—of danger, damage, and disease (Macleod 2009; Shefer and Ngabaza 2015; Bhana 2015; Ngabaza and Shefer 2019). African feminist scholars like Sylvia Tamale (2011, 30) have long called for a move beyond the "tired polemics of violence, disease and reproduction" which have dominated mainstream sexualities and HIV research in global Southern contexts (Moletsane 2010). Yet the association of sexuality with negative consequences seems to be prevalent in the sexuality education classroom in South Africa. Consequently, the ABC emphasis (abstain, be faithful, and condomise) has been a very strong component of both policy and practice (MacPhail and Campbell 2001). This emphasis has continued despite a global critique of and challenge to the effectiveness of this approach (Kirby 2008; Francis and DePalma 2014; Mathe 2013). Scholars and practitioners have rather called for addressing the challenges related to unequal gender relations and other dimensions of inequality that shape unsafe and coercive sexual practices among young people, arguing for a comprehensive sexuality education (CSE) approach (UNESCO 2009, 2018). This does not argue against possible benefits of sexual abstinence but centres the goal of providing accurate and accessible knowledge, such as contraception methods and procedures, disease-prevention methods (Kirby 2008; Francis and DePalma 2014; Willan 2013), and knowledge of sexual and reproductive rights. CSE has been globally promoted for its potential to reduce rates of unwanted early pregnancy and STIs/HIV while also facilitating young people's agency and capacity to make informed decisions about their sexual, reproductive, and general health and well-being (UNESCO 2009, 2018).

Alongside these arguments against the abstinence approach, researchers have pointed out the punitive and authoritarian way in which young people are taught about sexuality, with abstinence not only promoted but also assumed as normative for young people (Francis 2012; Ngabaza et al. 2016). The strong presence of a language of consequence is evident in the cautioning of young people to abstain from sexual practices or "face consequences" (Shefer and Macleod 2015; Francis and DePalma 2014; Macleod 2009). Sexuality continues to be primarily taught through its association with HIV/AIDS, STIs, violence and unwanted, early pregnancy, rather than any positive lenses of pleasure, relationality, care, and so on. It has been noted that teachers regularly show films that present graphic details of STIs, birthing, or sexual violence as part of LO (Shefer and Ngabaza 2015). In this way, sexuality education is deployed towards regulating young people's sexuality and bodies. Rather than open up spaces for young people's sexual agency and responsibility to direct their health, safety, and pleasure, lessons are directed at precautionary and punitive narratives that demonise young sexual desire and practice (Bhana et al. 2010; Ngabaza, Shefer, and Macleod 2016; Bhana et al. 2007). One of the participants in Jearey-Graham and Macleod's (2015, 19) qualitative study on sexuality education articulates this: "They (teachers) just say if you sleep with a boy you will get pregnant or you will get AIDS." The deterministic way in which sexuality is conflated with negative consequences was similarly summed up by another young woman reflecting on the sexuality education she received (Shefer and Ngabaza 2015, 68):

And I have been told that there is nothing fun about having sex while you are still in high school. It just brings down everything that you do you know because you are gonna get pregnant at the end of the day or you might contract one of the diseases and it is just not worth it.

The teaching of sexuality through this lens of danger, disease, and damage raises further concerns about the relationships between schooling and sexuality. Many scholars of sexuality and gender justice in schools have pointed out the entrenched stereotype of childhood as a phase of sexual *innocence* and the insistent denial of sexuality at school, while presenting the school as an asexual space (Bhana et al. 2010; Bhana 2016; Morrell et al. 2012). Ironically, young people are highly sexualised in school in the emphasis on sexual violence and the unitary representation of women as victims and men as perpetrators (Driscoll 2013; Renold and Ringrose 2013; Shefer and Macleod 2015). Yet, as emerges in research on pregnancy and parenting at schools (Morrell et al. 2012), schools are characterised as sanitised spaces where young sexual desire, practice, and parenthood are unimaginable. Researchers have documented punitive and "othering" responses to pregnant and parenting young people in schools which clearly illustrate this strong resistance towards acknowledging young people as sexual (Bhana et al. 2008; Nkani and Bhana et al. 2010). Shaming of young people, usually women, who disrupt this asexual picture by becoming pregnant, has been shown to be common, even in the LO classroom (Bhana et al. 2010; Ngabaza and Shefer 2013). Further, while constitutionally and legally prohibited, exclusion-ary and discriminatory practices towards pregnant and parenting women at school remain a challenge (Morrell et al. 2012; Shefer et al. 2013).

It remains concerning that young pregnant and parenting women at school are stigmatised and that this may be particularly promoted through the sexual-ity education class. Studies have reported cases where a pregnant or parenting learner was spoken about by a teacher during lessons on sexuality as a way of illustrating the "consequences" of transgressing prescribed rules of feminin-ity and sexuality at school (Morrell et al. 2012; Ngabaza and Shefer 2013). Thus, the nuances and complexities of negotiating safer and equitable sex among young people that shape the possibility of unplanned, unwanted preg-nancy are obfuscated by the dominant trope of young women's "irresponsible behaviour" (Smith and Harrison 2013). Rather, schools appear to reproduce an individualised ungendered and youth-*un*friendly context for engaging young people that is not facilitative of gender, sexual, and Reproductive Justice.

POLICING OF GENDER NORMS, HETERONORMATIVITY, AND PRO-FAMILY DISCOURSE

Although sexuality education has been promoted as a key vehicle for chal-lenging gender and sexual reproductive injustice, scholars continue to show how normative gender and sexual identities and practices are reinforced in the teaching and learning of the subject, as well as how HIV/AIDS and GBV are approached (Helleve et al. 2011; Bhana 2017; Epstein et al. 2004; Shefer and Macleod 2015; Pattman and Chege 2003). The positioning of sexuality education as a tool with which to "teach" and control gender norms and hege-monic rigid relations between sex, gender, and sexuality (Butler 1990) is seen throughout most scholarship on the subject.

Binaristic gender and sexual normativity, foregrounded in young people's experiences, show how a gendered language of consequence is the main form of communicating sexuality and SRH to young people. The deployment of consequences in such a manner deprives young people of accurate knowledge on managing their SRH. Young women, through what some scholars term "a discourse of responsibilisation" (Macleod et al. 2015), are continuously reminded how they are not only responsible for their sexuality but carry the burden of managing their male partners' sexual desires and practices as well (Kelly 2001; Kruger et al. 2015; Ngabaza et al. 2016). This recreates a gender binary logic that rationalises and reinforces oppositional gendered sexual roles. At the same time, this portrays women as submissive and inexorable victims open to exploitative masculine power, sexual risks, and violence, while men are positioned as problematic, dangerous, sexual predators.

Young women continue to receive lessons about feminised responsibility, in their prescribed role to police male sexuality, which consistently reiterates stereotypical notions of male irresponsibility and a general lack of care (Shefer and Macleod 2015). Simultaneously, such discourses reproduce and perpetuate gendered hierarchies in learning spaces. Scholarship in this area further shows how young female learners are continuously reminded of idealised heteronormative expectations as they describe how they are required to "talk," "dress," "walk," "sit" through stereotyped notions of feminine and masculine bodies and performance (Ngabaza et al. 2016). There is a general expectation that young women conform to set norms and standards of female respectability (Van Wyk 2015; Kehily 2012). The notion of female respectability necessitates rejecting and resisting male sexual advances and upholding a sexually restrained and obedient femininity instead (Kruger et al. 2015; Van Wyk 2015).

While educators declare tolerance of sexual diversity in teaching and learning spaces, empirical evidence points to how heteronormativity is encouraged while non-heterosexuality is condemned and stifled (Bhana 2014; Francis 2012; DePalma and Francis 2014). Further evident is how moralistic discourses are drawn on to undermine, shame, and challenge gender and sexual non-conforming identities and practices (Smith and Harrison 2013; Bhana 2014). The literature shows how homophobia silences learners with alternative desires, identification, and practices (Msibi 2012; Ngabaza et al. 2016; Mthatyana and Vincent 2015). South African scholars have also shown the extent and nature of heteronormativity and heterosexism in schools (Bhana 2014). Such research emphasises how heterosexuality is assumed normative and promoted within the heterosexual nuclear family, as well as in approaching HIV education. This excludes non-heterosexual learners, compromising young people's Reproductive Justice. As a female respondent in one recent local study shared, "So in Life Orientation they explain that sex is sleeping with a male" (Shefer and Ngabaza 2015, 58).

Compulsory heterosexuality renders any sexual intimacy or relationship outside of male–female nuclear partnering unimaginable. Scholars have indicated how this compulsory heteronormativity is a result of educators' inadequate knowledge of and resistance to gender-inclusive learning spaces (Wilmot and Naidoo 2014; Beyers 2012; Francis and Msibi 2011;

Bhana 2014). Some researchers attribute such resistance to educators' own moralities and culture-rationalised heteronormative convictions (Helleve et al. 2009; Helleve et al. 2011; Khau 2012; Baxen 2010; Johnson 2014; Baxen and Breidlid 2009).

Along with this, embedded within messages on HIV is a discourse that emphasises a particular set of family values that promote heterosexual marriage and the nuclear family (Ngabaza and Shefer 2019). Antecedents of the colonial politics of birth control are evident in reproductive health policies that continue to flag their entanglement with South Africa's settler political ideologies (Macleod 2003, 2009), carrying continued implications for Reproductive Justice. Eurocentric notions of the heterosexual nuclear family, and North American pro-family discourses in African countries (McEwen 2018), continuously shape narratives on sexuality and SRH in the public domain and find their way into the sexuality education curriculum. For most South Africans, a stereotypic nuclear family is not the norm, nor is it historically representative. However, the heterosexual nuclear family structure and other imagined moralities associated with it shape much of the sexuality education curriculum.

Further evidence from learners and educators points to how sexuality education assumes a heterosexual nuclear family, prescribing such values and sexual assumptions to judge young pregnant learners in schools. Educators tell learners to abstain from sexual activities until they are heterosexually married at an "appropriate" age (Ngabaza et al. 2016). This not only foregrounds the nuclear family as the only acceptable context for sexual desire, intimacy, and parenting but also stigmatises school-aged parents as not conforming to the assumed "model." Young parenting while at school continues to be pathologised and problematised in post-apartheid South Africa, even if this phenomenon is widely common (Mkhwanazi and Bhana 2017). Indeed, sexuality education is deployed as a space where a moral panic related to sex, gender, and reproduction is articulated. The space reproduces particular moral assumptions and norms about the family that may interfere with sexuality, gender justice, Reproductive Justice, and freedom for young people.

ADULT REGULATION OF YOUNG SEXUALITIES

Adult authority and control of how sexuality education is taught are normalised and enforced throughout most of the work on sexuality education. As illustrated, information directed at young people indicates that they require adult guidance. Such messages are supported by developmental psychology that constructs young people as living in a developmental flux towards responsible and mature adulthood (Shefer 2018). This representation of young people is strongly associated with the binaristic notions of child–adult in which adult privilege and child–youth subjugation characterise sexuality education. Scholars such as Hearn (2018, 47) call for critical studies on adult-hood (CRAS) to deconstruct such practices and wonder if this could be done "without reproducing or enhancing the power of adults and adulthood."

Literature further shows how messages related to young people in sexual-ity education are predominantly framed as a "civilising discourse" and are generally presented in didactic methodologies which tell young people what to do, while their voices are stifled and silenced. However, research on young people's narratives on sexuality education shows how some young people have resisted such adult expectations by not taking teachers' directions seri-ously, showing how futile disciplinary responses to young people's sexual desires and practices have been (Ngabaza et al. 2016; Jearey-Graham and Macleod 2015).

Work describing various constraints experienced by educators in sexuality education at school undermines this flawed didactic pedagogical approach. Some of these include poorly equipped educators due to a lack of training (Helleve et al. 2009; Shefer and Macleod 2015). Some studies point to more subjective challenges and discomforts that teachers could encounter, given their own experiences (or lack thereof) of sexuality education (Masinga 2009; Beyers 2013). At the same time, teachers' own convictions, norms, and values can pose challenges (Moult 2013; Thaver and Leao 2012), as they may have been products of authoritarian, conservative, and heteronormative ideologies on gender and sexuality (Bhana 2015; Francis 2012; Shefer and Ngabaza 2015). Research further shows that some of the challenges also stem from inconsistencies and a lack of clarity in policies (Kirby 2008), as well as discomfort associated with limited or inadequate understanding of what is expected of teachers as sexuality educators (Francis 2012; DePalma and Francis 2014).

In some cases, educators have struggled to position themselves as sexual-ity education practitioners (Beyers 2012; Johnson 2014; Diale 2016; Ahmed et al. 2009), given that teaching requires teachers to perform multiple roles. Helleve et al. (2011, 22) reported how teachers found themselves positioned as "a teacher, friend, parent and/or counsellor" and grappled with fulfilling these as they lacked the necessary experience to do so. The authors further show how the educators' own subjective histories and current discomfort in tackling topics related to sexuality impacted strongly on how they managed these classes.

At the same time, educators indicated how assuming a position of author-ity was critical for discipline (Helleve et al. 2011; Smith and Harrison 2013). Within the dominant teaching and learning spectrum, which relies on a notion of "expert-based" education, moralistic methods and hypercritical attitudes towards young people are promoted and expected. Young people are burdened with unidirectional messages on what they are expected to do or not do and the adverse consequences of "not paying attention." Some scholars have been critical of the deployment of adult authority, and how certain moralities and norms assumed by sexuality education teachers seem to dominate messages "conveying correct sex and sexuality" relayed to young people (Bhana 2013; Francis 2012).

In the previous section, we showed how educators construct gender and normative sexuality in authoritative ways in sexuality education classrooms through the assumption of "compulsory" heterosexuality and the endorsement of heteronormative prejudice. Such practices point to multiple gaps in sexuality educators' skills, knowledge, and understanding to facilitate constructive forms of sexuality education, undermining Sexual and Reproductive Justice for young people. Local researchers and practitioners of sexuality are increasingly challenging the dominance of adult authority in the teaching and learning of sexuality education, arguing for more participatory pedagogical methods. Methods that will position young people at the centre of their own learning, focussing on their narratives, experiences, needs, and desires in relation to sexuality and reproductive health and well-being in the LO sexuality education class are increasingly being promoted (Jearey-Graham and Macleod 2015; Francis and Msibi 2011; Pattman 2013).

CONCLUDING THOUGHTS

Sexuality education that serves youth Sexual and Reproductive Justice must be holistic, inclusive, honest, complete, and accurate. It must also work to normalise inclusive and safe patterns of sexual intimacies that uphold individual dignity and well-being (Le Grice and Braun 2018). Yet, our reading of contemporary research shows that sexuality education in South Africa remains characterised by complexities and challenges that undermine the goal of delivering socially just sexuality education to young people. This space emerges as strongly related to adult authority and the expected compliance of the young person, where young people's "irresponsible" sexualities are policed, regulated, and controlled. It is troubling that an emphasis on negative meanings of sexuality through narratives of disease, danger, damage, doomed futures, and violence appears to dominate in local sexuality education. It is also concerning that educators—seen as key for delivering sexuality education—face challenges of knowledge, capacity, comfort, and appropriate pedagogical approach in working with young people on this. Further, in the documented narratives emerging from young people and in critical analyses of the curriculum and pedagogical practices, the sexuality education class is also a space where gender hierarchies and binarisms are perpetuated and maintained, and where heteronormativity and pro-family ideologies are rationalised and reinstated.

Increasingly, the risk-focussed, authoritative, didactic framework of sexuality education is being challenged. Perhaps the assumption of school as the best space to teach sexuality should be interrogated. Further, whether it should be even "taught" and if so by whom? Some scholars argue that peer education is more successful than adult education in dealing with SRH, although this has also been contested given the probability of peer education reproducing the same messages and methodologies (Campbell and MacPhail 2002). Further, the inclusion of young people's voices in the classroom is not necessarily a panacea, especially if used as a confessional imperative, as highlighted by a growing body of feminist critique of mainstream notions of women's "agency" and "voice" (Hardon and Posel 2012; Ryan-Flood and Gill 2010).

Several scholars have called for opening a space to think differently about and experiment with alternative, creative, and novel approaches to sexuality education. For example, an approach that equips young people with comprehensive accurate knowledge on their SRH without judging, controlling, or policing their sexualities (UNESCO 2018) but also draws on dialogical and dynamic methods of pedagogy for inclusivity (Yang and MacEntee 2015). Participatory methods that facilitate young people's voices, sharing their concerns, challenges, joys, and pleasures, may open up a more productive space. The task of reconceptualising sexuality education in South Africa, to make it relevant to young people and their contexts, and to centre their needs, desires, and experiences, is a vital project.

Research has shown that learners' valuing of and positive engagement with sexuality education rested on the extent to which learners found the content relevant to their own circumstances (Adams et al. 2016). Thus, it is urgent to interrogate current practices, particularly from a reflexive, intersectional gender and youth-centred perspective, and to find ways to disturb dominant narratives and pedagogical orthodoxies in the teaching of sexuality. This means going beyond the now-popular call to "educate," better "prepare," or work with the discomfort of educators. Rather, we argue that ways must be sought to centre young people's stories and subjective and material realities in directing pedagogical practices in the sexuality education classroom. To better harness the potentially valuable space that sexuality education offers, far more critical reflection is needed. We therefore argue for the importance of re-thinking what is taught, the skills teachers need to promote gender and sexual justice, and how such teaching and learning should happen. Generating pedagogical practices that are based on and facilitate young people's agency, while also centring the challenges and opportunities they face and are "expert" on, seems imperative for a project of sexuality education that is truly committed to gender, sexual equality, and justice.

NOTE

1. This is a reworked version of an article that was initially published in a special issue of *Sex Education* in 2019. (Ngabaza, S., and T. Shefer. 2019. "Sexuality Education in South African Schools: Deconstructing the Dominant Response to Young People's Sexualities in Contemporary Schooling Contexts." *Sex Education* 19 (4): 422–435.

REFERENCES

Adams Tucker, Leigh, Gavin George, Candice Reardon, and Saadhna Panday. 2016. "'Learning the Basics': Young People's Engagement with Sexuality Education at Secondary sShools." *Sex Education* 16 (4): 337–52. http://dx.doi.org/10.1080/14681811.2015.1091768.

Ahmed, Nazeema, Alan J. Flisher, Catherine Mathews, Wanjiru Mukoma, and Shahieda Jansen. 2009. "HIV Education in South African schools: The Dilemma and Conflicts of Educators." *Scandinavian Journal of Public Health* 37 (2): 48–54. https://doi.org/10.1177/1403494808097190.

Allen, Louisa. 2007. "Denying the Sexual Subject: Schools' Regulation of Student Sexuality." *British Educational Research Journal* 33 (2): 221–34. https://doi.org/10.1080/01411920701208282.

———. 2008. "'They Think You Shouldn't Be Having Sex Anyway': Young People's Suggestions for Improving Sexuality Education Content." *Sexualities* 11 (5): 573–94. https://doi.org/10.1177/1363460708089425.

Bainame, Kenabetsho, Serai D. Rakgoasi, Mpho Keetile, and Motsholathebe Bowelo. 2016. "Sexuality Education and Men's Sexual and Reproductive Health Practices in a High HIV Prevalence Setting: Does Exposure to Sexuality Education Improve Sexual and Reproductive Health Outcomes in Botswana?." *African Population Studies* 30 (2): 2671–89. https://doi.org/10.11564/30-2-874.

Baxen, Jean. 2010. *Performative Praxis: Teacher Identity and Teaching in the Context of HIV/AIDS*. Oxford: Peter Lang.

Baxen, Jean, and Anders Breidlid, eds. 2009. *HIV/AIDS in Sub-Saharan Africa: Understanding the Implications of Culture & Context*. Juta and Company Ltd.

Beyers, Christa. 2012. "Picture That: Supporting Sexuality Educators in Narrowing the Knowledge/Practice Gap." *South African Journal of Education* 32 (4): 367–80. https://doi.org/10.15700/saje.v32n4a153.

———. 2013. "In Search of Healthy Sexuality: The Gap Between What Youth Want and What Teachers Think They Need." *TD: The Journal for Transdisciplinary Research in Southern Africa* 9 (3): 550–60. https://doi.org/10.4102/td.v9i3.197.

Bhana, Deevia. 2013. "Parental Views of Morality and Sexuality and the Implications for South African Moral Education." *Journal of Moral Education* 42 (1):114–28. https://doi.org/10.1080/03057240.2012.737314.

———. 2014. "Ruled by Hetero-norms? Raising Some Moral Questions for Teachers in South Africa." *Journal of Moral Education* 43 (3): 362–76. https://doi.org/10.1080/03057240.2014.922943.

———. 2016. *Gender and Childhood Sexuality in Primary School*. Springer.

———. 2017. "Love Grows with Sex: Teenagers Negotiating Sex and Gender in the Context of HIV and the Implications for Sex Education." *African Journal of AIDS Research* 16 (1): 71–9. https://doi.org/10.2989/16085906.2016.1259172.

Bhana, Deevia, Mary Crewe, and Peter Aggleton. 2019. "Sex, Sexuality and Education in South Africa." *Sex Education* 19 (4): 361–70. https://doi.org/10.1080/14681811.2019.1620008.

Bhana, Deevia, Robert Morrell, Jeff Hearn, and Relebohile Moletsane. 2007. "Power and Identity: An Introduction to Sexualities in Southern Africa." *Sexualities* 10 (2): 131–39. https://doi.org/10.1177/1363460707075794.

Bhana, Deevia, Robert Morrell, Tamara Shefer, and Sisa Ngabaza. 2010. "South African Teachers' Responses to Teenage Pregnancy and Teenage Mothers in Schools." *Culture, Health & Sexuality* 12 (8): 871–83. https://doi.org/10.1080/13691058.2010.500398.

Butler, Judith. 1990. *Gender Trouble: Feminism and the Subversion of Identity*. New York and London: Routledge.

Campbell, Catherine, and Catherine MacPhail. 2002. "Peer Education, Gender and the Development of Critical Consciousness: Participatory HIV Prevention by South African Youth." *Social Science & Medicine* 55 (2): 331–45. https://doi.org/10.1016/S0277-9536(01)00289-1.

DePalma, Renée, and Dennis Francis. 2014. "South African Life Orientation Teachers: (Not) Teaching about Sexuality Diversity." *Journal of Homosexuality* 61 (12): 1687–711. https://doi.org/10.1080/00918369.2014.951256.

Department of Basic Education (DBE). 2011. *National Curriculum Statement (NCS) Curriculum and Assessment Policy Statement. Futher Education and Training Phase Grades 10-12*. Pretoria, South Africa: DBE.

———. 2012. *Department of Basic Education Integrated Strategy for HIV, STIs and TB 2012 – 2016*. Pretoria, South Africa: DBE.

Diale, B. M. 2016. "Life Orientation Teachers' Career Development Needs in Gauteng: Are We Missing the Boat?" *South African Journal of Higher Education* 30 (3): 85–110. https://doi.org/10.20853/30-3-670.

Driscoll, Catherine. 2013. "The Mystique of the Young Girl." *Feminist Theory* 14 (3): 285–94. https://doi.org/10.1177/1464700113499847.

Epstein, Debbie, Robert Morrell, Relebohile Moletsane, and Elaine Unterhalter. 2004. "Gender and HIV/AIDS in Africa South of the Sahara: Interventions, Activism, Identities." *Transformation: Critical Perspectives on Southern Africa* 54 (1): 1–16. https://doi.org/10.1353/trn.2004.0017.

Fine, Michelle. 1988. "Sexuality, Schooling, and Adolescent Females: The Missing Discourse of Desire." *Harvard Educational Review* 58 (1): 29–54.

Francis, Dennis A. 2010. "Sexuality education in South Africa: Three Essential Questions." *International Journal of Educational Development* 30 (3): 314–19. https://doi.org/10.1016/j.ijedudev.2009.12.003.

———. 2011. "Sexuality Education in South Africa: Wedged Within a Triad of Contradictory Values." *Journal of Psychology in Africa* 21 (2): 317–22. https://doi.org/10.1016/j.ijedudev.2009.12.003.

———. 2012. "Teacher Positioning on the Teaching of Sexual Diversity in South African Schools." *Culture, Health & Sexuality* 14 (60): 597–611. https://doi.org/10.1080/13691058.2012.674558.

Francis, Dennis A., and Renée DePalma. 2014. "Teacher Perspectives on Abstinence and Safe Sex Education in South Africa." *Sex Education* 14 (1): 81–94. https://doi.org/10.1080/14681811.2013.833091.

Francis, Dennis, and Thabo Msibi. 2011. "Teaching about Heterosexism: Challenging Homophobia in South Africa." *Journal of LGBT Youth* 8 (2): 157–73. https://doi.org/10.1080/19361653.2011.553713.

Frohlich, Janet A., Nolunthando Mkhize, Rachael C. Dellar, Gethwana Mahlase, Carl T. Montague, and Q. Abdool Karim. 2014. "Meeting the Sexual and Reproductive Health Needs of High-School Students in South Africa: Experiences from Rural KwaZulu-Natal." *South African Medical Journal* 104 (10): 687–90. https://doi.org/10.7196/SAMJ.7841.

Haberland, Nicole A. 2015. "The Case for Addressing Gender and Power in Sexuality and HIV Education: a Comprehensive Review of Evaluation Studies." *International Perspectives on Sexual and Reproductive Health* 41 (1): 31–42. https://doi.org/10.1363/4103115.

Hardon, Anita, and Deborah Posel. 2012. "Secrecy as Embodied Practice: Beyond the Confessional Imperative." *Culture, Health & Sexuality* 14 (1): S1–S13. https://doi.org/10.1080/13691058.2012.726376.

Hearn, Jeff. 2018. "Personally Rememorizing Young People Differently: What Might Critical Adult Studies (Paradoxically) Have to do with Researching, and Engaging with, Young People." In *Engaging Youth in Activism, Research and Pedagogical Praxis: Transnational and Intersectional Perspectives on Gender, Sex, and Race,* edited by Tamara Shefer, Jeff Hearn, Kopano Ratele, and Floretta Boonzaier, 41–56. New York: Routledge.

Helleve, Arnfinn, Alan J. Flisher, Hans Onya, Wanjiru Mukoma, and Knut-Inge Klepp. 2009. "South African Teachers' Reflections on the Impact of Culture on Their Teaching of Sexuality and HIV/AIDS." *Culture, Health & Sexuality* 11 (2): 189–204. https://doi.org/10.1080/13691050802562613.

———. 2011. "Can Any Teacher Teach Sexuality and HIV/AIDS? Perspectives of South African Life Orientation teachers." *Sex Education* 11 (1): 13–26. https://doi.org/10.1080/14681811.2011.538143.

Jearey-Graham, Nicola, and Catriona Macleod. 2015. "A Discourse of Disconnect: Young People from the Eastern Cape talk about the Failure of Adult Communications to Provide Habitable Sexual Subject Positions." *Perspectives in Education* 33 (2):11–29. https://hdl.handle.net/10520/EJC171669.

Johnson, Bernadette. 2014. "The Need to Prepare Future Teachers to Understand and Combat Homophobia in Schools." *South African Journal of Higher Education* 28 (4):1249–68. https://doi.org/10.20853/28-5-417.

Kehily, Mary Jane. 2012. "Contextualising the Sexualisation of Girls Debate: Innocence, Experience and Young Female Sexuality." *Gender and Education* 24 (3): 255–68. https://doi.org/10.1080/09540253.2012.670391.

Kelly, Peter. 2001. "Youth at Risk: Processes of Individualisation and Responsibilisation in the Risk Society." *Discourse: Studies in the Cultural Politics of Education* 22 (1): 23–33. https://doi.org/10.1080/01596300120039731.

Khau, 'Mathabo. 2012. "'Our culture does not allow that': Exploring the challenges of Sexuality Education in Rural Communities." *Perspectives in Education* 3 (1): 61–69. https://doi.org/10.1080/14681811.2012.677210.

Kirby, Douglas B. 2008. "The Impact of Abstinence and Comprehensive Sex and STD/HIV Education Programs on Adolescent Sexual Behavior." *Sexuality Research & Social Policy* 5 (3): 18–27. https://doi.org/10.1525/srsp.2008.5.3.18.

Kruger, Lou-Marie, Antoinette Oakes, and Tamara Shefer. 2015. "'I could have done everything and why not?': Young Women's Complex Constructions of Sexual Agency in the Context of Sexualities Education in Life Orientation in South African Schools." *Perspectives in Education* 33 (2): 30–48. https://hdl.handle.net/10520/EJC171668.

Le Grice, Jade and Virginia Braun. 2018. "Indigenous (Māori) Sexual Health Psychologies in New Zealand: Delivering Culturally Congruent Sexuality Education." *Journal of Health Psychology* 23 (2): 175–87. https://doi.org/10.1177/1359105317739909.

Macleod, Catriona. 2003. "Teenage Pregnancy and the Construction of Adolescence: Scientific Literature in South Africa." *Childhood* 10 (4): 419–37. https://doi.org/10.1177/0907568203104003.

———. 2009. "Danger and Disease in Sex Education: The Saturation of 'Adolescence' with Colonialist Assumptions." *Journal of Health Management* 11 (2): 375–89. https://doi.org/10.1177/097206340901100207.

Macleod, Catriona, Dale Moodley, and Lisa Saville Young. 2015. "Sexual Socialisation in Life Orientation Manuals Versus Popular Music: Responsibilisation Versus Pleasure, Tension and Complexity." *Perspectives in Education* 3 (2): 90–107. https://hdl.handle.net/10520/EJC171664.

MacPhail, Catherine, and Catherine Campbell. 2001. "'I think Condoms are Good but, aai, I Hate Those Things': Condom Use Among Adolescents and Young People in a Southern African Township." *Social Science & Medicine* 52 (1): 1613–27. https://doi.org/10.1080/09540120500498203.

Makina, Ndinda, Mahua Mandal, Khou Xiong, Aiko Hattori, Milissa Markiewicz, Andy Beke, and Ilene Speizer. 2017. *Impact Evaluation of a School-Based Sexuality and HIV Prevention Education Activity in South Africa.* Baseline Survey Report. Chapel Hill, NC: Measure Evaluation.

Masinga, Lungile. 2009. "An African Teacher's Journey to Self-knowledge Through Teaching Sexuality Education." In *Making Connections: Self-study and Social Action*, edited by Kathleen Pithouse, Claudia Mitchell, and Relebohile Moletsane, 237–51. New York: Peter Lang.

Mathe, Sibonsile. 2013. "Love Is Good Even When it is Bad: Competing Sexuality Discourses in a Township High School in South Africa." *Agenda* 2 (3): 77–86. https://doi.org/10.1080/10130950.2013.842288.

McEwen, Haley. 2018. "The US Pro-Family Movement and Sexual Politics in Africa." PhD diss., University of the Witwatersrand, Johannesburg.

Mkhwanazi, Nolwazi, and Deevia Bhana eds. 2017. *Young Families: Gender, Sexuality and Care.* Cape Town: HSRC Press.

Moletsane, Relebohile. 2010. "Culture, Nostalgia, and Sexuality Education in the Age of AIDS in South Africa." In *Memory and Pedagogy*, edited by Claudia Mitchell, Teresa Strong-Wilson, Kathleen Pithouse, and Susann Allnutt, 209–44. New York and London: Routledge.

Morrell, Robert, Deevia Bhana, and Tamara Shefer eds. 2012. *Books and Babies: Pregnancy and Young Parents in Schools.* Cape Town: HSRC Press.

Moult, Kelley. 2013. "Talking Taboos: Teaching and Learning about Sexuality, Gender and Violence in Western Cape Schools." *Agenda* 27 (3): 67–76. https://doi .org/10.1080/10130950.2013.843893.

Msibi, Thabo. 2012. "'I'm Used to it Now': Experiences of Homophobia Among Queer Youth in South African Township Schools." *Gender and Education* 24 (5): 515–33. https://doi.org/10.1080/09540253.2011.645021.

Mthatyana, Andisiwe, and Louise Vincent. 2015. "Multiple Femininities in a 'Single Sex' School: Re-orienting Life Orientation to Learner Lifeworlds." *Perspectives in Education* 33 (2): 49–62. https://hdl.handle.net/10520/EJC171667.

Mturi, Akim J., and Andre L. Bechuke. 2019. "Challenges of Including Sex Education in the Life Orientation Programme Offered by Schools: The Case of Mahikeng, North West Province, South Africa." *African Journal of Reproductive Health* 23 (3): 134–48. https://doi.org/10.29063/ajrh2019/v23i3.12.

Ngabaza, Sisa, and Tamara Shefer. 2013. "Policy Commitments vs. Lived Realities of Young Pregnant Women and Mothers in School, Western Cape, South Africa." *Reproductive Health Matters* 21 (41): 106–13. https://doi.org/10.1016/S0968 -8080(13)41683-X.

———. 2019. "Sexuality Education in South African Schools: Deconstructing the Dominant Response to Young People's Sexualities in Contemporary Schooling Contexts." *Sex Education* 19 (4): 422–35. https://doi.org/10.1080/14681811.2019 .1602033.

Ngabaza, Sisa, Tamara Shefer, and Ida Macleod Catriona. 2016. "'Girls Need to Behave Like Girls You Know': The Complexities of Applying a Gender Justice Goal Within Sexuality Education in South African Schools." *Reproductive Health Matters* 24 (48): 71–78. https://doi.org/10.1016/j.rhm.2016.11.007.

Nkani, Frances Nomvuyo, and Deevia Bhana. 2010. "No to Bulging Stomachs: Male Principals Talk about Teenage Pregnancy at Schools in Inanda, Durban." *Agenda* 24 (83): 107–13. https://doi.org/10.1080/10130950.2010.9676297.

Pattman, Rob. 2013. "Learning from the Learners about Sexuality in a Participatory Interview in a South African School." In *Sexuality, Society and Pedagogy*, edited by D. Francis, 121–33. Stellenbosch: SUN Press.

Pattman, Rob, and Fatuma Chege. 2003. "'Dear Diary I Saw an Angel, She Looked Like Heaven on Earth': Sex Talk and Sex Education." *African Journal of AIDS Research* 2 (2):103–12. https://doi.org/10.2989/16085906.2003.9626565.

Potgieter, Cheryl, and Finn C. G. Reygan. 2012. "Lesbian, Gay and Bisexual Citizenship: A Case Study as Represented in a Sample of South African Life Orientation Textbooks." *Perspectives in Education* 30 (4): 39–51. https://hdl .handle.net/10520/EJC128205.

Renold, Emma, and Jessica Ringrose. 2013. "Feminisms Re-figuring 'Sexualisation', Sexuality and 'the Girl'." *Feminist Theory* 14 (3): 247–54. https://doi.org/10.1177 /1464700113499531.

Ryan-Flood, Róisín, and Rosalind Gill, eds. 2013. *Secrecy and Silence in the Research Process: Feminist Reflections*. Routledge. https://doi.org/10.4324/9780203927045.

SANAC (South African National Aids Council). 2017. *National Strategic Plan 2017-2022*. South Africa: SANAC.

Sham, Fatimah, Wan Nur Atiqah Wan Mohd Zaidi, Zariq Nadia Zahari, Ajau Danis, and Salmi Razali. 2020. "Sexuality Means 'Sex': Opinions of Parents on Sexuality Education in Malaysia." *International Journal of Caring Sciences* 13 (3): 1818–25.

Shefer, Tamara. 2018. "South African Research and Practice Directed at Young People's Sexualities and Genders: The Political Effects of Current Responses in Local and Transnational Contexts." In *Engaging Youth in Activism, Research and Pedagogical Praxis: Transnational and Intersectional Perspectives on Gender, Sex, and Race,* edited by Tamara Shefer, Jeff Hearn, Kopano Ratele, and Floretta Boonzaier, 25–40. New York: Routledge. https://doi.org/10.4324 /9781315270470-2.

Shefer, Tamara, Deevia Bhana, and Robert Morrell. 2013. "Teenage Pregnancy and Parenting at School in Contemporary South African Contexts: Deconstructing School Narratives and Understanding Policy Implementation." *Perspectives in Education* 31 (1): 1–10. https://doi.org/10.4324/9781315270470-2.

Shefer, Tamara, Lou-Marie Kruger, Catriona Macleod, Jean Baxen, and Louise Vincent. 2015. "'… a huge monster that should be feared and not done': Lessons Learned in Sexuality Education Classes in South Africa." *African Safety Promotion: A Journal of Injury and Violence Prevention* 13 (1): 71–87.

Shefer, Tamara, and Sisa Ngabaza. 2015. "'And I have been told that there is nothing fun about having sex while you are still in high school': Dominant Discourses on Women's Sexual Practices and Desires in Life Orientation Programmes at School." *Perspectives in Education* 33 (2): 63–76.

Shefer, Tamara, and Catriona Macleod. 2015. "Life Orientation Sexuality Education in South Africa: Gendered Norms, Justice and Transformation." *Perspectives in Education* 33 (2): 1–10. https://hdl.handle.net/10520/EJC171670.

Smith, Kelley Alison, and Abigail Harrison. 2013. "Teachers' Attitudes Towards Adolescent Sexuality and Life Skills Education in Rural South Africa." *Sex Education* 13 (1): 68–81. https://doi.org/10.1080/14681811.2012.677206.

Stern, Erin, Rosemarie Buikema, and Diane Cooper. 2016. "South African Women's Conceptualisations of and Responses to Sexual Coercion in Relation to Hegemonic

Masculinities." *Global Public Health* 11 (1-2): 135–52. https://doi.org/10.1080/17441692.2015.1032993.

Strode, A., and Z. Essack. 2017. "Facilitating Access to Adolescent Sexual and Reproductive Health Services Through Legislative Reform: Lessons from the South African Experience." *South African Medical Journal* 107 (9): 741–44. https://doi.org/10.7196/samj.2017.v107i9.12525.

Tamale, Sylvia ed. 2011. "Researching and Theorising Sexualities in Africa." In *African Sexualities: A Reader*, 11–36. Cape Town: Pambazuka Press.

Thaver, Lerissa, and Astrid Leao. 2009. "Sexual and HIV/AIDS Education in South African Secondary Schools." *A Journal on African Women's Experiences* 3: 87–90.

UNESCO. 2009. *International Technical Guidance on Sexuality Education: An Evidence-Informed Approach for Schools, Teachers and Health Educators. The Rationale for Sexuality Education.* Paris, France: UNESCO.

———. 2018. *International Technical Guidance on Sexuality Education: An Evidence-Informed Approach*, revised ed. Paris, France: UNESCO.

Van Wyk, Sherine B. "" It's hard work to be a girl": Adolescent Girls' Experiences of Girlhood in Three Low-Income Communities in South Africa." PhD diss., Stellenbosch: Stellenbosch University, 2015.

Willan, Samantha. 2013. *A Review of Teenage Pregnancy in South Africa– Experiences of Schooling, and Knowledge and Access to Sexual & Reproductive Health Services,* 1–63. Report Commissioned by Partners in Sexual Health (PSH).

Wilmot, Mark, and Devika Naidoo. 2014. "'Keeping Things Straight': The Representation of Sexualities in Life Orientation Textbooks." *Sex Education* 14 (3): 323–37. https://doi.org/10.1080/14681811.2014.896252.

Yang, Kyung-Hwa, and Katie MacEntee. 2015. "'Use Condoms for Safe Sex!' Youth-led Video Making and Sex Education." *Sex Education* 15 (6): 613–25. https://doi.org/10.1080/14681811.2015.1051179.

Zulu, Joseph Mumba, Astrid Blystad, Marte E. S. Haaland, Charles Michelo, Haldis Haukanes, and Karen Marie Moland. 2019. "Why Teach Sexuality Education in School? Teacher Discretion in Implementing Comprehensive Sexuality Education in Rural Zambia." *International Journal for Equity in Health* 18 (1): 1–10. https://doi.org/10.1186/s12939-019-1023-1.

Chapter 12

Infanticide and Reproductive (In)Justice in the South Pacific

The Construction of Pacific Women in Criminal Trials

Kate Burry, Kristen Beek, Bridget Haire, and Heather Worth

Reproductive Justice moves beyond narrow choice-based rhetoric or individual rights-based conceptualisations of reproductive health and rights (Unnithan and Pigg 2014; Luna and Luker 2013; Ross 2017; Jolly 2016). Rather, Reproductive Justice "requires analysis of reproductive issues through an intersectional lens that considers the simultaneous operations of a person's statuses such as race, class, gender, sexuality, and ability" (Luna and Luker 2013, 330). As Unnithan and Pigg (2014, 1183) articulate, "while rights-based protocols are powerful as they promote and reinforce autonomy and self-determination of individuals, they are limited precisely in that they obscure other modes of being, belonging, connections, obligations and affiliations generated by overlapping collectivities" and the impact of these on the right not to have children, to have children under chosen conditions, and to parent children one already has under safe and healthy conditions (SisterSong 2007, see also Morison and Mavuso, this volume).

In this chapter, we apply a Reproductive Justice lens to analyse judicial files from 63 infanticide and concealment of birth cases brought to criminal courts in the Pacific region. We argue that these offences largely occur as an extreme outcome of sexual and reproductive injustice, including socio-economic inequity. Given that the law of infanticide pertains only to *women* who kill their biological infants, it is also clear that infanticide in these contexts represents "a rare instance of the overt gendering of the legal subject" (Loughnan 2012, 202). Thus, the trials analysed for this chapter are a reflection of reproductive injustice towards Pacific women through the "active construction of the defendant's character and identity" (Gurevich 2008, 518), particularly in relation to gender, motherhood, and class narratives.

A BRIEF HISTORY OF SEXUAL AND REPRODUCTIVE HEALTH AND GENDER IN THE PACIFIC

In some areas of the Pacific, colonial administrations implemented policies around fertility practices, drawing on moralistic and demographic anxieties regarding perceived population decline. Population decline was linked to birthing and infant feeding practices, fertility control methods, including abortion and infanticide, which reportedly occurred under particular circumstances in parts of the Pacific (Brewis 1995; Jolly 1991, 1998), and alleged "maternal insouciance" or indifference (George 2010, 93). In response to this perceived maternal incompetence, from the late 1800s until the 1930s colonial administrators and missionaries in Fiji and Vanuatu implemented various programmes, including surveillance of maternal behaviour such as inquests into miscarriages, stillbirths, and infant deaths (Jolly 1998).

From the mid-1800s until the early 1900s, Christian missionaries played a role in influencing gender roles, promoting female domesticity and other pro-natal practices such as earlier marriage, conjugal relations and cohabitation of men and women after marriage, and a decrease in post-partum abstinence (Bayliss-Smith 1974; Jolly 1998). Dureau (1993) notes of the Western Solomon Islands (as does Jolly (1991) of Vanuatu) the increased recognition of nuclear family structures as they pertain to women's roles, increasing women's workload as tasks related to the household, crop harvesting, cooking, and child rearing became less and less the collective responsibility of extended family networks.

There is some evidence to suggest that the extended period of engagement with missionaries and colonial administrators from the mid-19th and into the 20th century shaped the Christian values attached to motherhood and the maternal domesticated identity in the contemporary Pacific (Jolly 1998, 1991). The focus on motherhood as encompassing women's core value and legitimacy in contemporary Pacific society can be used by women to claim their importance in the social order, but this obscures the physiological, social, psychological, and emotional toll of Pacific women's reproductive labour, and the ongoing pressures of child rearing (George 2010; Dureau 1993). In addition to this, debates on other issues that affect women are often centred on the mother's failure to uphold family values to protect themselves and their children (George 2010). Among these concerns are sexual abuse and incest which relate to "less palpable truths about the circumstances of motherhood in the region" (George 2010, 91). The perpetrator of such violence is largely overlooked and absolved of guilt (George 2010). In this way, Pacific women are often blamed not just for others' assaults on them but also for the broader degeneration of the family unit and, therefore, society (George 2010; Cummings 2008). This blaming of women for broader societal shifts echoes colonial era denunciation of "other mothers"—mothers who did not fit the idealised White middle-class version of motherhood—and "bad mothering" for broader socio-economic, demographic, social, and political concerns (Jolly 1998; Roberts 1995).

The centrality of motherhood to Pacific Island women's identities and their socio-cultural and political value, tied to colonial and missionary influence, can be understood as complicating overt efforts to limit reproduction (George 2010; Segeral 2018; White, Mann, and Larkan 2018). The historical transition of gender roles also translates to decisions regarding reproduction and contraceptive use, with men who assume the role of household head often (but not always) making decisions on contraception and using threats of violence when women insist on their use (Family Planning New Zealand 2019; Family Planning International New Zealand 2009; Dureau 1993). This gendered inequity in reproductive decision-making alongside other barriers (e.g., insufficient contraceptive supplies, geographical remoteness, high rates of gender-based and sexual violence, and misinformation and stigma attached to sexual and reproductive health) results in low rates of contraceptive prevalence and high levels of unmet need in the Pacific (Brewis 1994; Family Planning New Zealand 2019; Rallu, Rogers, and Reay-Jones 2010; Dureau 1993; Family Planning International New Zealand 2009). Ultimately, these historical, gendered, socio-cultural, political, and practical factors constrain Pacific women's freedom to make sexual and reproductive choices.

LEGAL TERMINOLOGY AND RELEVANT STATUTES

Infanticide is both a distinct homicide offence and a partial defence for murder in cases where a woman causes the death of her biological child under 12 months of age by any wilful act or omission, and where, at the time of the act or omission, "the balance of her mind was disturbed" due to her not having fully recovered from the effect of childbirth, or due to the effect of lactation (Loughnan 2012). However, the "open-textured nature" (Loughnan 2012, 203) of such psychiatric labels as "disturbed," often encompassing not just the lethal act but also the woman's character and her broader circumstances, "overlaid with the social meanings accorded to childbirth and motherhood" (Loughnan 2012, 203), is well established in infanticide trials.

Most Pacific states and territories are "effectively common law jurisdictions" (Aleck 1991, 138) derived from colonial legislation and jurisprudence and with a continued reliance on case law from these countries (Rousseau 2008; Forsyth 2004), despite "some measure of legal recognition of the custom or customary practices of the local indigenous inhabitants" (Aleck 1991, 138).[1] The law pertaining to the offence/defence of infanticide is a legacy of British colonisation in the Pacific (included in the criminal legislation of all jurisdictions relevant to the cases in this chapter, except for Vanuatu),[2] more or less replicating the British Infanticide Act 1922 (amended in 1938). (For more on this Act, see Oberman 2002; Kramar and Watson 2006). Most women convicted under the British Infanticide Act are sentenced to probation plus counselling, as opposed to prison sentences (Oberman 2002). Although once a capital offence, the offence of concealment of the birth of a dead infant through secret disposal of its body, also a legacy of British colonial law, holds a maximum penalty of two years' imprisonment (Loughnan 2012; Oberman 2002). A summary of the convictions and sentences for all 63 cases is included in table 12.1.

Table 12.1   Legal Outcomes and Number of Women Receiving Each Outcome

Legal Outcome	No. of Women
Conviction	N = 59
Infanticide	27
Murder	9
Intentional homicide	8
Concealment of birth	8
Attempted murder	1
Unintentional arm causing death	2
Manslaughter	2
Failing to provide necessities of life	2
Sentence	
Life imprisonment	8
Prison sentence (ranging from 1 month to years)	27 (12 wholly/ partially suspended)
Probation/community sentence	14
Fine	1
Acquitted/Released	7
Prosecution permanently stayed	7
Appeals	12
Total appealed	12
Appeal dismissed	2
Conviction/sentence reduced	8
Counselling order	10

NB: One woman received three convictions (incest (not counted), infanticide and concealment of birth). Four convictions, seven sentences, and two appeal outcomes were not found.
Twelve women spent time in custody (from one month to a year) awaiting trial, including some who were released or received community sentences.

OUR STUDY

In this chapter, we analyse judicial files from court cases of Pacific Island women charged with killing or concealing the birth of their dead infants from 1961 until 2019. Our aim is to explore (1) what the enforcement of these laws in criminal courts in Pacific Island jurisdictions reveals about these women's lives and the contextual factors underpinning their crimes and (2) how women—and gender and maternity more broadly—are constructed in the arguments put forward by these courts. We have close working or familial relationships in Pacific Island nations but do not identify as Pacific Islanders so acknowledge our position as cultural outsiders (Ritchie 2001; Hesse-Biber and Leavy 2006).

All court documents were sourced from the Pacific Islands Legal Information Institute (University of the South Pacific School of Law 2020) using the key words "infanticide" and "concealment of birth." This search produced documents from 63 cases, including: 27 from Fiji, 11 from Papua New Guinea, 6 from Samoa, 7 from the Solomon Islands, 1 from Tonga, and 11 from Vanuatu. We took a feminist and social constructionist approach to our analysis of these documents to "theorize the sociocultural contexts, and structural conditions" of the women's lives (Braun and Clarke 2006, 85). We undertook an inductive thematic analysis of the court documents, with "the data provid[ing] the bedrock for identifying meaning and interpreting [the] data" (Terry et al. 2017, 9) as opposed to imposing "a priori categories and concepts" theorised separately (Pope and Mays 1995, 44).

The judicial files that we sourced and analysed did not contain the full subjective accounts from the women themselves but largely included summing up and sentencing by judges. As Tsing (1990, 285) describes, explanations or "stories" of the crime and the woman who is charged, presented by the defence and prosecution, "must be tailored for persuasion within dominant or emergent community standards." Summing up and sentencing by judges "introduces several opportunities for [. . .] narrativisation" (Heffer 2010, 213), including "by fitting the defendant's individual conduct within a more general moral sanction against certain behaviour in society" (Heffer 2010, 215). Thus, our analysis of these judicial documents from the Pacific takes an intersectional lens, rooted in Reproductive Justice, that pay particular attention to the narratives of gender, motherhood, and class used in the trials in constructing convincing accounts of the women, informing the type of evidence drawn out by the counsels, and the "more general moral sanction" of women's and mothers' behaviour (Heffer 2010, 215).

EVIL WOMEN, DISTURBED WOMEN, AND OBJECTS OF PITY: THE CONSTRUCTION OF PACIFIC WOMEN IN CRIMINAL TRIALS

Women who kill their infants often do so in circumstances of gender-based sexual and reproductive oppression, isolation, fear, and other socio-economic inequities (Oberman 2002; Spinelli 2002; Vellut, Cook, and Tursz 2012). In line with other literature on infanticide, key recurring socio-economic features of the lives of women in these cases include young age; abandonment from the father of the infant; limited financial means or independence alongside significant parenting and economic obligations; little or no social and emotional support; isolation; abuse from a male partner or family member; and lack of assistance as solo parents (Oberman 2002; Vellut, Cook, and Tursz 2012; Spinelli 2002). Additionally, prior convictions were only reported for two women in these cases.

   Below we describe three key themes from our analysis of the construction of women (and gender and maternity more broadly) in these court cases: women's "failure" to conform to medical standards in pregnancy and birth; corrupted motherhood; and attempts to reconcile femininity in the offenders. These themes are analysed in relation to recurring contextual factors in the women's lives, such as socio-economic inequities and gender-based violence. Although the names of most of the defendants were used in the judicial files that are available publicly, we have chosen not to use these to minimise public exposure.

Secret Pregnancies, Unattended Births, and Ambiguous Deaths: Failure to Conform to Medical Standards

All 63 women in these cases attempted to keep their pregnancies secret from their families and communities, did not receive any antenatal care, and all except one gave birth unattended by a skilled practitioner. These factors were treated by the courts in one of two ways. First, in some trials the defendant's secrecy regarding their pregnancy and non-attendance of antenatal care was used as evidence of their "disturbed" mind which was the result of socio-economic factors (Wilczynski 1991). Second, the defendant was constructed as naïve or "simple," confused, "uneducated," "unsophisticated," rural, or irrational (Briggs and Mantini-Briggs 2000; Chunn and Menzies 1990).[3] For example, in the Fijian case State v S (2014), the defendant's concealment of her pregnancy and her giving birth alone was taken as evidence by the judge of her disturbed mind, aggravated by her "lack of seeking medical attention and counselling," therefore supporting an infanticide conviction rather than one of murder.

In other instances, women were constructed as deceiving, conniving individuals who concealed their pregnancies and failed to conform to medical
standards during pregnancy and birth as part of their broader plot to eventually kill their babies, thus proving criminal intent (Tsing 1990; Gurevich
2008; Briggs and Mantini-Briggs 2000).[4] In the Vanuatu case Public
Prosecutor v B (2004), the fact that the defendant "made all endeavours to
cancel [*sic*] her pregnancy" and "perpetuated a lie to everyone [. . .] that she
was not pregnant" was taken as evidence that the murder was premeditated.

All but one of the women gave birth alone. In 13 cases, this led to unclear
circumstances surrounding the infant's death and, in some others, women's
"confessions" were also unclear and were composed of the words and claims
of others (Tsing 1990; Briggs and Mantini-Briggs 2000).[5] Giving birth away
from a clinic or hospital was constructed in some trials as an effort to undermine the safety and well-being of the infant but overlooked the woman's
safety and well-being and the reasons these facilities were inaccessible (Tsing
1990). In the Solomon Islands case, Regina v P (2019), the defendant's
multiple "failures" to seek assistance were constructed as evidence of her
criminal intention by the judge:

Deliberate omission on her part to assist the smooth delivery of the child—She
did not seek any help or assistance from her mother, aunties or relatives. [. . .]
she deliberately failed to inform anyone about it [the pregnancy]. [. . .] Hence,
while I agree that she was in no proper state of mind, the actions leading up to
the offence speaks volume on her criminal culpability.

In the initial trial of M (2011) in Vanuatu, the judge goes further in establishing the defendant's criminality from the concealment of her pregnancy
and failure to seek assistance, while dismissing her account of her stepfather's threat should she fail to kill her newborn, stating:

You deliberately concealed deliveries and births of your children. You could
easily have talked to your church pastor, village chief or elder or your mother
about your situations but you did not. And the only explanation you have provided to the police on interview is that your step-father threatened to "spearem
mi wetem knife" ["stab me with a knife"].

The stepfather who threatened to stab her had sexually abused her over
many years, impregnating her three times. This judge's arguments reveal a
lack of insight into the power inequities that likely manifest in M's fear of
further threats to her safety, as well as the impacts of trauma from five years
of sexual abuse (Crosson-Tower 2014).

Several other pregnancies occurred in the context of actual or threatened
abuse, including sexual abuse. In one case from Tonga (Court of Appeal v

K, 1990–1991), a young woman was sentenced to four years of imprisonment on charges of incest, concealment of birth, and infanticide. This young
woman was sexually abused by her biological father over many years and
during her trial was blamed for her abuse survival by the judge who reasoned
that if she "had not taken part [in the incest] of her own free will, it could
not have gone on so long," and she "had a favoured position in the family
as a result."

The women's isolation and socio-economic circumstances (most as single
mothers) meant their sexualities (often expressed out of wedlock) and resul-
tant pregnancies were subject to social and moral scrutiny and rejection.
Compounding this is the fact that the women were largely unable to access
antenatal care, assisted births, or legal and safe abortions in these contexts.
The result is that women were deprived of their right to decide to have, not to
have, or to parent and care for their children under safe conditions (SisterSong
2007, see also Morison & Mavuso, this volume). These women's "failure" to
comply with medical standards, undermining their socially assigned duty to
protect their infants, was constructed as evidence of their mental incapacity or
murderousness, outweighing their experiences of economic hardship, trauma,
stigma, and disenfranchisement (Loughnan 2012; Tsing 1990).

Corruption of the Maternal Ideal

As described earlier, the maternal ideal in the Pacific has been largely influenced by the colonial and missionary (middle class) feminine ideal of the
domesticated, modest wife and child bearer (Jolly 1998). These cases reveal
many contradicting points in a seeming struggle to reconcile feminine identity. Many of the women were cast as evil, their role as givers and destroyers
of life a violation of normative motherhood.

Several courts focussed on the corruption of idealised motherhood, upon
whom "nature usually bestows motherly compassion, affection and caring
comfort" (Fiji, State v Mw 2010), and who, above all else, have a "duty to
protect" (Fiji, State v L, 2017) foetuses and infants in all circumstances, as
such is "normal human nature" (Samoa, Police v L, 2005). The women's
failure to protect life was often framed as evil, "unnatural," or "contrary to
human nature," with these women showing an obvious "distaste for life" or
significant mental disturbance.[6] In the Vanuatu case of Public Prosecutor v M
(2011) described above, the defendant's account of her survival of prolonged
sexual abuse and killing two of her infants under threat of serious assault was
minimised by the judge, and she was morally condemned as neglecting her
"duty of care" and committing "a breach of trust as a mother." In this way, the
judge exhibits an uncritical prioritising of maternal ideals without reflection
on the context of abuse, violence, and intimidation (George 2010).

In some cases, the woman's unborn child and current dependents were referenced as lessening or influencing the terms of her sentence, so that she might not fail any further in her maternal duties.[7] In the Fijian case State v Mw (2010), for example, the judge ordered "the prison authorities to submit the prisoner to constant medical counselling and keep her under observation both during and after pregnancy." The notion that women are deeply embedded in their social, economic, and gendered environments and are intimately aware of their parental responsibilities seems to be absent from these narratives, or considered then put aside in favour of broader judgements relating to anti-maternal rhetoric (Briggs and Mantini-Briggs 2000). The example above speaks to the ongoing reproductive injustice faced by this defendant. She appears to have been subjected to constant surveillance during and after her pregnancy, presumably with little or no protection of her rights to decide how to manage her pregnancy and birth, and to parent the child in a safe and healthy environment (SisterSong 2007, see also Morison & Mavuso, this volume).

In addition to the positioning of these women as failed and corrupt maternal figures and alongside their non-compliance with medical standards in pregnancy and birth (discussed above), some women's prevailing socio-economic circumstances were framed as contributing to their disturbance of mind (Wilczynski 1991). For instance:

> I accept the social pressures brought to bear upon you especially the fact that you were not well-liked by your relatives due to the fact that you had become pregnant and that the child was an illegitimate child. Those matters clearly must have affected your mind sufficiently to reduce the culpability from that of murder. At the same time, I cannot see how your actions resulting in the death of an innocent child can be anything less than a deliberate and callous act. (Solomon Islands, Regina v I, 1992)

The logic in this example, and the wording in the final sentence, is replicated in another Solomon Islands case, Regina v J (2017). Here we begin to uncover a core struggle over ideology, where the realities of women's socio-economic and gendered inequities—including experiences of abuse, ostracism, and abandonment—are overcome by the essentialist narrative that any woman who is implicated in the death of an infant, or, in some cases, who tries to bury a dead infant without others knowing, must be innately degenerate.

Even where the notion of mental "disturbance" was advanced in the trial, essentialised markers of gender may be used as measurements for "normal." In the Fijian case State v R (2007), for example, the expert witness, a psychiatrist, "described the symptoms of post-partum depression as including a failure to care for the child, lack of communication and unkempt grooming." The maternal ideal in the Pacific is constructed through colonial and missionary ideals of women as agreeable, domesticated child bearers and wives (Jolly 1998), yet here this maternal ideal is presented as innate, intuitive, and a measurement for normal. Women who do not fit this construction are therefore abnormal and mentally ill (Chunn and Menzies 1990). In these constructions there also appears to be a failure to recognise that pregnancy, childbirth, and child rearing occur "within a specific network of social relations" and institutions (Browner 2000, 774). Instead, only the mother's behaviour, social presentation, and acceptability are under scrutiny (Nations and Rebhun 1988).

The cases of women who conceived in the context of sexual abuse (including incest) and domestic violence (including from [usually male] family members) starkly reveal this essentialising of the maternal ideal in the trials.[8] One case from Fiji, D v State (2010–2014), where the defendant drowned her 20-day-old infant and her 1-year and 9-month-old daughter and attempted to drown herself, is particularly revealing. In this case, the defendant's experiences of her husband's intimidation; verbal, physical, and sexual abuse; humiliating and derogatory treatment of her; criticisms of her and her family; "exhortations for her to end her life" (which she attempted twice); as well as social isolation and financial vulnerability were all detailed in her account. Despite these reports and her fear for her own and her children's safety, the judge reduced her "reactions" and depressive symptoms to a de-contextualised, vindictive decision:

> The failure of her husband to return home with baby diapers is a farfetched excuse to take two lives of innocent small girls and to rely on "diminished responsibility." On the other hand, such a claim is a serious insult to the mothers who go through the mill with their children having high expectations of creating a better tomorrow for them.

This last sentence suggests that the defendant's response to her experiences of daily abuse and her associated suicide attempts are an insult to the social institution of motherhood. This is a clear instance of victim blaming and fails to address the unsafe circumstances in which this woman was trying to parent (George 2010). The role of the father (and, by extension, other abusers), whose persistent terrorising of the family led to the woman's fear and suicidality, is rendered invisible. The implication here is "that a woman's obligation to her children always takes precedence over her own interest in independence and physical safety" (Roberts 1995, 107). Mothers are entirely responsible for the well-being of their children, including protecting them from others' maltreatment, and for the broader social goal of preserving sacred motherhood, regardless of the context of abuse.

The court's lack of analysis of gendered constraints and power inequities is also seen in the Papua New Guinea case Regina v Y & A (1961). In this case, A compelled his daughter, Y, to kill her infant because of the shame the infant (conceived illegitimately) brought him. The power inequity between Y and her father was noted, with Y described as having become a "domestic woman servant in his power" after her mother's death. Despite this, the judge maintained:

> She knew and understood what she was doing and why, and exercised her own choice as to the actual time and means of carrying out her father's orders. [. . .] [I]t is clear from [Y]'s own evidence that her actions were not caused by anything relating to the processes of birth or lactation. She made up her mind to obey her father before the child was born, and her actions were clearly premeditated.

While infanticide law requires a link (at least temporally (Loughnan 2012)) between the offence, the defendant's reproductive functions, and mental disturbance, this case reveals a more nuanced picture of power inequities and how they constrain women's choices. Put simply, either women's reproductive bodies render them mentally incapable and, to use the wording in Fijian case State v Mw, unable to "perceive any rational thought" or they act on free choice (Browner 2000). This leaves no room for analysing ways that socioeconomic, gender, and other power inequities constrain women's agency (Walker and Gill 2019; Roberts 1995).

A "GOOD MOTHER" WHO ACTED "OUT OF CHARACTER": ATTEMPTS TO RECONCILE FEMININE IDENTITY

When the act or omission that caused the death of these women's babies (even if unclear or accidental) could not be incorporated within any normative gender framework, courts often had to look to other indicators of the women's character to make moral inferences (Chunn and Menzies 1990; Wilczynski 1991). Evidence of women's successful performance as mothers with other dependents played a significant role in garnering sympathy and was an important mitigating factor in sentencing. In other cases, alternate indicators of appropriate feminine behaviour were referenced, such as a change to the defendant's relationship status from single to partnered (Wilczynski 1991; Amon et al. 2020). Furthermore, some judges in their sentencing determined that the woman had been punished enough by divergence from her naturalised maternal identity.

Evidence of women's maternal behaviour was often important in creating a more morally acceptable image. Having other dependants and, for some, being currently pregnant were regularly brought in as mitigating factors during trials (Roberts 1995).[9] In a Fijian case, State v E (2011), the fact that the defendant had four other children was sufficient evidence of her fulfilling her maternal (and gendered) duties: "There is no evidence before this Court that you are not a fit and proper person to be a mother. You have four young children depended on you." In another Fijian case, State v K (2018), details of maternal capability were provided, such as that she "wrapped the baby properly" (she knows how to perform childcare tasks), and "she held her child and she loved him" (displaying essentialised maternal instincts). In these cases, the offence was constructed as "out of character" in relation to evidence of other maternal behaviour.[10]

The defendant's actual or anticipated realisation of her involvement (however tenuous) in her baby's death (or the concealment of it) and her corruption as a woman or maternal figure was sometimes constructed as sufficient punishment by the court (Loughnan 2012). For example, in a case in Fiji (State v N, 1990) of attempted suicide and infanticide, the judge argued, "There cannot possibly be a greater punishment to a mother than finding herself in such a predicament through her own act." In a Papua New Guinea case, State v E (2007), the judge suggested that, as a result of the infanticide, the defendant "may well be emotionally scarred, ridden with guilt and shame by what she has done, for the rest of her life." The notion that the women had "suffered enough" and would have to live with the memory, shame, and guilt was raised in several cases.[11] This argument by the courts links to the notion of motherhood as essentialised, not contested (Roberts 1993), and frames women's family responsibilities as providing sufficient social control over their lives and behaviour by reinforcing gender roles (Roberts 1995). Yet, to quote Gurevich (2008, 532), "No one, however, remarked how well or poorly the women were situated to fulfil those obligations, nor were the obligations themselves put to question but rather treated as universal and incontrovertible standards of care and behavior."

Establishing the argument that these women behaved "out of character" when they killed or concealed their dead infant depoliticises and decontextualises women's responses to the injustice they face and does nothing to address these factors (Kramar and Watson 2006; Roberts 1995). It rather presents the "incident" as an anomaly in an otherwise socially acceptable life of good domestic and maternal behaviours which are natural and normal and, in some cases, ought to continue unhindered. This is despite these pregnancies occurring in systems of oppression, isolation, sexual and physical abuse, and socio-economic and gender inequity (Wilczynski 1991).

CONCLUSION

Women in the Pacific face "intersecting oppressions" (Ross 2017, 288) regarding their sexual and reproductive health and lives, including experiencing high rates of violence, economic inequality, social stigma, and patriarchal control. These oppressions link directly to the offences analysed in this chapter (Razali, Fisher, and Kirkman 2019). This injustice is grounded in a history of surveillance, condemnation, "instruction," and criminalisation of Pacific women's behaviour (particularly as mothers) (Briggs and Mantini-Briggs 2000), reducing socially sanctioned maternal behaviour to colonial middle-class ideals of modest, Christian, domesticated carers, and linking to their exclusion from emerging capitalism and national politics (Jolly 1991; 1998; Dureau 1993; Roberts 1995; George 2010).

These trials of women convicted over the death or concealment of the birth of their dead infants reveal the multiple injustices operating in these women's lives: many were socially isolated, economically vulnerable, had survived abuse, and were treated with suspicion and contempt. They were also denied access to the resources and power to render their situation any different. Yet, the "court's power to impose identities and regulate the conduct of individuals in keeping them is augmented when a person is not seeking legal protection but has been charged with a crime" (Briggs and Mantini-Briggs 2000, 306). As such, maternity was constructed by the courts in complex ways to transcend history, consciousness, and the daily struggles of these women (Tsing 1990; Roberts 1993). Anti-maternal behaviour was either a symptom of irrationality or "disturbance" (thus falling under the offence/ defence of infanticide) or of unfettered wicked intention. Women's agency appeared to be recognised only in the context of idealised motherhood (or anti-motherhood from medical and social standpoints) as the only socially and politically relevant realm in which a woman can act, while simultaneously obscuring paternal, communal, and state responsibilities (Gurevich 2008; Tsing 1990). Their broader agency was restricted through the courts' denial of women's sexuality and minimising of coercive control and violence. This was compounded by the lack of access to education and employment during pregnancy, and the limited freedom to make choices regarding reproductive care, contraception, and safe and legal abortion. These factors were largely discounted by the courts despite their power to shape women's sexual and reproductive lives and decisions (Browner 2000; Ross 2017; Tsing 1990). Institutional forces such as sexism, colonialism, and poverty underlie the crimes of the women discussed in this chapter (Ross 2017, 291; see also Morison & Mavuso, this volume), and these forces were largely sustained by the courts through relaying gender stereotypes, maternal ideologies, and through silence in the face of reproductive injustice.

Our analysis of these trials argues for an understanding of motherhood, and of maternal health (including mental health), from the lens of Reproductive Justice, taking proper account of the nuanced nature of women's lives, their capacity for reproductive autonomy, and the contexts in which they are trying to parent. This requires an analysis of motherhood as not simply "natural" and innate but as political and shaped by historical, gendered, socio-cultural, political, and practical factors that enable or constrain women's freedom to make sexual and reproductive choices.

NOTES

1. Judges of Pacific Island descent appear to make up the majority of the justices that presided over the trials analysed in this chapter. Customary contexts, beliefs, and reconciliation practices were taken into account in a few of these cases (Rousseau 2008). However, it is beyond the scope of this chapter to analyse this in detail (for further discussion of Indigenous jurisprudence, "custom," and "*kastom*" in legal practice in the Pacific, see Rousseau 2008; Aleck 1991; Forsyth 2004; Powles 1997).

2. The Fiji Crimes Act 2009 has the most extensive law regarding infanticide, including as a cause of mental disturbance and considers not only physiological factors related to birth and lactation but also "any other matter, condition, state of mind or experience associated with her pregnancy, delivery or post-natal state that is proved to the satisfaction of the state" (Republic of Fiji Islands Government 2009). Fiji is also the only context in which judges of infanticide trials, in their summing up and sentencing, made explicit mention of "social" and "cultural failures," as well as the defendants' "emotional failures" as underpinning the defendants' acts/omissions (State v K, 2018, State v R, 2007, and State v L, 2017).

3. For example, in the Fiji cases State v S (2014), State v R (2007), State v A (2015), State v E (2011), State v Ak (1990), and State v K (2018); the Papua New Guinea cases State v K (2000) and State v M (2008); and the Vanuatu cases Public Prosecutor v A (2014) and Public Prosecutor v R (1995).

4. For example, in the Vanuatu case Public Prosecutor v L (2015) and the Fijian case State v M (2018).

5. For example, Fijian case State v T (2002).

6. For example, State v V (Fiji, 2010), State v J (Papua New Guinea, 1992), and Police v L (Samoa, 2005).

7. For example, in the Vanuatu case Public Prosecutor v T (2014).

8. For example, Tonga, Court of Appeal v K (1990–1991); Vanuatu, Police Prosecutor v A (2014), Police Prosecutor v M (2011), and Police Prosecution v N (2010); Samoa, Police v P (2008).

9. For example, in the Fijian cases State v C (2014) and State v Mw (2010).

10. For example, Papua New Guinea, State v M (2008); Samoa, Police Prosecution v T (2014); Vanuatu, Public Prosecutor v N (2010); Fiji, State v L (2017).

11. For example, Solomon Islands, Regina v H (2004) and Regina v P (2019); Vanuatu, Public Prosecutor v N (2010) and Public Prosecutor v R (1995), including cases of concealment of birth (e.g., Samoa, Police Prosecution v N (2013)).

REFERENCES

Aleck, Jonathan. 1991. "Beyond Recognition: Contemporary Jurisprudence in the Pacific Islands and the Common Law Tradition South Pacific Law Section." *Queensland University of Technology Law Journal* 7: 137–44.

Amon, Sabine, Claudia M. Klier, Hanna Putkonen, Ghitta Weizmann Henelius, and Paula Fernandez Arias. 2020. "Neonaticide in the Courtroom—Room for Improvement? Conclusions Drawn from Austria and Finland's Register Review." *Child Abuse Review* 29 (1): 61–72. https://doi.org/10.1002/car.2589.

Bayliss-Smith, Tim. 1974. "Constraints on Population Growth: The Case of the Polynesian Outlier Atolls in the Precontact Period." *Human Ecology* 2 (4): 259–95.

Braun, Virginia, and Victoria Clarke. 2006. "Using Thematic Analysis in Psychology." *Qualitative Research in Psychology* 3 (2): 77–101. https://doi.org/10.1191/1478088706qp063oa.

Brewis, Alexandra A. 1994. "Reproductive Ethophysiology and Contraceptive Use in a Rural Micronesian Population." *The Journal of the Polynesian Society* 103 (1): 53–74.

———. 1995. "Fertility and Analogy in Pacific Palaeodemography." *Asian Perspectives* 34 (1): 1–20.

Briggs, Charles L., and Clara Mantini-Briggs. 2000. "'Bad Mothers' and the Threat to Civil Society: Race, Cultural Reasoning, and the Institutionalization of Social Inequality in a Venezuelan Infanticide Trial." *Law & Social Inquiry* 25 (2): 299–354. https://doi.org/10.1111/j.1747-4469.2000.tb00964.x.

Browner, Carole. H. 2000. "Situating Women's Reproductive Activities." *American Anthropologist* 102 (4): 773–88. https://doi.org/10.1525/aa.2000.102.4.773.

Chunn, Dorothy E., and Robert J. Menzies. 1990. "Gender, Madness and Crime: The Reproduction of Patriarchal and Class Relations in a Psychiatric Court Clinic." *The Journal of Human Justice* 1 (2): 33–54. https://doi.org/10.1007/BF02627465.

Crosson-Tower, Cynthia D. 2014. *Confronting Child and Adolescent Sexual Abuse.* Thousand Oaks: SAGE Publications. http://ebookcentral.proquest.com/lib/unsw/detail.action?docID=5165183.

Cummings, Maggie. 2008. "The Trouble with Trousers: Gossip, Kastom, and Sexual Culture in Vanuatu." In *Making Sense of AIDS: Culture, Sexuality, and Power in Melanesia,* edited by Leslie Butt and Richard Eves, 133–49. Honolulu: University of Hawai'i Press.

Dureau, Christine. 1993. "Nobody Asked the Mother: Women and Maternity on Simbo, Western Solomon Islands." *Oceania* 64 (1): 18–35.

Family Planning International New Zealand. 2009. *A Measure of the Future: Women's Sexual and Reproductive Risk Index for the Pacific.* Family Planning

International New Zealand and Secretariat of the Pacific Community. https://pacificwomen.org/resources/a-measure-of-the-future/.

Family Planning New Zealand. 2019. *Planem Gud Famili Blong Yumi: Knowledge, Access and Barriers to Family Planning in Rural Vanuatu*. Wellington: Family Planning New Zealand.

Forsyth, Miranda. 2004. "Beyond Case Law: Kastom and Courts in Vanuatu." *Victoria University of Wellington Law Review* 35: 427–46.

George, Nicole. 2010. "'Just like Your Mother?' The Politics of Feminism and Maternity in the Pacific Islands." *Australian Feminist Law Journal* 32 (1): 77–96. https://doi.org/10.1080/13200968.2010.10854438.

Gurevich, Liena. 2008. "Patriarchy? Paternalism? Motherhood Discourses in Trials of Crimes Against Children." *Sociological Perspectives* 51 (3): 515–39. https://doi.org/10.1525/sop.2008.51.3.515.

Heffer, Chris. 2010. "Narrative in the Trial: Constructing Crime Stories in Court." In *The Routledge Handbook of Forensic Linguistics*, edited by Malcolm Coulthard and Alison Johnson, 199–217. London: Taylor & Francis Group. http://ebookcentral.proquest.com/lib/unsw/detail.action?docID=487985.

Hesse-Biber, Sharlene Nagy, and Patricia Leavy. 2006. "In-Depth Interviewing." In *The Practice of Qualitative Research*, edited by Sharlene Nagy Hesse-Biber and Patricia Leavy, 119–47. Thousand Oaks: SAGE Publications.

Jolly, Jallicia. 2016. "On Forbidden Wombs and Transnational Reproductive Justice." *Meridians* 15 (1): 166–88. https://doi.org/10.2979/meridians.15.1.09.

Jolly, Margaret. 1991. "'To Save the Girls for Brighter and Better Lives': Presbyterian Missions and Women in the South of Vanuatu: 1848-1870." *The Journal of Pacific History* 26 (1): 27–48.

———. 1998. "Other Mothers: Maternal 'Insouciance' and the Depopulation Debate in Fiji and Vanuatu, 1890–1930." In *Maternities and Modernities: Colonial and Postcolonial Experiences in Asia and the Pacific*, edited by Kalpana Ram and Margaret Jolly, 177–212. Cambridge: Cambridge University Press. https://doi.org/10.1017/CBO9780511621826.008.

Kramar, Kirsten Johnson, and William D. Watson. 2006. "The Insanities of Reproduction: Medico-Legal Knowledge and the Development of Infanticide Law." *Social & Legal Studies* 15 (2): 237–55. https://doi.org/10.1177/0964663906063579.

Loughnan, Arlie. 2012. "Gender, 'Madness', and Crime: The Doctrine of Infanticide." In *Manifest Madness: Mental Incapacity in the Criminal Law*, 202–25. Oxford: Oxford University Press. http://oxford.universitypressscholarship.com/view/10.1093/acprof:oso/9780199698592.001.0001/acprof-9780199698592-chapter-8.

Luna, Zakiya, and Kristin Luker. 2013. "Reproductive Justice." *Annual Review of Law and Social Science* 9 (1): 327–52. https://doi.org/10.1146/annurev-lawsocsci-102612-134037.

Nations, Marilyn K., and L. A. Rebhun. 1988. "Angels with Wet Wings Won't Fly: Maternal Sentiment in Brazil and the Image of Neglect." *Culture, Medicine and Psychiatry* 12 (2): 141–200. https://doi.org/10.1007/BF00116857.

Oberman, Michelle. 2002. "A Brief History of Infanticide and the Law." In *Infanticide: Psychosocial and Legal Perspectives on Mothers Who Kill*, edited by Margaret G. Spinelli and Ann E. Norwood, 3–18. Washington, DC: American Psychiatric Publishing.

Pope, Catherine, and Nick Mays. 1995. "Reaching the Parts Other Methods Cannot Reach: An Introduction to Qualitative Methods in Health and Health Services Research." *BMJ: British Medical Journal* 311 (6996): 42–45.

Powles, Guy. 1997. "Common Law at Bay? The Scope and Status of Customary Law Regimes in the Pacific." *Journal of Pacific Studies* 21: 61–82.

Rallu, Jean-Louis, Godfrey Rogers, and Robert Reay-Jones. 2010. "The Demography of Oceania from the 1950s to the 2000s: A Summary of Changes and a Statistical Assessment." *Population (English Edition, 2002-)* 65 (1): 8–115.

Razali, Salmi, Jane Fisher, and Maggie Kirkman. 2019. "'Nobody Came to Help': Interviews with Women Convicted of Filicide in Malaysia." *Archives of Women's Mental Health* 22 (1): 151–58. https://doi.org/10.1007/s00737-018-0832-3.

Republic of Fiji Islands Government. 2009. *Crimes Act 2009. Penal.* 10 (5). https://laws.gov.fj/Acts/DisplayAct/798.

Ritchie, J. 2001. "Not Everything Can Be Reduced to Numbers." In *Health Research*, edited by Catherine Anne Berglund, 149–73. Melbourne, Victoria, and Oxford: Oxford University Press.

Roberts, Dorothy E. 1993. "Racism and Patriarchy in the Meaning of Motherhood." *Journal of Gender and the Law* 1 (1): 1–38.

———. 1995. "Motherhood and Crime." *Social Text* 42: 99–123. https://doi.org/10.2307/466666.

Ross, Loretta J. 2017. "Reproductive Justice as Intersectional Feminist Activism." *Souls* 19 (3): 286–314. https://doi.org/10.1080/10999949.2017.1389634.

Rousseau, Benedicta. 2008. "'This Is a Court of Law, Not a Court of Morality': Kastom and Custom in Vanuatu State Courts." *Journal of South Pacific Law* 12 (2): 15–27.

Segeral, Nathalie. 2018. "(Re-)Inscribing the South Pacific in the Francophone World: (Non-) Motherhood, Gendered Violence, and Infanticide in Three Oceanian Women Writers." *Contemporary French and Francophone Studies* 22 (2): 238–47. https://doi.org/10.1080/17409292.2018.1469718.

SisterSong. 2007. *Reproductive Justice Briefing Book: A Primer on Reproductive Justice and Social Change.* Pro-Choice Public Education Project (PEP) and SisterSong Women of Color Reproductive Justice Collective. https://www.law.berkeley.edu/php-programs/courses/fileDL.php?fID=4051.

Spinelli, Margaret G. 2002. "Neonaticide: A Systematic Investigation of 17 Cases." In *Infanticide: Psychosocial and Legal Perspectives on Mothers Who Kill*, edited by Margaret G. Spinelli and Ann E. Norwood, 105–18. Washington, DC: American Psychiatric Publishing.

Terry, Gareth, Nikki Hayfield, Victoria Clarke, and Virginia Braun. 2017. "Thematic Analysis." In *The SAGE Handbook of Qualitative Research in Psychology*, edited by Carla Willig and Wendy Stainton Rogers, 17–36. London: SAGE Publications.

Tsing, Anna Lowenhaupt. 1990. "Monster Stories: Women Charged with Perinatal Endangerment." In *Uncertain Terms: Negotiating Gender in American Culture*, edited by Faye Ginsburg and Anna Lowenhaupt Tsing, 282–99. Boston: Beacon Press.

University of the South Pacific School of Law. 2020. "Pacific Islands Legal Information Institute." November 27. http://www.paclii.org/.

Unnithan, Maya, and Stacy Leigh Pigg. 2014. "Sexual and Reproductive Health Rights and Justice – Tracking the Relationship." *Culture, Health & Sexuality* 16 (10): 1181–87. https://doi.org/10.1080/13691058.2014.945774.

Vellut, Natacha, Jon M. Cook, and Anne Tursz. 2012. "Analysis of the Relationship between Neonaticide and Denial of Pregnancy Using Data from Judicial Files." *Child Abuse & Neglect* 36 (7): 553–63. https://doi.org/10.1016/j.chiabu.2012.05 .003.

Walker, Samantha, and Aisha K. Gill. 2019. "Women Who Kill: Examining Female Homicide through the Lens of Honour and Shame." *Women's Studies International Forum* 75 (July): 102247. https://doi.org/10.1016/j.wsif.2019.102247.

White, Ashley L., Emily S. Mann, and Fiona Larkan. 2018. "'You Just Have to Learn to Keep Moving On': Young Women's Experiences with Unplanned Pregnancy in the Cook Islands." *Culture, Health & Sexuality* 20 (7): 731–45. https://doi.org/10 .1080/13691058.2017.1371336.

Wilczynski, Ania. 1991. "Images of Women Who Kill Their Infants: The Mad and the Bad." *Women & Criminal Justice* 2 (2): 71–88. https://doi.org/10.1300/ J012v02n02_05.

Chapter 13

The Contraceptive Paradox, Contraceptive Agency, and Reproductive Justice

Women's Decision-Making about Long-Acting Reversible Contraception

Tracy Morison, Yanela Ndabula,
and Catriona Ida Macleod

The "contraceptive paradox" refers to the ways in which contraception can be a source of empowerment and agency for some and a source of oppression for others. Historically, contraception has simultaneously been a source of personal control or autonomy *and* wielded by those in power to control women's[1] fertility, sometimes without their knowledge or consent (Gomez, Mann, and Torres 2018). Long-acting reversible contraception (LARC) (viz., injectables, intra-uterine devices (IUDs), and subdermal implants) in particular is seen as the epitome of the contraceptive paradox (Takeshita 2010). These provider-administered, potentially imposable, contraceptives have historically been central to population control strategies and maintaining oppressive reproductive politics. In recent years a new generation of LARC has been widely taken up in public health and linked to targeted promotion efforts focussed on "at-risk" populations, including young and poor women and Women of Colour (Grzanka and Schuch 2020).

In response to the history of reproductive oppression in a range of contexts, the question of reproductive and contraceptive autonomy has subsequently been highlighted in global policy and research. Reproductive autonomy is understood as refraining from compelling or coercing anyone into (particular) contraceptive usage, and ensuring that patients are "fully empowered agents in their reproductive needs and decisions and to access reproductive health services without interference or coercion" (Senderowicz and Higgins 2020, 81).

However, some Reproductive Justice scholar-activists have questioned researchers' use of the notion of reproductive autonomy, highlighting its reliance on an individualised, rational economic model of choice (Gomez, Mann, and Torres 2018). The emphasis on choice neglects the socially embedded character of personhood, the power relations and inequities within which people are located, and the complex, at times "irrational," nature of decision-making (Madhok 2013). While some research on reproductive autonomy does broaden the focus to include wider contextual factors (e.g., Senderowicz 2019), it views these factors mostly as external to the individual, thereby reinforcing a view of self-outside-society (Donchin 1995).

We argue that understanding how the contraceptive paradox operates within the healthcare nexus requires a different conceptualisation of women's freedom to act in this space—one that considers the irreducibly social nature of human subjectivity and social interconnection. As such, our work takes a feminist poststructuralist view and recognises the interconnection of the individual, interpersonal, and social processes involved in contraceptive decision-making. We therefore use the concept of "contraceptive agency" rather than "contraceptive autonomy" to differentiate our approach (as explained further below) and to show how the contraceptive paradox plays out in reports of healthcare interactions in contraceptive consultations in which LARC was discussed or offered. Our analysis shows how, despite overt acknowledgement of women's right to choose, the contraceptive paradox (subtly and not-so subtly) complicates and undermines power and agency in decision-making.

CONCEPTUALISING CONTRACEPTIVE AGENCY

The role of agency in decision-making has largely been overlooked in contraceptive research, especially in relation to those from marginalised groups (Carvajal and Zambrana 2020). Where agency has been considered, it is often conceptualised in much the same way as what the notion of reproductive autonomy has been, as discussed above: in an individualistic sense as the autonomous, rational, calculation of self-interest (Beynon-Jones 2013).Some even use these terms ("autonomy" and "agency") interchangeably. This individualised conceptualisation has prompted attempts to measure contraceptive agency (e.g., Senderowicz 2020), an exercise criticised by critical scholars who argue that "the over-focus on clear, measurable 'agentic actions' ignores the strategies and actions that women take in challenging contexts" (Willan et al. 2020, 2).

The problems with an individualistic conceptualisation of contraceptive agency are highlighted in the critical literature on LARCs (e.g., Mann and Grzanka 2018; Grzanka and Schuch 2020; Gomez, Mann, and Torres 2018). Given that LARCs are an effective means of preventing and reducing unintended pregnancies, in many public health circles their use is presented as *the* rational choice in cases where people do not wish to conceive (Mann and Grzanka 2018). However, qualitative studies highlight how women's decision-making with respect to LARCs is shaped by their own agendas, preferences, needs, and desires, such as the importance of sexual pleasure (Higgins et al. 2015, 2016), the question of personal control afforded by a method (Gomez, Mann, and Torres 2018), or ambivalence about pregnancy (Higgins 2017; Coombe, Harris, and Loxton 2018). Accordingly, Alspaugh et al. (2020, 82) argue that the "desire for contraceptive agency may be more important than the perceived effectiveness as understood by her health care provider."

Importantly, this emerging body of critical work also highlights how contraceptive agency is constrained by contextual issues, especially intersecting inequities such as race/ethnicity, class, and sexuality (Carvajal and Zambrana 2020; Grzanka and Schuch 2020). For instance, Grzanka and Schuch's (2020) research with young women in the USA shows how participants' experiences of LARC were shaped by privilege and marginalisation so that "participants exercised conditional agency, whereby contraceptive decisions were differentially constrained depending on how each woman was situated" (24).

In line with this idea (of conditional or situated agency) we adopt a feminist poststructuralist conceptualisation of contraceptive agency as the socioculturally mediated ability to act and decide on contraception (Ahearn 2001). From this perspective, individuals are never *outside* socio-cultural forces or discursive practices but, always subject to them, regulated by the range of socially sanctioned subject positions, or the "ways of being" made available to them by the discourses operating in a given social context (Davies 1991).

While individuals are unable to transcend the limits of their context, they can creatively transform language, discourse, and tradition. Action is therefore *regulated* but not *determined* (Madhok 2013) or, as Butler (1990) puts it, is discursively constrained. It involves the "taking up of the tools where they lie, where the very 'taking up' is enabled by the tool lying there" (Butler 1990, 145). This contextual or situated conceptualisation of agency simultaneously considers the self as "a collection of social prescriptions and processes" *and* "an agent with differing levels of access to freedom" (Vera-Gray 2016, 44).

Proceeding from this conceptualisation, we illustrate how the contraception paradox plays out in complex ways in women's personal accounts of contraceptive care in South Africa and Aotearoa (New Zealand).[2] Our data are drawn from a project on LARC provision and use that included contraceptive service users and healthcare providers in these two countries; our focus in this chapter is on the service users' accounts.

Background of Contraceptive Care in the Two Countries

Why use data from two seemingly disparate countries? The answer lies in the historical legacies underpinning current contraceptive practices, although the current landscape of contraceptive care today is rather different in each location. As former colonies, Aotearoa and South Africa share histories of racially motivated contraceptive provision founded upon colonialist concerns, White nationalism, and eugenic thinking.

In South Africa, fears of "White race suicide" and the so-called Black threat (or "*Swart gevaar*") drove the apartheid government's attempts at race-based population control, which included family planning programmes targeting Black and sometimes poor White women. Black women were disproportionately prescribed long-acting, provider-controlled methods (usually the injectable *Depo Provera*[3]) and sometimes subject to coercive practices (e.g., forced sterilisation). In contrast, White women's fertility was encouraged, especially among the middle-class and Afrikaner women, who were dubbed "mothers of the [White Afrikaner] nation." Unlike Black women, these middle-class White women were more often prescribed the user-controlled oral contraceptive pill, which could be discontinued at will, rather than long-acting, provider administered methods (Mkhwanazi 2014).

In Aotearoa, similar anxieties about the degeneration of the "White race" were evident at the turn of the last century. These were central to eugenic efforts to restrict the "lower classes'" reproduction. The *Commission of Inquiry into Mental Defectives and Sexual Offenders*, for example, deemed certain White women a threat to their "race." Measures to curb their fertility were justified by labelling them "unfit," "feebleminded," "oversexed," or "immoral" and casting them as prolific breeders of defective or "sub-normal" children (Wanhalla 2007). Strengthening the "racial vigour" of those of settler heritage reinforced the colonial idea of Aotearoa as a White and British country; tellingly Māori did not feature in these policies, rendering them invisible as reproductive citizens (Green 2011).

Racialised patterns in family planning have not disappeared in either country. Differential contraceptive care and use is still evident in South Africa cutting largely along racial categorisations (Lince-Deroche et al. 2016). This situation is exacerbated by the bifurcation of healthcare into public and private sectors. Poorer, uninsured, largely Black women access contraceptives in public facilities—encountering long waiting times, method bias (notably towards injectables), lack of guidance, method stock-outs, negative staff attitudes, and abuse. Wealthier, largely White women are able to afford medical aid and so access private providers are presented with greater method choice (Lince-Deroche et al. 2016).

In Aotearoa, public concerns about high unintended pregnancy rates have focussed on Māori and Pasifika as "at-risk" groups (Morison and Herbert 2018). This forms part of a larger practice of Othering in public discussion of health and related social issues, in which epidemiological discourse is deployed to effect "the continual unfavourable comparison between Māori and 'everyone else,' as well as the repeated positioning of Māori and Pasifika as 'the other'" (Morison and Herbert 2019, 440). In sexual and reproductive health, much attention has been given to the intersecting issues of teenage pregnancy and welfare assistance, centring on and problematising young (unmarried) Indigenous mothers on welfare (Ware, Breheny, and Forster 2017). Consequently, LARC has received much enthusiasm as a potential solution to a range of social issues, especially welfare dependency and poverty (Parker 2015).

South Africa now has rights-based enabling policies and guidelines for contraceptive service provision, with generally high knowledge and uptake. Nonetheless, the history of racialised population control and HIV/AIDS epidemic have shaped the country's priorities and programming. The oral contraceptive pill is generally more available through private healthcare. Male/external condoms and injectable contraceptives are the most readily accessible and widely used forms of contraception. Other than injectables, LARC measures such as the subdermal implant and modern versions of the IUDs were introduced relatively later and usage remains low relative to other methods (Lince-Deroche et al. 2016).

In Aotearoa, the targeting of "at-risk groups" for LARC use coheres with the country's sexual and reproductive health policy that strongly relies on neoliberal risk discourse, emphasising individualised risk and responsibility with little to no attention to rights. Particular targets are women on welfare assistance or with children in state custody, many of whom are Māori or Pasifika (Green 2011, Morison and Herbert 2018). Currently, fully subsidised long-acting methods include the implant (*Jadelle*), copper IUD, and *Mirena* IUD system. Government funding and a range of sexual and reproductive health services, programmes, and initiatives usually keep costs low. Non-governmental organisations also offer services, though usually only in larger urban centres. Still, access to care differs due to variable costs of contraceptives and services, as well as the shift of services to primary health spaces where doctor shortages create long waiting times and discontinuity of care (McGinn, Mount, Fulcher 2021).

OUR STUDY

In each country, a site-based approach was used to locate a diverse range of reproductive-aged women who had used contraceptive services where they had been offered an LARC in the process of contraceptive decision-making. Women were eligible to participate whether they had ended up using an LARC or not, since it was the process of decision-making that was of interest. In South Africa, participants were recruited from rural and urban settings through (i) advertisements displayed at ten health centres and (ii) from family planning meetings at clinics in the two districts of the Eastern Cape Province. In Aotearoa, posters and flyers were displayed in rural and urban healthcare facilities (e.g., hospitals, public health organisations, family planning clinics) and community spaces (e.g., university, library) in the lower North Island. Online advertisements were also circulated through the social media channels of relevant sexual health/family planning organisations, universities, and community groups with a national reach. In both countries snowballing and referrals were also used.

A total of 90 women participated in this research and their characteristics are summarised belin table 13.1.

Narrative interviews were conducted in which participants were asked about their experiences of contraceptive care and about how they came to use an LARC or not. In South Africa, Yanela (a young Black Xhosa woman) conducted interviews in a combination of English and Xhosa. Xhosa speech was translated by Yanela and a professional bi-lingual transcriber/translator. In Aotearoa all interviews were in English. Tracy (a White South African woman, resident in the country since 2016) interviewed non-Māori/Pākehā participants.

Table 13.1 Participant Characteristics

		South Africa (n = 53)	Aotearoa (n = 37)
Age	Range	18–49	19–44
(years)	Average	27.2	28.8
"Race"/		42 Black South African	18 Māori, Kiwi
ethnicity and		8 White South African	17 Pākehā/
nationality		1 Black Nigerian,	White, Kiwi
		migrant	1 White Irish,
		1 Black Somalian,	migrant
		migrant	1 White British,
		1 Black Namibian,	resident
		migrant	
Parity	Nulliparous	19	22
	Parous	21	2
	Multiparous	13	13
Sexuality	Heterosexual	41	32
	Unreported	12	0
	Bisexual	-	5
Relationship	Single/divorced Dating/	12	10
	partnered (with man)	41	27

Note: Pākehā is a Māori term denoting any non-Indigenous citizens. "Kiwi" is widely used to refer to all citizens of Aotearoa (though is not entirely unproblematic).

Two research assistants interviewed Māori participants; both are Māori young women proficient in tikanga Māori (appropriate indigenous practices).

Our analysis takes a discursive approach informed by feminist post-structuralism. In this view, talk is viewed as constitutive: people construct versions of social reality (events, identities, experiences) by drawing on shared sets of prevailing socio-cultural meanings, which we term scripts. A "script" denotes a socially established way of speaking/lines of argument delimiting what can be said about a topic, each one identifiable by its pattern of familiar themes, motifs, or truisms (Speer 2001). We use "scripts" to foreground the discursive constraint on action as "scripts establish what is [discursively] possible and acceptable, but also may be improvised upon" (Morison and Macleod 2015, 35). Thus, specific scripts enable and constrain situated agency. Accordingly, speakers can draw on and negotiate existing scripts to construct and negotiate (non)agentic social identities as they position themselves/others in particular ways in their talk.

Data from each site were first analysed by the researchers from the respective countries. We then discussed the analyses and identified patterns of talk resonating across contexts. Here we focus on three decision-making scripts drawn on by participants in each country, with a specific interest in their implications for women's contraceptive agency and the contraceptive paradox.

DECISION-MAKING SCRIPTS AND CONTRACEPTIVE AGENCY

The three scripts identified construct interactive processes within contraceptive counselling sessions differently, assigning the locus of decision-making variously to providers, patients, or a combination. Each rendition has implications for the patient's contraceptive agency. We summarise their main features in table 13.2 below, before discussing each one, using anonymised data extracts for illustration.

EXPERT-DIRECTED DECISION-MAKING SCRIPT

The expert-directed script reflects familiar interactive roles in healthcare and is therefore, unsurprisingly, the most common script across the data. According to this script, decision-making is largely driven by providers, with little input from patients. Its hallmark is, therefore, "the failure to achieve mutuality" (Pilnick and Dingwall 2011, 1375). This uneven patient-provider positioning is supported by the biomedical discourse, which values expert medical knowledge, based on scientific evidence, over lay knowledge (Berndt

Table 13.2 Overview of Decision-Making Scripts

Script	Contraceptive Agency Enabled	Based on
Expert-led	Passive	• Expert knowledge; client ignorance • Expert knowledge extends to knowing what is best for the individual
	Muted	• Nominally given a choice • Discredit patient input
	Covertly resistant	• Inability to engage and indirect resistance
Patient-led	Active neoliberal subject	• Responsibilisation • Self-education
Collaborative	Interactive knowledge-seeking	• Sharing information • Health service provider listens
	Located subject (situated agency)	• Unique experiences and contexts considered in dialogue

and Bell 2021). The latter is considered, at best, supplementary and, at worst, irrelevant or a hindrance to the provider's job. As we show below, the contraceptive agency enabled through this interactive script is (i) passive (lay knowledge, irrelevant), (ii) muted (lay knowledge, supplementary), or (iii) resistant (evade/exit specific interaction or ignore directives).

Passive Contraceptive Agency

Counselling was commonly depicted as a top-down process, with providers delivering expert information, as illustrated by the following extracts.

Extract 1, Kiara (22, White, Pākehā, NZ)
It really was a lot of doctor/nurse-led: "This is what we think is gonna be best for you. You should give this a go." [. . .] Like, if I had said to my doctor, then, "No, I want to be on the jab." They would have been like "Well . . . We don't think that's the best option for you." And when a doctor says "we don't think that's a good option" you kind of just nod and agree.

Extract 2, Abosede (42, Black, Nigerian, SA)
Well, based on the advice of the doctor . . . he told me that this [method] will fit because when he wanted to (.) when he started a lecture on contraception, he told me all the various options. He didn't just talk about the IUD. He told me all the various options, telling me the side effects, the pros and cons of each one of them. And after the lecture, he now said, "this one," because he is my gynae. I don't know what made him, but he said based on my structure, everything concerning me, that this will best fit with me.

In these extracts, the providers are positioned not only as expert knowers of contraception but also of the optimal choice for the patient ("best option for you"; "best fit for me"). The participants note that in this expert-led, "lecture"-like interactive space, they are trapped in the position of compliant, docile patient who must accept provider recommendations ("just nod and agree"). Kiara's hypothetical scenario of disputing recommendations demonstrates that she expects such a conversation to be closed. Dispute is therefore construed as futile; instead, the patient simply becomes the passive recipient of expert directives.

Participants described providers' preferences for specific methods. For instance, reporting having "had the pill pushed on me" (Hailey, 31, Pākehā, Aotearoa) or that a particular method "wasn't given to me as an option . . . [I was told] this is what we give" (Zoe, 26, Pākehā, Aotearoa). This was especially evident in South African participants' accounts of public providers' tendency to prescribe injectable contraceptives, which require minimal provider expertise and user adherence, resonating with other South African research findings (Lince-Deroche et al. 2018).

The expert status of providers, along with possible time constraints, means that "doctor/nurse-led" or "lecture"-like interactions may allow little information exchange. For instance, participants said that providers "semi-explained it to me" (Stacey, 22, Pākehā, Aotearoa) or "didn't tell me anything else . . . they sort of give you a brief rundown . . . after they put it in" (Kiara, 22, Pākehā, Aotearoa). A scenario is constructed where a contraceptive agency is rendered passive by limited information—often simply brochures, photocopied leaflets, and cursory explanations.

The hierarchical expert-patient power relations and associated client passivity were depicted as exacerbated by race and age, pointing to racist and adultist profiling of women as "irresponsible" and "risky" reproducers. For instance:

Extract 3, Lisa (21, White, Pākeha, Aotearoa)
You get your rights almost taken away from you because you don't (.) you wouldn't know any better because you're just a baby. So, you basically do what you're told [. . .] there's no collaboration when you're younger.

Extract 4, Sandra (24, Māori, Aotearoa)
I think I didn't have a choice in the end because I was Māori and young and out of school . . . Like I'm just gonna be another one [unplanned teenage pregnancy].

Extract 5, Kuhle (25, Black, Xhosa, SA)
Obviously, when you are being discharged from hospital, they do inject you. In fact, they don't tell you and don't beg you, especially if you are a child and you have a child. They don't beg you. They don't ask you if you want it or not.

Here young women, deemed incapable of decision-making due to their age, are obliged to submit to providers' directives and "do what you're told." The participants attribute coercive intervention to healthcare providers' dismissal of young patients as ignorant ("don't know any better") and unreliable ("gonna be another one"). In extract 4, this positioning is coupled with racist positionings of young Māori women as more prone to unplanned ("teenage") pregnancy; this rests upon the embedded colonial view of Indigenous' and Women of Colour's reproductive capacities as risky and a threat to public health and economic "development" (Grzanka and Schuch 2020; Ware et al. 2017).

Similarly, South African participants reported that young women attending public healthcare facilities are administered post-partum contraception as a matter of course. This is supported by other research with providers (Holt et al. 2018). Participants expressed the belief that this practice is "standard procedure for the Department of Health . . . not a choice" (Zimkitha, 25, Xhosa, SA). As Siyasanga (SA) explained, "I thought after giving birth a person has to get that injection so that's why I did not say no."

Muted Contraceptive Agency

Expert biomedical knowledge generally secures authority, requiring patients' deference and compliance (Pilnick and Dingwall 2011). Nevertheless, providers were also portrayed as offering choices, suggesting their cognisance of the need to provide options or the rhetoric of contraceptive choice, as seen below.

Extract 6, Qaqamba (24, Black, Xhosa, SA)
No, there is no conversation. They just ask you what you want? "What are you going to inject? The *Petogen*[4]?" They inject and then you leave.

Extract 7, Khanya (29, Black, Xhosa, SA)
It wasn't a personalised conversation. It was very much a professional, tick-a-box, *PowerPoint* presentation of what this thing is. "If you can't do this, do that. If you can't do this, do that" blah blah.

As with the passive positioning discussed above, here decision-making is depicted as top-down and directive—an impersonal "tick-a-box," one-size-fits-all approach that is narrowly focussed on biomedical issues. Yet, providers are also depicted as asking questions or providing options. These choices are, of course, limited and restrictive (e.g., choosing between types of injectables). They are still choices, however. The general reproductive health emphasis on clients' contraceptive decision-making is thus evident, even in expert-led interactions.

Berndt patient participation is, nonetheless, limited and therefore muted. Participants frequently recounted how, when they did provide inputs, these were disregarded or dismissed. For example, participants described being disbelieved when reporting negative side effects. The providers in Marion's (44, Pākehā,

Aotearoa) account indicated that she was "imagining things" and in Suzanne's (32, Māori, Aotearoa) were reported to have said, "Oh no, that can't happen . . . it's not as bad as what you're making out." Some Aotearoa participants described "condescending" (Eva, 35, Pākehā, Aotearoa) providers and "being treated like I was quite stupid" (Kath, 32, Pākehā, Aotearoa). As part of this, participants in Aotearoa described providers who refused certain methods for non-medical reasons, were reluctant to reverse a long-acting method, or declined such requests. South African participants also told how providers imposed their views about specific contraceptives so that other contraceptive measures went undiscussed. The privileging of biomedical knowledge over lay/embodied knowledge positions patients as having little to offer in contraceptive counselling: their inputs and agency are muted. This echoes international research findings (Waller, Tholander, and Nilsson 2017; Amico et al. 2016; Berndt and Bell 2021).

Covert Resistance

Patient deference, as Pilnick and Dingwall (2011) highlight, is not simply the imposition of the healthcare professional's agenda since patients actively submit to providers, as shown in Kiara's positioning of herself as agreeing to "go along with" expert recommendations (extract 1). Clients are therefore not unaware of the power relations taking place. Rather, silence, secrecy, and inaction can serve a self-protective function at an individual level in disempowering contexts where women's voices have no institutional or collective power (Madhok, Phillips, and Wilson 2013).

In the case of contraceptive care, asymmetrical provider-patient power relations may be co-constructed to the extent that deference is necessary to secure care. For example, South African participants depicted provider-directed decision-making as speeding up clinic visits in oversubscribed public facilities. Olwethu (25, Xhosa, SA) maintained that "when you go to the clinic you just want them to help you with what you want and then leave" implying that very little information exchange is expected.

Despite some expressions of discomfort (e.g., "just looking at you as a walking reproductive system" Eva, 35, Pākehā, Aotearoa), participants' accounts construed challenging practitioners about practices they disliked or questioning providers as impossible or not even considered. Instead, several South African participants related how they took matters into their own hands if side effects did not subside and/or providers did not offer solutions, mostly by independently discontinuing contraceptive use. Similarly, Aotearoa participants described changing providers or services, independently stopping/removing contraceptives, or avoiding specific providers. Thus, resistance to expert-led interactions is rendered as possible only through covert actions *outside* the consultation, not within it.

Patient-Led Decision-Making Script

In contrast to the previous script, the patient-led script positions the patient as primarily responsible for contraceptive decision-making. This script rests heavily on dominant neoliberal "self-health" practice (Johnson 2014). The ideal patient is "a reflexive subject concerned with health and lifestyle and . . . geared towards practices of active health, lifestyle, self-assessment, and self-education" (Johnson 2014, 334), which Johnson (2014) terms "the expert patient ideal" (332).

A notable feature of this script is its association with the performance of competence in relation to reproductive health, as illustrated in the extract below where Lunathi answers a question about her experience of contraceptive counselling.

Extract 8, *Lunathi* (28, Black, Xhosa, SA)
So, very easy. . . . I think also being an older student gives me more confidence. I was like "Lady, may I please have a contraceptive" and she's like, "Have you been on it [before]?" "No, it's my first time can you take me through it?" She was like "OK. Ja [yes]." I was like, "No, [I want the] two-month one [injection]." Needle. Done.

This account invokes the neoliberal "ideal young woman as the 'can-do' girl" who uses contraception to secure a promising future (Mann and Grzanka 2018). Lunathi describes how she directed the consultation, instructing the provider to present her with further information. She positions herself as proactively seeking contraception; she is in control of the counselling interaction and, more broadly, her reproductive health. The depiction of herself as mature, "confident," and assertive is indicative of how participants commonly used this script to position themselves as having and expressing clear preferences and being assertive ("confident in what I want," Faith, Aotearoa; "empowered," Eva and Anna, Aotearoa).

Contraceptive use was frequently constructed as the responsible choice, part of the wider responsibility for managing one's health, as summed up by Terina (28, Māori, Aotearoa): "it's your health, it's your wellbeing, it's your body, and you need to own it . . . don't be afraid to ask or stand up for what you want in your health." Being proactive about contraception was therefore constructed as taking charge of one's health and part of the responsibility for making good "lifestyle choices" (Eva, 35, Pākehā, Aotearoa).

In the patient-led script, women "are expected to adopt a highly reflexive, intentional and carefully researched orientation to the consumer market catering to pregnancy and parenting" (Johnson 2014, 331), as illustrated in the extract below where Sinead recounts a negative experience with the copper IUD.

Extract 9, Sinead (27, White, European, Aotearoa)
I was a bit disappointed with (.) first of all, maybe, just myself, for being uninformed. I felt like I could have been a more informed consumer . . . I hadn't done any proper reading about it beforehand. [. . .]/*Tracy*: [. . .] So, what is it about contraception that makes you feel like you needed to be more prepared?/[. . .] I guess because it's something that you're supposed to have personal responsibility over. That's how you feel as a woman. It's something that you're supposed to have, personal responsibility to look after your contraception if you don't want to get pregnant. That's the information you need to gather, to make sure it doesn't need to happen. That's on you.

Here Sinead attributes her negative experience to being an "uninformed consumer," positioning herself, rather than the provider, as responsible for information and preparation related to the fitting of an IUD. She positions herself as having failed to present as the "expert patient [who] is expected to negotiate their healthcare with careful research and self-education" (Johnson 2014, 331). Tracy's question prompts further discussion, which illuminates associated gendered discourses related to pregnancy prevention and the gendered nature of responsibilisation, as Sinead positions herself as responsible "as a woman" for preventing unintended pregnancy.

Aotearoa participants frequently reported having "done my homework" or "done the research," constructing self-education as part of the "personal responsibility" for "managing" pregnancy prevention, especially since in a digital age "information is readily available" (Marie, 35, Pākehā, Aotearoa). Among South African participants, the expert-patient subjectivity was more commonly taken up by those who had obtained IUDs and implants through private services. For example, Nomawabo (Black, SA) said, "I also had some knowledge from *Google* so that I come with my own information, but it's great to hear it from someone else." Similarly, Emma (26, White, SA) reported, "I did some basic research, you know like, *WebMD* and stuff like that, where they just tell you the pros and cons."

This responsibilisation of the patient, of course, removes responsibility from providers. Participants drawing on this script typically described foreclosed counselling in which service providers gave information only about methods patients explicitly mentioned, without introducing other methods, guiding the conversation, or participating in decision-making. The drawback of foreclosed counselling is highlighted by accounts of negative outcomes (mostly side effects or discomfort) and anger or regret at not receiving more information or options. It was only in such instances that providers' lack of input was named and questioned. Generally, the "informed consumer" subjectivity was favourably cast and largely taken for granted.

Collaborative Decision-Making Script

The collaborative decision-making script contrasts with both preceding scripts as *both* caregivers and patients are positioned as active in decision-making:

> *Extract 10, Gladys* (40, Black, Xhosa, SA)
> She explains to you. She doesn't do anything without talking to you and giv[ing] you options so that you choose. She educates you a lot. . . . So, she talks to you. She has a discussion and I made the decision because I was informed. I never felt I didn't know what it was going to do. Even with the implant . . . she explained everything to me.

> *Extract 11, Jolene* (34, Māori, Aotearoa)
> There was that little bit of collaboration or a recommendation based on my medical needs. So, that absolutely made a difference. I remember saying to someone just afterwards "Oh they actually listened to what I was saying and didn't just recommend a standard sort of contraceptive" (.) I appreciate that, but generally speaking, yeah, it hasn't always been that way.

These extracts show how the collaborative decision-making script establishes less hierarchical power relations than the traditional expert-led decision-making script. Although caregivers are still positioned as experts who "educate," "inform," "explain," and "recommend," they are also described as taking the time to provide enough information and, importantly, to *engage in discussion*. Contraceptive agency is enabled by interactive knowledge-sharing in this script. In these extracts, especially extract 10, the patient does not simply defer to expert recommendation but actively chooses ("you choose," "I made the decision").

This contrasts with the generic, one-size-fits-all approach many participants criticised and associated with the expert-directed decision-making script. Above Jolene refers to the provider tailoring recommendations to her "medical needs." Similarly, Sandra (24, Māori, Aotearoa) recounted how she valued contraceptive care involving "spending time with me, talking to me about my story and coming up with a plan through that." Her comment shows appreciation for being viewed as a located subject, with a unique set of experiences that are valued and factored into decision-making.

The approach captured by the collaborative decision-making script was often described as the preferred approach to contraceptive counselling. At the same time, however, it was viewed as "rare" (Mere, 43, Aotearoa) or occurring if one is "really lucky" (Kath, 32, Pākehā, Aotearoa). Indeed, this script was drawn on far less across the dataset.

CONCLUDING DISCUSSION

We have focussed on women's contraceptive agency, framed against the broad background of the contraceptive paradox: the simultaneous enablement and disempowerment of specific persons in contraceptive decision-making. Proceeding from a feminist poststructuralist understanding of contraceptive agency, our analysis of accounts of contraceptive counselling interactions illuminates how the contraceptive paradox plays out in this interactive space. The scripts we focussed on—the expert-directed, patient-led, and collaborative decision-making scripts—have implications for patients' contraceptive agency.

The dominant expert-directed script—supported by a biomedical discourse and characterised by patient deference—invokes a compliant contraceptive user who is passively obedient or muted and only able to enact agency through covert resistance. This can potentially enable coercive practices. These positions do little to support reproductive health. Passive or muted subjects may be prescribed contraception that does not holistically meet needs or causes unanticipated complications; the covertly resistant subject may discontinue contraception and ultimately end up without the contraception she may want or need.

The counter to this script is the patient-led script that ascribes the locus of decision-making to patients, offering them greater interactive power and enabling resistance to traditional practitioner-patient power relations. Indeed, many participants framed this script positively and depicted the subject position of the empowered "expert consumer" as one to be aspired to. Yet, the neoliberal underpinnings of this script work to place responsibility for contraceptive knowledge and use on women, reinforcing the patriarchal imperative of women as wholly responsible for reproductive outcomes (Wigginton et al. 2014). The limitation of this positioning is, as many accounts demonstrated, that patients may not have sufficient knowledge for making fully informed choices or managing unfavourable outcomes (e.g., contraceptive failure, side effects) and if these do transpire, they can be deemed responsible.

Finally, the collaborative decision-making script—the most preferred option yet least referred to in participants' accounts—contrasts with both preceding scripts. It constructs decision-making as a negotiation between patient and provider that balances providers' medical knowledge with patients' situated, embodied knowledge. Dialogue is construed as centring on biomedical knowledge *and* the unique situations and preferences of each patient. These findings support international research showing the benefits of shared decision-making strategies focussed on eliciting and responding to patient preferences, needs, and values in contraceptive counselling (Holt, Dehlendorf, and Langer 2017). They also align with findings indicating that in contraceptive care "shared decision making seems to be an exception rather than a rule" (Waller, Tholander, and Nilsson 2017, 3).

Supporting shared decision-making requires a shift in perspective towards what Holt and colleagues (2020) call a person-centred approach, which is underpinned by values of patient agency and health equity. A major focus of a person-centred approach is on locating the person in context, as embedded in community and social contexts. Significantly, this approach is attuned to issues of power, calling for the shifting of traditional patient-provider power relations by, for instance, tasking providers with making space for interactive information sharing and deliberation, limiting inappropriate influence over decision-making processes, and being aware of their agenda (of pregnancy prevention) or role in creating barriers (Amico et al. 2016).

This approach can promote Reproductive Justice aligned counselling praxis, to counter the problematic positioning of certain women (young, of colour, poor) as "risky." Instead, this approach recognises that contraceptive efficacy and pregnancy prevention may not be a woman's first/only consideration. Instead, patient preferences, needs, and agency are prioritised above the public health aim of pregnancy prevention, which drives much of the LARC promotion and can encourage coercive practices, regardless of provider intention.

Effecting such an approach is not simply about healthcare provider training, however. Policy framings (e.g., the language of risk and responsibility in contraceptive policies in Aotearoa), material constraints (e.g., contraceptive stock-outs in South Africa), and institutional dynamics (e.g., oversubscribed health facilities) may lead to consultations that dissuade dialogue. It is in this context that the holistic, intersectional nature of a Reproductive Justice approach is important so as to enable contraceptive consultations that do not err on the side of disempowerment/coercion (expert-led consultations) or neoliberal, responsibilising autonomy (patient-led consultations) but rather empower women through decision-making that rests on a *combination* of biomedical, contextual, and embodied knowledge.

NOTES

1. Not all those who seek/use contraception are cisgender women, but we focus on this group because as the targets of LARC promotion efforts.
2. We use the indigenous country name in line with moves to decolonisation.
3. *Depo Provera* is an injectable contraceptive.
4. Customary practices or behaviours.

REFERENCES

Ahearn, Laura M. 2001. "Language and Agency." *Annual Review of Anthropology* 30: 109–37. https://doi.org/10.1007/978-3-030-04681-1_8.

Alspaugh, Amy, Julie Barroso, Melody Reibel, and Shannon Phillips. 2020. "Women's Contraceptive Perceptions, Beliefs, and Attitudes: An Integrative Review of Qualitative Research." *Journal of Midwifery and Women's Health* 65 (1): 64–84. https://doi.org/10.1111/jmwh.12992.

Amico, Jennifer R., Ariana H. Bennett, Alison Karasz, and Marji Gold. 2016. "'She Just Told Me to Leave It': Women's Experiences Discussing Early Elective IUD Removal." *Contraception* 94 (4): 357–61. https://doi.org/10.1016/j.contraception.2016.04.012.

Berndt, Virginia Kuulei, and Ann V. Bell. 2021. "'This Is What the Truth Is': Provider-Patient Interactions Serving as Barriers to Contraception." *Health* 25 (5): 613–629. doi:10.1177/1363459320969775.

Beynon-Jones, Siân M. 2013. "'We View That as Contraceptive Failure': Containing the 'Multiplicity' of Contraception and Abortion within Scottish Reproductive Healthcare." *Social Science and Medicine* 80: 105–12. https://doi.org/10.1016/j.socscimed.2012.12.004.

Butler, Judith. 1990. *Gender Trouble: Feminism and the Subversion of Identity.* London and New York: Routledge.

Carvajal, Diana N., and Ruth Enid Zambrana. 2020. "Challenging Stereotypes: A Counter-Narrative of the Contraceptive Experiences of Low-Income Latinas." *Health Equity* 4 (1): 10–16. https://doi.org/10.1089/heq.2019.0107.

Chen, Margaret, Alexa Lindley, Katrina Kimport, and Christine Dehlendorf. 2019. "An In-Depth Analysis of the Use of Shared Decision Making in Contraceptive Counseling." *Contraception* 99 (3): 187–91. https://doi.org/10.1016/j.contraception.2018.11.009.

Coombe, Jacqueline, Melissa L. Harris, and Deborah Loxton. 2018. "Accidentally-on-Purpose: Findings from a Qualitative Study Exploring Pregnancy Intention and Long-Acting Reversible Contraceptive Use." *BMJ Sexual and Reproductive Health* 44 (3): 207–13. https://doi.org/10.1136/bmjsrh-2018-200112.

Davies, Bronwyn. 1991. "The Concept of Agency: A Feminist Poststructuralist Analysis." *Social Analysis* 30: 42–53.

Donchin, Anne. 1995. "Reworking Autonomy: Toward a Feminist Perspective." *Cambridge Quarterly of Healthcare Ethics* 4 (1): 44–55. https://doi.org/10.1017/S0963180100005636.

Gomez, Anu Manchikanti, E. S. Mann, and V. Torres. 2018. "'It Would Have Control over Me Instead of Me Having Control': Intrauterine Devices and the Meaning of Reproductive Freedom." *Critical Public Health* 28 (2): 190–200. https://doi.org/10.1080/09581596.2017.1343935.

Green, Alison. 2011. "A Discursive Analysis of Māori in Sexual and Reproductive Health Policy." Masters Thesis, University of Waikato.

Grzanka, Patrick R., and Elena Schuch. 2020. "Reproductive Anxiety and Conditional Agency at the Intersections of Privilege: A Focus Group Study of Emerging

Adults' Perception of Long-Acting Reversible Contraception." *Journal of Social Issues* 76 (2): 270–313. https://doi.org/10.1111/josi.12363.

Higgins, Jenny A. 2017. "Pregnancy Ambivalence and Long-Acting Reversible Contraceptive (LARC) Use Among Young Adult Women: A Qualitative Study." *Perspectives on Sexual and Reproductive Health.* https://doi.org/10.1363/psrh .12025.

Higgins, Jenny A., Renee D. Kramer, and Kristin M. Ryder. 2016. "Provider Bias in Long-Acting Reversible Contraception (LARC) Promotion and Removal: Perceptions of Young Adult Women." *American Journal of Public Health* 106 (11): 1932–37. https://doi.org/10.2105/AJPH.2016.303393.

Higgins, Jenny A., Jessica N. Sanders, Mari Palta, and David K. Turok. 2016. "Women's Sexual Function, Satisfaction, and Perceptions after Starting Long-Acting Reversible Contraceptives." *Obstetrics & Gynecology* 128 (5): 1143–51. https://doi.org/10.1097/AOG.0000000000001655.

Higgins, Jenny A., Kristin Ryder, Grace Skarda, Erica Koepsel, and Eliza A. Bennett. 2015. "The Sexual Acceptability of Intrauterine Contraception: A Qualitative Study of Young Adult Women." *Perspectives on Sexual and Reproductive Health* 47 (3): 115–22. https://doi.org/10.1363/47e4515.

Holt, Kelsey, Christine Dehlendorf, and Ana Langer. 2017. "Defining Quality in Contraceptive Counseling to Improve Measurement of Individuals' Experiences and Enable Service Delivery Improvement." *Contraception* 96 (3): 133–37. https://doi.org/10.1016/j.contraception.2017.06.005.

Holt, Kelsey, Icela Zavala, Ximena Quintero, Doroteo Mendoza, Marie C. McCormick, Christine Dehlendorf, Ellice Lieberman, and Ana Langer. 2018. "Women's Preferences for Contraceptive Counseling in Mexico: Results from a Focus Group Study." *Reproductive Health* 15 (1): 128–39. https://doi.org/10.1186 /s12978-018-0569-5.

Johnson, Sophia. 2014. "'Maternal Devices', Social Media and the Self-Management of Pregnancy, Mothering and Child Health." *Societies* 4 (2): 330–50. https://doi.org /10.3390/soc4020330.

Lince-Deroche, Naomi, Jane Harries, Deborah Constant, Chelsea Morroni, Melanie Pleaner, Tamara Fetters, Daniel Grossman, Kelly Blanchard, and Edina Sinanovic. 2018. "Doing More for Less: Identifying Opportunities to Expand Public Sector Access to Safe Abortion in South Africa through Budget Impact Analysis." *Contraception* 97 (2): 167–76. https://doi.org/10.1016/j.contraception.2017.07 .165.

Lince-Deroche, Naomi, Melanie Pleaner, Jane Harries, Chelsea Morroni, Saiqa Mullick, Cindy Firnhaber, Masangu Mulongo, Pearl Holele, and Edina Sinanovic. 2016. "Achieving Universal Access to Sexual and Reproductive Health Services: The Potential and Pitfalls for Contraceptive Services in South Africa." In *South African Health Review 2016*, edited by Ashnie Padarath, J. King, E. Mackie, and J. Casciola, 95–108. Durban: Health Systems Trust. https://www.hst.org.za/publica-tions/South African Health Reviews/SAHR 2016.pdf.

Madhok, Sumi. 2013. *Rethinking Agency: Developmentalism, Gender and Rights.* India: Routledge.

Madhok, Sumi, Anne Phillips, and Kalpana Wilson. 2013. "Introduction." In *Gender, Agency, and Coercion*, 1–13. Basingstoke: Palgrave Macmillan.

Mahmood, Saba. 2011. *Politics of Piety: The Islamic Revival and the Feminist Subject*. Princeton University Press.

Mann, Emily S., and Patrick R. Grzanka. 2018. "Agency-without-Choice: The Visual Rhetorics of Long-Acting Reversible Contraception Promotion." *Symbolic Interaction* 41 (3): 334–56. https://doi.org/10.1002/symb.349.

Mcginn, Orna, Vicki Mount, and Helen Fulcher. 2021. "Increasing Access to Contraception in New Zealand: Assessing the Impact of a New Funding Initiative." *New Zealand Medical Journal* 15: 1528. www.nzma.org.nz/journal.

Morison, Tracy, and Catriona Macleod. 2015. *Men's Pathways to Parenthood: Silence and Heterosexual Gender Norms*. Cape Town, South Africa: HSRC Press.

Morison, Tracy, and Sarah Herbert. 2018. "Rethinking 'Risk' in Sexual and Reproductive Health Policy: The Value of the Reproductive Justice Framework." *Sexuality Research and Social Policy*, 1–12. https://doi.org/10.1007/s13178-018-0351-z.

Parker, George. 2015. *Coerced Contraception: A Reproductive Justice Perspective*. Auckland: Women's Health Action. http://womens-health.org.nz/coerced-contraception-a-reproductive-justice-perspective/.

Pilnick, Alison, and Robert Dingwall. 2011. "On the Remarkable Persistence of Asymmetry in Doctor/Patient Interaction: A Critical Review." *Social Science and Medicine* 72 (8): 1374–82. https://doi.org/10.1016/j.socscimed.2011.02.033.

Senderowicz, Leigh. 2020. "Contraceptive Autonomy: Conceptions and Measurement of a Novel Family Planning Indicator." *Studies in Family Planning* 51 (2): 161–76. https://doi.org/10.1111/sifp.12114.

Speer, Susan A. 2001. "Reconsidering the Concept of Hegemonic Masculinity: Discursive Psychology, Conversation Analysis and Participants' Orientations." *Feminism & Psychology* 11 (1): 107–35. https://doi.org/10.1177/0959353501011001006.

Takeshita, Chikako. 2010. "The IUD in Me: On Embodying Feminist Technoscience Studies." *Science as Culture* 19 (1): 37–60. https://doi.org/10.1080/09505430903558021.

Vera-Gray, Fiona. 2016. *Men's Intrusion, Women's Embodiment: A Critical Analysis of Street Harassment*. Routledge.

Waller, Rosalind, Michael Tholander, and Doris Nilsson. 2017. "'You Will Have These Ones!': Six Women's Experiences of Being Pressured to Make a Contraceptive Choice That Did Not Feel Right." *Social Sciences* 6 (4). https://doi.org/10.3390/socsci6040114.

Ware, Felicity, Mary Breheny, and Margaret Forster. 2017. "The Politics of Government 'Support' in Aotearoa/New Zealand: Reinforcing and Reproducing the Poor Citizenship of Young Māori Parents." *Critical Social Policy* 37 (4): 499–519. https://doi.org/10.1177/0261018316672111.

Wigginton, Britta, Melissa L. Harris, Deborah Loxton, Danielle L. Herbert, and Jayne Lucke. 2014. "The Feminisation of Contraceptive Use: Australian Women's

Accounts of Accessing Contraception." *Feminism & Psychology* 25 (2): 178–98. https://doi.org/10.1177/0959353514562802.

Willan, Samantha, Andrew Gibbs, Inge Petersen, and Rachel Jewkes. 2020. "Exploring Young Women's Reproductive Decision-Making, Agency and Social Norms in South African Informal Settlements." Edited by Susan A. Bartels. *PLOS ONE* 15 (4): e0231181. https://doi.org/10.1371/journal.pone.0231181.

Chapter 14

Directive Counselling Undermines "Safe" Abortion

A Critical Discursive Psychology Approach to Reproductive Justice

Jabulile Mary-Jane Jace Mavuso,
Catriona Ida Macleod, and Ryan du Toit

The World Health Organisation (WHO) (2019) considers abortion "unsafe" when carried out by persons lacking necessary skills, in an environment that does not conform to minimal medical standards, or both. Its updated definition of "safe" abortion includes procedures supported (but not necessarily performed) by trained persons, or where those having a medical abortion have access to accurate information or trained providers. This update was the result of Brazilian feminist work that inspired feminist movements across the globe (Assis and Larrea 2020). Working in/from contexts with restrictive abortion legislation that make legal abortion largely inaccessible, these movements pushed for the recognition of the safety of self-administered and self-managed medical abortion outside of healthcare facilities.

Although the updated definition of safe abortion is now more inclusive than before, it refers to only one aspect of the service: the physical procedure (whether administered in person or supported by a trained provider). Where counselling is mentioned in relation to unsafe abortion, it is only to indicate that mandatory counselling and/or the provision of misleading information may lead to seeking unsafe abortions (WHO 2019).

The WHO's concentration on the physical safety of abortion relates to mortality and morbidity associated with unsafe abortion. Health complications of unsafe abortion mentioned by the WHO include haemorrhage, infection, and injury to the genital tract and/or internal organs. While the physical sequelae of unsafe abortion are clearly of utmost importance, Macleod (2012) highlights the general lack of emphasis on the psychological outcomes of unsafe abortion.

Indeed, the WHO's understandings of the un/safety of abortion show limited engagement with the role counselling can play. A WHO (2015) document on the roles of healthcare practitioners in providing safe abortion emphasises the provision of scientifically accurate, easy-to-understand information in voluntarily non-directive counselling. Accurate, non-directive counselling is deemed "a core element of good quality abortion services" (WHO 2015, 56). In this chapter we argue that understandings of the provision of accurate and non-directive voluntary abortion counselling must be extended to the *safety*, not just the quality, of abortion services. If, as indicated by the WHO (2019, non-paginated), abortion-seekers "may experience a range of harms that affect their quality of life and well-being" following unsafe abortion, and if unsafe/safe abortion is viewed as a continuum (from least to most safe, as suggested by the WHO), then psychological or emotional harms as a *result of abortion counselling services* should be included in the definition of the safety of abortion.

Research on abortion experiences (when the abortion is performed under legal circumstances) demonstrates that people's emotional and psychological experiences of abortion vary greatly. Those who have abortions may experience relief, happiness, and a sense of empowerment, sadness, loss, grief, trauma symptoms, and/or ambivalence; and for those who do experience them, trauma symptoms may dissipate from two months to two years following an abortion (Kimport, Foster, and Weitz 2011; Major et al. 2009). Further, this research demonstrates that the experience of psychological distress and/ or trauma symptoms depends on various factors, *including* abortion stigma which is in turn socio-culturally produced through dominant understandings of abortion, pregnancy, and (cis) womanhood (Beynon-Jones 2017; Kimport et al. 2011; Kumar et al. 2009; O'Donnell, O'Carroll, and Toole 2018). Recent research and scholarship on abortion counselling points to how directive anti-abortion counselling may exacerbate or even produce distress around abortion by constructing abortion as dangerous, unsafe, irresponsible, detrimental, and immoral (Ely, Polmanteer, and Kotting 2018; Mavuso 2018; Mavuso and Macleod 2019).

Nonetheless, the WHO's (2019) definition of un/safe abortion does not consider the psychological distress that may be exacerbated or produced during the provision of legal abortion services that would otherwise be deemed "safe." This, we argue, hampers efforts to ensure the complete safety of legal abortion services. In this chapter, we show how directive anti-abortion counselling is effected within the context of abortion services that would, according to the WHO, nevertheless be deemed safe. Drawing on critical discursive psychology and Reproductive Justice approaches, we analyse recordings of abortion counselling sessions and interviews with (cis) women about their experiences of the counselling at three public facilities in the Eastern Cape province of South Africa. While not all recorded interactions or experiences were negative, we concentrate here on discursive counselling practices that, first, undermine Reproductive Justice principles (the right to not have children, to have children under conditions of one's choosing, and to parent children in safe and healthy communities), and, second, escalate or produce psychological or emotional harms. We call for a further expansion of understandings of the safety of abortion services.

ABORTION IN SOUTH AFRICA

The Choice on Termination of Pregnancy Act (No. 92 of 1996) (hereafter CTOP Act) legislates abortion in South Africa, framing abortion as a reproductive right afforded to "women."[1] Under the Act, abortion may be performed on demand during the first trimester by a nurse or midwife, for a broad range of circumstances and by a doctor during the second trimester, and thereafter only on restricted grounds. The Act further stipulates that abortion counselling should be voluntary and non-directive but does not specify the content of non-directive counselling nor how providers should implement this important stipulation.

Several barriers greatly limit access to legal abortion services, rendering these services inaccessible for many, particularly in the public sector where health services are free and on which a majority rely for their healthcare (Hodes 2016; Trueman and Magwentshu 2013). These barriers include anti-abortion attitudes (which at best indicate tolerance or conditional support) (Mosley et al. 2020), a dearth of providers willing to perform abortions, a dire shortage of functioning designated public sector abortion facilities, and long waiting lists at facilities that are functioning (Hodes 2016; Jewkes et al. 2005).

Research on abortion counselling in South Africa is scarce. Analysing semi-structured questionnaire responses from 60 (cis) women attending a public facility, Birdsey et al. (2016) reported that all clients described providers as respectful and non-judgemental. Some felt that the group counselling they received did not address their specific support needs around intimate partner violence which was an important context for their abortion requests. Our own research (Mavuso and Macleod 2019) shows contradictions in (cis) women's experiences of abortion counselling, with some expressing an appreciation of non-directive and empathic counselling and the provision of information, and others indicating that the counselling was upsetting and hurtful.

The paucity of research on abortion counselling experiences is concerning, given fears that counselling may in fact be directive, despite the stipulations of the CTOP Act (Vincent 2012). These concerns arise in response to research on abortion services in general. This work has found that healthcare providers and other personnel deploy various shaming tactics (Mookamedi, Mogotlane, and Roos 2015). Some abortion-seekers avoid legal abortion services from fear of providers' disapproval and hostile treatment (Harries et al. 2015). Furthermore, several international studies on abortion counselling point to or document directive practices (e.g., Beynon-Jones 2013 and Hoggart 2015 in the United Kingdom; Beckman 2016 in the United States; Möller et al. 2012 in Nepal). Thus, rather than being dismissed as "fears" or presumed to rarely occur, the prospect of directive abortion counselling in South Africa bears serious consideration and an adequate response.

The consequences of directive abortion counselling further underscore the need to adequately respond to and prevent directive abortion counselling. For anti-abortion counselling, these consequences may include forced pregnancy (Ely et al. 2018), resorting to illegal and unsafe providers (Harries et al. 2015), and, as we shall show, psychological distress. Psychological distress potentially resulting from directive anti-abortion counselling may go unaddressed due to socio-economic inequities. Systems of oppression create inequitable access to psychological (and other) healthcare, so that (quality) healthcare is largely inaccessible to black, working class, poor, and rural communities (as well as other marginalised communities) in South Africa (Bantjes, Kagee, and Young 2016; Pillay and Barnes 2020) and globally (see Gaffney and McCormick 2017 for the US context). In the Eastern Cape province, where our research was conducted, health inequities may be particularly marked due to the province having the lowest health service delivery coverage in South Africa (Morris-Paxton, Reid, and Ewing 2020).

OUR STUDY

The findings we discuss in this chapter are based on research conducted at three public hospitals in the Eastern Cape province of South Africa. Sites 1 and 2 are in the same city. In addition to serving the surrounding urban/peri-urban communities, site 1 also serves township[2] and rural communities. Site 3 is in a different city to the other research sites and serves both peri-urban/urban and township communities. At two of the sites (1 and 3) counselling was conducted by registered midwives employed at the hospital. At the remaining site (site 2), an external Christian non-governmental organisation volunteered lay counsellors to counsel abortion-seekers at the hospital free of charge.

Following ethics clearance from *Rhodes University*'s Ethics Committee, two inter-related sets of data were collected: (1) audio-recordings of 28 abortion counselling sessions (21 individual sessions and 7 group counselling sessions, average counselling duration was 16:08 minutes), and (2) semi-structured interviews with 30 black (cis) women (ranging in age from 17 to 38) and 4 healthcare workers about their experiences of the counselling. After informed consent procedures and with permission from providers and clients, counselling sessions were recorded, and interviews were conducted on site in English and/or isiXhosa by the first author and co-researchers. Participants in the recordings are not necessarily the same as those who were interviewed.

A narrative-discursive approach (Mavuso 2018; Taylor and Littleton 2006) was used to analyse the data. Our analysis consisted of two major tasks. First, we investigated the discursive resources drawn on by counsellors and nurses in the abortion counselling recordings. Discourses, in this understanding, are socio-culturally available systems of statements, images, and symbols that cohere around common meanings (Taylor and Littleton 2006). Second, we analysed the interview data for the construction of micro-narratives: localised "small stories." These micro-narratives are generated in short bursts during question and answer interactions (O'Donovan 2006) and deploy various discursive resources in constructing sequence and consequence (Taylor and Littleton 2006). Building on previous research (Beynon-Jones 2017; Kimport et al. 2011) and applying this to abortion counselling, we argue that this critical discursive psychology approach, which is rooted in poststructuralist theory, makes the operation of dominant discourses and power relations in directive anti-abortion counselling visible.

FINDINGS

In our analysis, we first present instances of counselling sessions, identifying the common discourses deployed in these interactions, namely, awfulisation of abortion discourse, foetal personhood and motherhood–womanhood discourses, and a religious discourse. Then, in the following section, we show how these discourses underpinned interview participants' micro-narratives recounted during talk about their experiences of counselling. We present anonymised extracts of three, often interwoven, micro-narratives, namely: (i) "I was ready to say I'm cancelling/I have doubts," (ii) "I was so hurt," and (iii) "It was hard, but I don't have a choice."

Recordings: Discourses Deployed in Directive Counselling

Collectively, the discourses deployed by providers—the awfulisation of abortion discourse, foetal personhood and motherhood–womanhood discourses, and a religious discourse—construct abortion as irresponsible and implicitly immoral, harmful to abortion-seekers and their foetus/child, and as antithetical to (biological and gestational) motherhood and cis womanhood. We discuss each discourse with exemplars from the data below.

Awfulisation of Abortion

In the awfulisation discourse, abortion is constructed as a threat and dangerous, on multiple levels, to cis women (Hoggart 2015; Sparrow 2004). In the recorded sessions, counsellors spoke of: (disputed) physical risks, in particular developing breast cancer, becoming infertile, and dying/death; the probability of psychological trauma; and the horrible nature of the procedure.

> *Tracy* (Counsellor, site 2, 4 years counselling experience)
> You [sic] also exposing yourself to the possibility of developing breast cancer as you get older. So there—these are very real side-effects.

> *Buhle* (Nurse, site 1, 4 months abortion provision experience)
> You are 20-years old and your future is still long. You will get married and want children, get a job, and have your own money and want children, and children will not come. And [you will] not be able to get any children [. . .] Or your womb might get injured while it is being cleaned. Do you understand these things?

> *Tracy* (Counsellor, site 2, 4 years counselling experience)
> So there's that option, then there's of course termination which is risky to your body. You can see in the consent form it says you can die.

> *Buhle* (Nurse, site 1, 4 months abortion provision experience)
> Even psychological, and trauma. You might get mentally disturbed. And we might see you being a little maniac here because of this.

> *Linda* (Counsellor, site 2, 3.5 years counselling experience)
> They push the metal tube into the vagina, into the cervix, into the uterus and they suck the baby out. The baby comes out in bits and pieces.

Despite substantial evidence to the contrary (e.g., "pregnancy loss [is] not associated with later cancer development") (Mikkelsen 2019, 80), these counsellors deploy various rhetorical techniques to persuade the clients about the "awful nature" of abortion. Tracy uses formal health language ("side effects") and an official form ("consent form") to establish legitimacy in her claims that abortion leads to cancer and bodily risk. Nurse Buhle stokes fears of an uncertain future, damage to the womb, and infertility ("you will want children, and children will not come"). From a position of expertise, she predicts bad psychological outcomes ("being a little maniac"). Counsellor Linda uses graphic descriptions to depict the procedure as horrendous.

Foetal Personhood Discourse Paired with Motherhood–womanhood Discourse

In the pre-abortion counselling interaction providers intricately construct the foetus/child as a person. As a process, "person-making" (Michael and Morgan 1999, 6) involves a wide range of practices that construct the foetus/child as separate from the body of the pregnant person.

> *Linda* (Counsellor, site 2)
> The baby is already this size. This is a little model, just to show you exactly the size of your baby. The baby's already got the formations of legs. It's got little arms. It's already got a head that's forming. And so, it is vitally important to know that what comes out is not just cells that look like blood clots, they are in fact the baby that you have already conceived.

> *Buhle* (Nurse, site 1)
> That whole process of giving birth will happen to you. The baby will come out the same way a baby would have come out. Do you understand? You will see him [or] her.

In these extracts, the construction of foetal personhood is achieved through symbolic representation (showing a foetal model), listing various physiological features ("legs," "little arms," and "a head") and describing abortion as akin to giving birth to a fully formed baby. However, we wish to note that foetal person-making is not itself at issue; pregnant people (including abortion-seekers) have varying relationships to their pregnancies (Millar 2017). Rather, at issue is the providers' deployment of foetal personhood to regulate how abortion-seekers *should* relate to their pregnancies, themselves, and their foetuses/children.

Vulnerability is conferred on the foetus/child: as a "little" "baby" who needs caring. A particular relationship between the pregnant person and the foetus/child is therefore conjured and circumscribed. As such, the foetal personhood discourse dovetails with and inevitably invokes the motherhood–womanhood discourse. The latter discourse has several features. Motherhood is constructed as a valuable and fulfilling experience, thus operating as a "powerful incentive for [women] to procreate" (Morison 2011, 183). Simultaneously, motherhood is a duty centred on the nurturance and protection of vulnerable children and extends to pregnancy, such that pregnancies *should* end with childbirth and parenthood. Biological and gestational motherhood is thus naturalised and foregrounded as the essential "motherhood experience," which *should* be desired by and is also expected of cis women. Indeed, cis womanhood is ultimately fulfilled through becoming a (preferably biological) mother (Bimha and Chadwick 2016).

The motherhood–womanhood discourse is cis-normative. Cis-normativity regulates who should reproduce, including gestationally, by imagining pregnant people, indeed anyone with the capacity to gestate, as cis/non-trans women and as not intersex, and by understanding pregnancy as integral and essential to cis womanhood (Moseson et al. 2020; Radi 2020; Weissman 2017). In this discourse, abortion-seekers are therefore necessarily and invariably assumed to be women, so that "women" (within this discourse defined cis-normatively and as endosex/non-intersex) commonly shadows "abortion" whenever abortion is spoken/written about. However, this discourse belies the gender and sex diversity of people with uteri (Riggs et al. 2020) and of abortion service users (Moseson et al. 2020, 2022; Nixon 2013), a diversity which is visibilised through scholarship on the reproductive experiences of trans men, trans masculine, non-binary, and intersex people, for example.

Religious Discourse

In providers' talk, a religious discourse references key religious activities—such as prayer/praying, blessings, reading the Bible, and doing God's will—in constructing specific understandings of (im)morality and the meaning of pregnancy, abortion, and motherhood. Independent counsellors either explicitly positioned themselves as Christian ("I am a Christian") or through the use of a religious discourse.

> *Linda* (Counsellor, site 2)
> You need to just go home and be quiet ((sniffing)) and ((slight laughter)) just really absorb all this knowledge now. These special gifts because I mean not many everyone's blessed with a baby and to be blessed with two, is a double blessing.

> *Tracy* (Counsellor, site 2)
> To become the mother that God has planned for your life. You may have not wanted this pregnancy, but if you didn't want it seriously you would have made sure you used proper prevention. Now you have this baby and now you gotta make a decision with this baby.

> *Linda* (Counsellor, site 2)
> I have counselled so many girls of every culture, my own culture, that struggled with—after terminations 'cause when God puts that baby in your stomach, He also puts it in your heart and now it's babies.

As these extracts illustrate, a religious discourse served to reinforce the foetal personhood and motherhood–womanhood discourses. Counsellors who drew on the religious discourse tended to construct the foetus/child as "precious," "special," a "blessing," and a "gift" from God. Constructing the foetus/child as a gift evokes normative understandings of gift-giving as a celebration of a special event and gift-receiving as expressing gratitude. In the above extract the gift-giver is God who can bestow the gift of life, in this case the "baby." To decline the gift (i.e., opt for abortion) or alternatively to go against God's plan for motherhood is to commit a sin. Committing the sin of abortion is linked in the last quote to emotional consequences ("struggled . . . after terminations"), thereby linking the religious and awfulisation of abortion discourses. These extracts illustrate a complex web of discursive practices that undermine reproductive autonomy.

Micro-Narratives

We turn in this section to some of the micro-narratives constructed by (cis) women in interviews about their counselling experiences. Alluding to the discourses described above, participants' accounts point to doubt and emotional harms resulting from counselling sessions.

"I Was Ready to Say I'm Cancelling/I Have Doubts"

Some participants spoke about having doubts about their decision *after* the counselling. Through the providers' discursive practices, abortion was ultimately *delegitimised* as a safe, appropriate, and responsible decision and form of care.

Zimkhitha (site 1)
The scary *thing*[3] is the counselling *can* make us run away. So, I didn't feel comfortable about what they talked about, the *disadvantages* of abortion, because no one is there to motivate you in bad or good things. So, at least getting a *motivator* to tell you, "OK, even though this is a bad thing, something *good* might come out of it."

Nokubonga (site 2)
I did say to her she will not counsel me again, right? She will not see me again here. Then now, about her saying that I am risking my life, I really became scared. So, I explained to her that she will not see me again here doing an abortion.

Both Zimkhitha and Nokubonga take up (to varying degrees) the awfulisation of abortion discourse in their micro-narratives ("disadvantages of abortion"; "risking my life"). They relate how constructing abortion as awful created anxiety ("the scary thing"), uncertainty ("can make us run away"), or a promise to not return for another abortion ("she will not see me again here"). During her interview, Zimkhitha expressed frustration at the admonitory approach used by the nurse at site 1 and was especially upset and frustrated at the lack of any positive framing of abortion. Echoing Zimkhitha, Nokubonga explains how she "really became scared" after having been warned that she was "risking" her life. This construction of legal abortion as life-threatening shames Nokubonga for "risking" her own life and therefore, it is implied, for being "irresponsible." The disclosure of her promise not to return reveals the limited possibilities for recuperating a positive identity from within an awfulisation of abortion discourse. Below, Lisa talks about how the discussion of abortion created doubts for her:

> *Lisa* (site 1)
> Another thing she told me is [. . .] [about] *physical* damages is that for the future I may go without having children. Other people, they say because they have seen the child, they cannot erase that image. The image does not go away, and they end up having problems in their mind [. . .] So, that is what made me, like, I have doubts.

Here Lisa mentions having received information around the risk of infertility, through which abortion is constructed as "physically damaging." In addition, she describes the nurse's implicit reference to so-called inevitable and permanent psychological trauma resulting from having been shown "the child" after the abortion procedure. Reference to "the child" implicitly positions Lisa as a mother. It is this positioning that renders the possibility of infertility and the experience of seeing "the child" traumatic, and in this way the foetal personhood and motherhood–womanhood discourses mutually reinforce the construction of abortion as inevitably harmful and to be avoided.

"I Was So Hurt"

The participants spoke of negative emotions following counselling, as illustrated below.

> *Zipho* (site 3)
> I felt *down [depressed]* because I never expected it. I never expected the things that were discussed. I thought, I think I thought, like, it was a game/joke. But when they told me, I felt down [depressed]. But I do not have an option of not doing it.

> *Nziweni* (site 2)
> Things like, *when* you are twelve weeks and *above* it is now a person that has a soul, you see? So, if [the abortion] is done there, you are given pills to

take. You expel a *person*, a child. What is left is blood, but the feet are there, the hands you see them; they are there. Then, how will you take the pills and expel it when it is still breathing? You need to wait even for it to pass out of you, you give birth to it. Yes, you are watching everything. So, other things like that that make you feel painful.

In her micro-narrative, Zipho explains that she felt "down" because of the counselling. Ultimately the intended effect of providing this "information" is that abortion-seekers change their minds about having the abortion. However, when abortion is the only option, as it was for Zipho, the result is emotional turmoil that must be dealt with *outside* of the abortion counselling context where it was produced or, at the very least, exacerbated.

In the detailed and graphic information Nziweni describes being given during the counselling, the foetal personhood and motherhood–womanhood discourses are interlinked and work together to position abortion-seekers as cis women who are always already mothers. This positioning serves to shame them into changing their minds about having an abortion and taking up the mother position. Those who continue with the procedure are shamed for failing to take up this role. Nziweni's emotional turmoil is clear when she asks, "how will you take the pills and expel it when it is still breathing?" Implicitly, then, abortion is also framed as "murder" of a person by an already mother.

The negative emotions invoked in the deployment of these discourses extended not only to pain, hurt, or "feeling down" but also to moral uncertainty. In the extract below, the participant's confusion is related to the combined deployment of the awfulisation of abortion, foetal personhood, and motherhood–womanhood discourses in counselling sessions.

Sbongiseni (site 2)
They explained how dangerous it could be and I could get infected with some *cancer*. Yes, and then um maybe it's my first and *last* child; I will *never* have another one. Then I, I was *confused* I felt like, I felt like I'm doing something *wrong*.

Here, like Lisa's micro-narrative above, Sbongiseni relates how the negative information provided in counselling contradicted her own understandings ("I was confused"), leading to moral uncertainty ("like I'm doing something wrong"). The position of immorality and subsequent shaming is achieved through the combined effect of the awfulisation of abortion, foetal personhood, and motherhood–womanhood discourses. In the end, the positioning of the counsellor as the expert results in her claim that she "felt like I'm doing something wrong."

"It Was Hard, but I Don't Have a Choice"

In this micro-narrative, the "I was so hurt" narrative is paired with a lack of choice in having an abortion. Participants described an impossible situation: no avenue for retreat from the "inevitable, negative" consequences of abortion, the shame of refusing a motherhood role, and disregarding God's gift or plan.

> *Vanessa* (site 2)
> I think it was just from the *whole* "this is what the procedure is gonna be," you know, and then "this is what the risks are" and that. What *really* got to me is when they said, "*God* created this." And that was the way I was feeling as well, that this happened and, you know, who are *you* to play God? Because that's what you're doing. And then it was "Ok, if you *don't* want the baby why don't you keep it and *give* it up?" And that's not an option.

> *Nziweni* (site 2)
> I was so hurt I don't want to lie but I had already taken a decision that I want to do this, you see? And I have to because of the situation, you see? Yes, so, getting hurt there, I was hurt. And then I feel bad about what I'm going to do, because I've never done this before; it's my first time to do it. Yes, I was so hurt, man, because I even cried and, can it be that I save this child? Or what do I do? I didn't have a choice. I can't carry the baby for nine months and give her or him away. No.

Vanessa's account points to the joint deployment of the awfulisation of abortion and religious discourses that position her as over-stepping her bounds by "playing God," as a "sinner" for violating the "sanctity" of life and motherhood, as "ungrateful" for not recognising the "gifts" she has been given, and as a "bad mother" and "bad woman." Adoption is framed as an option that is always already available. Contrary to the lay counsellor's construction, however, Vanessa asserts that adoption placement is "not an option" for her. Similarly, Nziweni resists the lay counsellor's framing of adoption as a viable option and a preferable and uncomplicated alternative to abortion. Nziweni's micro-narrative demonstrates that this framing is predicated on the interweaving of the foetal personhood discourse, which positions the foetus/child as vulnerable and in need of saving, and the motherhood–womanhood discourse, which positions Nziweni as a(cis) woman/mother. Instead, like Vanessa, Nziweni asserts her own authority in knowing what is and is not a viable option. The negative emotional effects of having to do so, however, in a counselling session in which her decision is delegitimised and criticised, are evident: she feels "hurt" (repeated multiple times), "bad," and cries.

CONCLUDING DISCUSSION

We have used two data sources to illustrate how directive anti-abortion counselling that draws on particular discursive practices may negatively impact those receiving it. Our analysis visibilised the network of discourses and attendant positionings, underpinning the instances of directive anti-abortion counselling practices participants described as deployed in these settings. Awfulisation of abortion, foetal personhood, motherhood–womanhood, and religious discourses work together to: (1) position abortion-seekers as cis women who are always already actual or potential mothers, (2) construct abortion as harmful and detrimental to both the foetus/child and service users, (3) construct abortion as immoral and abortion-seekers as sinful, and ultimately (4) delegitimise abortion as a resolution to a pregnancy. Our analysis of the micro-narratives about counselling experiences shows the conflict, doubt, and hurt produced by the directive anti-abortion counselling practices described, thereby enabling a recognition of these counselling practices as *harm*.

These directive anti-abortion counselling practices perpetuate and are shaped by patriarchal relations of power in healthcare that patronisingly position abortion-seekers as needing three things from counselling. First, (instructive) guidance about what is in their own "best interests." Being ignorant, the abortion service user must be informed about the "dangers" of abortion. Second, they need to be responsibilised into "proper" reproductive subjects. Patriarchal anti-abortion discourses imagine people with uteri and abortion service users necessarily as cis women and therefore as always already mothers (Radi 2020), and construct abortion as antithetical to biological and gestational motherhood and cis womanhood (Kumar et al. 2009; Millar 2017). Third, abortion-seekers need to be "rescued" from themselves, specifically their "ignorance" of the "awful nature" of abortion.

Returning to our initial discussion of the WHO (2019) definition of the safety of abortion, we have noted that while directive abortion counselling is discouraged, it is not recognised as (potentially) psychologically *harmful* to abortion-seekers. Such counselling may create or exacerbate doubt, decisional and moral conflict, emotional turmoil, and psychological distress, as seen in our findings. Most people who present at abortion clinics have already decided on the pregnancy outcome and for many, terminating the pregnancy is the only option (Brown 2013; Kumar et al. 2004). Thus, counsellors'—who carry the weight of expert authority in the clinic setting—presentation of adoption or parenting as inherently preferable and viable options disregards clients' knowledge of their own circumstances, and what clients' desires might be. The construction of this "alternative" serves simply to create anguish and to place the abortion-seeker (presumed(cis) woman) in a conflictual situation where forgoing abortion is constructed as the only way to reconcile this conflict.

The safety of legal abortion services is undermined through the harms created by directive anti-abortion counselling identified in our analysis. We argue that this harm must be recognised and, more importantly, adequate steps for prevention need to be laid out. How may such prevention be effected following Reproductive Justice principles and critical discursive approaches? We argue that it may be achieved through policies and guidelines and abortion care curricular and training that recognises:

- directive counselling as a threat to the safety of legal abortion;
- that the discourses underpinning directive anti-abortion counselling act as a form of psychological reproductive control that regulates reproductive decision-making by delegitimising abortion as a safe, moral, common, beneficial, and appropriate way to resolve a pregnancy. In doing so, abortion-seekers' rights not to have children, to have children and parent them under conditions of their choosing, and to have an abortion with *dignity* are violated and undermined;
- that, in the context of inequitable access to healthcare, directive abortion counselling in the public sector adds to the racialised, classed, and gendered burden of injustices. Abortion-seekers from black, poor, and rural communities will be disproportionately burdened by the harms of directive counselling and then by lack of access to psychological support that might address these harms. Likewise, black, poor, and rural abortion-seekers bear the greater burden of infertility or death from illegal abortion. Anti-abortion counselling in the public sector may contribute to this where abortion-seekers have no recourse to private abortion care which may or may not be non-directive;
- the violence/harm and inaccessibility of cis-normative patriarchal reproductive healthcare for trans, non-binary, gender non-conforming, and intersex people with uteri (InterAct and Lambda Legal 2018; Luvuno, Ncama and Mchunu 2019; Strand and Smit n.d.; Moseson et al. 2020, 2022; Riggs et al. 2020) and that dominant cis-normative understandings of abortion may create further burdens of injustice and harm for black, low-income and poor, and rural abortion seekers who are trans, non-binary, gender non-conforming, and/or intersex.

A Reproductive Justice perspective underscores the duty of the state and societies/communities to remove the burden of injustice by creating conditions for reproductive freedom, and dignity (Ross 2017). Regarding safe legal abortion, this requires international bodies such as the WHO and states such as South Africa to acknowledge the harms of directive abortion counselling and to commit resources and training to ensure that abortion providers conduct non-mandatory, client-centred, feminist abortion counselling. To that effect, we developed a step-by-step guide to non-directive abortion counselling based on the broader findings of this study (Mavuso et al. 2018).

In the guide, we present abortion counselling that supports abortion service users' reproductive autonomy and dignity, affirms their decision-making capacity, is responsive to their varying needs, and recognises abortion-seekers' gender and sexual diversity. Specifically, non-directive abortion counselling is envisioned where providers: (1) use gender-inclusive terms[4] instead of "women" to refer to service users; (2) enable service users to opt in/out of abortion counselling and, for those who do opt in, to choose the kind of counselling that would support their needs, including opting in/out of specific discussions or "information"; (3) are attentive to and adopt the discursive frames and narratives abortion-seekers use to describe their pregnancies and relationships to them; (4) recognise and exclude normative anti-abortion discourses (e.g., abortion as an interruption of desirable motherhood) from counselling; (5) counter abortion stigma by normalising abortion as a safe, moral, beneficial, and common reproductive practice and form of care, and by validating abortion-seekers' diverse experiences of abortion; and (6) presenting factually accurate information when requested by the client (e.g., that abortion performed safely does not, in and of itself, lead to increased psychological distress compared to taking an unwanted pregnancy to term).

NOTES

1. This is a direct quote; "women" are the imagined abortion service users in the CTOP Act.

2. Townships are urban areas designated from the late 1800s until the end of apartheid for "non-white" residents who were to serve as labour to adjacent "white" cities and towns. They generally continue to be under-resourced and under-serviced compared to historically white residential areas.

3. Italics indicates emphasis.

4. This is only one of several changes necessary to create sex- and gender-affirming abortion care for all. See Moseson et al. (2020) for a list of such changes.

REFERENCES

Assis, Mariana. P, and Sara Larrea. 2020. "Why Self-Managed Abortion Is So Much More Than a Provisional Solution for Times of Pandemic." *Sexual and Reproductive Health Matters* 28 (1): 1–3. https://doi.org/10.1080/26410397.2020 .1779633.

Bantjes, Jason, Ashraf Kagee, and Charles Young. 2016. "Counselling Psychology in South Africa." *Counselling Psychology Quarterly* 29 (2): 171–83. https://doi.org/10.1080/09515070.2015.1128401.

Beckman, Linda J. 2016. "Abortion in the United States: The Continuing Controversy." *Feminism & Psychology* 27 (1): 101–13. https://doi.org/10.1177/0959353516685345.

Beynon-Jones, Siân M. 2013. "Expecting Motherhood? Stratifying Reproduction in 21st-century Scottish Abortion Practice." *Sociology* 47 (3): 509–25. https://doi.org/10.1177/0038038512453797.

———. 2017. "Untroubling Abortion: A Discourse Analysis of Women's Accounts." *Feminism & Psychology* 27 (2): 225–42. https://doi.org/10.1177/0959353517696515.

Bimha, Primrose Z. J., and Rachelle Chadwick. 2016. "Making the Childfree Choice: Perspectives of Women Living in South Africa." *Journal of Psychology in Africa* 26(5): 449–56. https://doi.org/10.1080/14330237.2016.1208952.

Birdsey, Graeme, Tamaryn L. Crankshaw, Sean Mould, and Serela S. Ramklass. 2016. "Unmet Counselling Need Amongst Women Accessing an Induced Abortion Service in KwaZulu-Natal, South Africa." *Contraception* 94: 473–77. https://doi.org/10.1016/j.contraception.2016.07.002.

Brown, Sally. 2013. "Is Counselling Necessary? Making the Decision to Have an Abortion. A Qualitative Interview Study." *The European Journal of Contraception & Reproductive Health Care* 18 (1): 44–48. https://doi.org/10.3109/13625187.2012.750290.

Choice on Termination of Pregnancy Act No. 92. 1996. *South African Government Gazette* 377 (17602). Cape Town.

Ely, Gretchen E., Rebecca S. R. Polmanteer, and Jenni Kotting. 2018. "A Trauma-Informed Social Work Framework for the Abortion Seeking Experience." *Social Work in Mental Health* 16 (2): 172–200. https://doi.org/10.1080/15332985.2017.1369485.

Gaffney, Adam, and Danny McCormick. 2017. "The Affordable Care Act: Implications for Health-Care Equity." *Lancet* 389 (10077): 1442–52. https://doi.org/10.1016/S0140-6736(17)30786-9.

Harries, Jane, Caitlin Gerdts, Mariette Momberg, and Diane G. Foster. 2015. "An Exploratory Study of What Happens to Women Who Are Denied Abortions in Cape Town, South Africa." *Reproductive Health* 12: 21–26. https://doi.org/10.1186/s12978-015-0014-y.

Hodes, Rebecca. 2016. "The Culture of Illegal Abortion in South Africa." *Journal of Southern African Studies* 42 (1): 79–93. https://doi.org/10.1080/03057070.2016.1133086.

Hoggart, Lesley. 2015. "Abortion Counselling in Britain: Understanding the Controversy." *Sociology Compass* 9 (5): 365–78. https://doi.org/10.1111/soc4.12256.

InterAct and Lambda Legal. 2018. Providing ethical and compassionate healthcare to intersex patients: Intersex-affirming hospital policies. https://www.lambdalegal

.org/sites/default/files/publications/downloads/resource_20180731_hospital-poli-cies-intersex.pdf

Jewkes, Rachel K., Tebogo Gumede, Margaret S. Westaway, Kim Dickson, Heather Brown, and Helen Rees. 2005. "Why are Women Still Aborting Outside Designated Facilities in Metropolitan South Africa?" *BJOG: An International Journal of Obstetrics and Gynaecology* 112: 1236–42. https://doi.org/10.1111/j.1471-0528.2005.00697.x.

Kimport, Katrina, Diane G., Foster, and Tracy A. Weitz. 2011. "Social Sources of Women's Emotional Difficulty After Abortion: Lessons from Women's Abortion Narratives." *Perspectives on Sexual and Reproductive Health* 43 (2): 103–09. https://doi.org/10.1363/4310311.

Kumar, Anuradha, Leila Mitchell, and Ellen M. H. Hessini. 2009. "Conceptualising Abortion Stigma." *Culture, Health & Sexuality: An International Journal for Research, Intervention and Care* 11 (6): 625–39. http://dx.doi.org/10.1080/13691050902842741.

Kumar, Usha, Paula Baraitser, Sheila Morton, and Helen Massil. 2004. "Decision Making and Referral Prior to Abortion: A Qualitative Study of Women's Experiences." *BMJ Sexual & Reproductive Health* 30 (1): 51–54. http://dx.doi.org/10.1783/147118904322702009.

Luvuno, Zamasomi P. B., Busisiwe Ncama, and Gugu Mchunu. 2019. "Transgender Population's Experiences with Regard to Accessing Reproductive Health Care in KwaZulu-Natal, South Africa: A Qualitative Study." *African Journal of Primary Health Care & Family Medicine* 11 (1): a1933. https://doi.org/10.4102/phcfm.v11i1.1933.

Macleod, Catriona. 2012. "Feminist Health Psychology and Abortion: Towards a Politics of Transversal Relations of Commonality." In *Advances in Health Psychology,* edited by C. Horrocks and S. Johnson, 153–68. Basingstoke: Palgrave Macmillan.

Major, Brenda, Mark Appelbaum, Linda Beckman, Mary A. Dutton, Nancy F. Russo, and Carolyn West. 2009. "Abortion and Mental Health: Evaluating the Evidence." *American Psychologist* 64 (9): 863–90. http://dx.doi.org/10.1037/a0017497.supp.

Mavuso, Jabulile M. J. 2018. "Narrated Experiences of the Pre-Termination of Pregnancy Counselling Healthcare Encounter in the Eastern Cape Public Health Sector." Unpublished doctoral thesis. Rhodes University, Makhanda, South Africa. http://hdl.handle.net/10962/62928.

Mavuso, Jabulile M. J., and Catriona I. Macleod. 2019. "Contradictions in Womxn's Experiences of Pre-Abortion Counselling in South Africa: Implications for Client-Centred Practice." *Nursing Inquiry.* https://doi.org/10.1111/nin.12330.

Mavuso, Jabulile M. J., Ryan du Toit, Catriona I. Macleod, and Marion Stevens. 2018. *Abortion Counselling in South Africa: A Step-By-Step Guide for Providers.* http://srjc.org.za/wpcontent/uploads/2017/06/Abortion_Counselling_Guide_Version_1-1.pdf.

Mikkelsen, Anders P., Pia Egerup, Julie F. M. Ebert, Astrid M. Kolte, Henriette S. Nielsen, and Øjvind Lidegaard. 2019. "Pregnancy Loss and Cancer Risk: A

Nationwide Observational Study." *EClinicalMedicine* 15: 80–88. https://doi.org /10.1016/j.eclinm.2019.08.017.

Millar, Erica. 2017. *Happy Abortions: Our Bodies in the Era of Choice*. London: Zed Books Ltd.

Möller, Amanda, Sofie Öfverstedt, and Karin Siwe. 2012. "Proud, Not Yet Satisfied: The Experiences of Abortion Service Providers in the Kathmandu Valley, Nepal." *Sexual and Reproductive Healthcare* 3 (1): 135–40. http://dx.doi.org/10.1016/j .srhc.2012.10.003.

Mookamedi, Ramaite E., Sophie M. Mogotlane, and Janetta H. Roos. 2015. "The Experiences of Women Who Undergo Termination of Pregnancy in Mpumalanga Province, South Africa." *Africa Journal of Nursing and Midwifery* 17 (1): 146–61. https://hdl.handle.net/10520/EJC186337.

Morgan, Lynn M., and Meredith Michaels eds. 1999. *Fetal Subjects, Feminist Positions*. Philadelphia: University of Pennsylvania Press.

Morison, Tracy. 2011. "'But What Story?': A Narrative-Discursive Analysis of 'White' Afrikaners' Accounts of Male Involvement in Parenthood Decision-Making." Unpublished doctoral thesis, Rhodes University, South Africa.

Morris-Paxton Angela A., Stephen Reid, and Rose-Marie G. Ewing. 2020. "Primary Healthcare Services in the Rural Eastern Cape, South Africa: Evaluating a Service-Support Project." *African Journal Primary Health Care & Family Medicine* 12 (1): a2207. https://doi.org/10.4102/phcfm.v12i1.2207.

Moseson, Heidi, Noah Zazanis, Eli Goldberg, Laura Fix, Mary Durden, Ari Stoeffler, Jen Hastings, Lyndon Cudlitz, Bori Lesser-Lee, Laz Letcher, Aneidys Reyes, and Juno Obedin-Maliver. 2020. "The Imperative for Transgender and Gender Nonbinary Inclusion." *Obstetrics & Gynecology* 135 (5): 1059–68. https://doi.org /10.1097/AOG.0000000000003816.

Moseson, Heidi, Laura Fix, Caitlin Gerdts, Sachiko Ragosta, Jen Hastings, Ari Stoeffler, Mitchell Lunn, Annesa Flentje, Matthew Capriotti, Micah Lubensky, and Juno Obedin-Maliver. 2022. "Abortion attempts without clinical supervision among transgender, nonbinary and gender-expansive people in the United States." *BMJ Sexual and Reproductive Health* 48: e22–e30.

Mosley, Elizabeth A., Amy J. Schulz, Lisa H. Harris, and Barbara A. Anderson. 2020. "South African Abortion Attitudes from 2007-2016: The Roles of Religiosity and Attitudes Toward Sexuality and Gender Equality." *Women & Health* 60 (7): 806–20. https://doi.org/10.1080/03630242.2020.1746951.

Nixon, Laura. 2013. "The right to (trans) parent: A Reproductive Justice Approach to Reproductive Rights, Fertility, and Family-Building Issues Facing Transgender People." *William & Mary Journal of Race, Gender, and Social Justice* 20 (1): 73–103. https://scholarship.law.wm.edu/wmjowl/vol20/iss1/5.

O'Donnell, Aisling T., Tara O'Carroll, and Natasha Toole. 2018. "Internalized Stigma and Stigma-Related Isolation Predict Women's Psychological Distress and Physical Health Symptoms Post-Abortion." *Psychology of Women Quarterly* 42 (2): 220–34. https://doi.org/10.1177/0361684317748937.

O'Donovan, Dennis. 2006. "Moving Away From 'Falling boys' and 'Passive girls': Gender Meta- Narratives in Gender Equity Policies for Australian Schools and why Micro-Narratives Provide a Better Policy Model." *Discourse: Studies in the Cultural Politics of Education* 27 (4): 475–95. https://doi.org/10.1080/01596300600988655.

Pillay, Anthony L., and Brendon R. Barnes. 2020. "Psychology and COVID-19: Impacts, Themes and Way Forward." *South African Journal of Psychology* 50 (2): 148–53. https://doi.org/10.1177/0081246320937684.

Radi, Blas. 2020. "Reproductive Injustice, Trans Rights, and Eugenics." *Sexual and Reproductive Health Matters* 28 (1): 1824318. https://doi.org/10.1080/26410397.2020.1824318.

Riggs, Damien W., Carla A. Pfeffer, Ruth Pearce, Sally Hines, and Francis R. White. 2020. "Men, Trans/Masculine, and Non-Binary People Negotiating Conception: Normative Resistance and Inventive Pragmatism." *International Journal of Transgender Health.* https://doi.org/10.1080/15532739.2020.1808554.

Ross, Loretta J. 2017. "Reproductive Justice as Intersectional Feminist Activism." *Souls* 19 (3): 286–314. https://doi.org/10.1080/10999949.2017.1389634.

Sparrow, Margaret J. 2004. "A Woman's Choice." *Australian and New Zealand Journal of Obstetrics and Gynaecology* 44: 88–92.

Strand, Mia, and Estian Smit. n.d. *Trans Rural Narratives: Perspectives on the Experiences of Rural-Based Trans and Gender Diverse Persons in South Africa.* Gender DynamiX.

Taylor, Stephanie, and Karen Littleton. 2006. "Biographies in Talk: A Narrative-Discursive Research Approach." *Qualitative Sociology Review* 2 (1): 22–38. http://www.qualitativesociologyreview.org/ENG/Volume3/abstracts.php#art2.

Trueman, Karen A., and Makgoale Magwentshu. 2013. "Abortion in a Progressive Legal Environment: The Need for Vigilance in Protecting and Promoting Access to Safe Abortion Services in South Africa." *American Journal of Public Health* 103: 397–99. https://doi.org/10.2105/AJPH.2012.301194.

Vincent, Louise. 2012. "Shaking a Hornets' Nest: Pitfalls of Abortion Counselling in a Secular Constitutional Order – A View from South Africa." *Culture, Health & Sexuality: An International Journal for Research, Intervention and Care* 14 (2): 125–38. http://dx.doi.org/10.1080/13691058.2011.627469.

Weissman, Anna L. 2017. "Repronormativity and the Reproduction of the Nation-State: The State and Sexuality Collide." *Journal of GLBT Family Studies* 13 (3): 277–305. https://doi.org/10.1080/1550428X.2016.1210065.

World Health Organisation. 2015. *Health Worker Roles in Providing Safe Abortion Care and Post-Abortion Contraception.* https://www.who.int/reproductivehealth/publications/unsafe_abortion/abortion-task-shifting/en/.

———. 2019. *Preventing Unsafe Abortion: Evidence Brief.* https://apps.who.int/iris/bitstream/handle/10665/329887/WHO-RHR-19.21-eng.pdf.

Conclusion

Jabulile Mary-Jane Jace Mavuso and Tracy Morison

Since its inception in the 1990s, the concept of Reproductive Justice has steadily gained traction and is widely used as a framework for social justice activism. In more recent years, scholars across a range of disciplines have also begun engaging with the concept to explore a variety of social issues related to sexuality and reproduction (Luna and Luker 2013; Ross 2017). Discussing its growing uptake among scholars, Ross and Solinger (2017, 71) comment that Reproductive Justice has served as "an open source code that people have used to pursue fresh critical thinking regarding power and powerlessness . . . [and] an important contribution to political and social analysis of reproductive politics."

Echoing this assertion, Eaton and Stephens (2020, 4) point to the value of this conceptual framework for psychologists in particular, in their recent editorial on psychology's engagement with Reproductive Justice. This framework, they assert, "offers the opportunity to redefine and revolutionise our field—moving us from making incremental contributions to knowledge to taking leaps of understanding in established and new domains of inquiry." Inspired by these insights, and our own work and thinking about Sexual and Reproductive Justice, we set out to edit a book that builds on the important contribution(s) that the Sexual and Reproductive Justice framework has made, and continues to make, to knowledge production and activism.

We have brought together diverse perspectives on issues that have to date not been (sufficiently) explored from a Sexual and Reproductive Justice perspective, as well as work from locations beyond the Global North where much of the Sexual and Reproductive Justice scholarship is produced. Our aim is not only to add new knowledge but also to purposefully push against the global politics of location and knowledge production that privilege certain voices and perspectives over others. We thus attend to voices and groups not ordinarily featured in scholarship taking a Sexual and Reproductive Justice perspective.

Our decision to title this volume *From the margins to the centre* is intentional and political. Indeed, the book is the culmination of us asking: What possibilities for, engagements with and understandings of Sexual and Reproductive Justice will be made visible and amplified by centring peripheried perspectives? Returning to these questions in this final chapter, we discuss the contributions to this volume in terms of how they can push understandings of sexual and reproductive injustices, and the conditions needed to achieve justice.

We reflect on the chapters in terms of the contributions they make to: (1) understanding in/exclusions within RJ as a movement/theory/praxis, (2) expanding the lens by incorporating issues of sexuality, (3) Sexual and Reproductive Justice for young people, (4) the right to supportive conditions for birthing and parenting, and (5) reproductive decision-making and the right to *not* have a child. Although we discuss the chapters in this way, many straddle these distinctions. Indeed, a strength of this volume is that it showcases the interconnections between issues and injustices.

IN/EXCLUSIONS IN SEXUAL AND REPRODUCTIVE JUSTICE SCHOLARSHIP AND MOVEMENTS

Sexual and Reproductive Justice: From the Margins to the Centre, as a collection, sheds light on the experiences of those who are normatively disregarded as sexual and/or reproductive subjects (sometimes even within Sexual and Reproductive Justice scholarship). Equally, many of the contributions challenge normative assumptions, patterns, and practices about who knowledge producers are. In doing so, they invite critical reflection about the conditions that produce sexual and reproductive oppressions, and the conditions needed to secure sexual and reproductive justice that is broad and wide-ranging enough to be fully inclusive of all people and groups and that is therefore fully *just*.

The scholarship brought together in this volume speaks to a range of violence perpetrated by the state, and individuals, enacted through oppressive policies, laws, and practices that regulate sexual and reproductive capacities, freedoms, dignity, and integrity. Much of this work focusses on oppressive healthcare and legislation, showcasing these as key sites of sexual and reproductive injustice. These chapters call us to think critically about the very limited and harmful kinds of "*health*" and "*care*" supported through the health and legal systems. As such, they invite serious consideration of *whose* and *which* rights are recognised and valued through our laws and democracies, and the implications this entails for our efforts to engender Sexual and Reproductive Justice through human rights frameworks.

Outside of healthcare and law enforcement, some of the contributions illuminate injustices produced in/through workplaces, communities, families, and intimate partnerships. Several chapters speak to the sexual and reproductive injustices produced through neoliberal governance and/or the ways in which neo-liberalism quite simply cannot engender sexual and reproductive justice. Collectively, the contributions in this volume show how eradicating sexual and reproductive injustices necessarily relies on the eradication of intersecting classist, racist, colonial, ciscentric, hetero-patriarchal, ableist, ageist, and other power relations— with which sexual and reproductive injustices are interconnected.

Several chapters contribute to the decolonial project of deconstruction and reconstruction, which entails "reclaiming our humanity; rebuilding our territorial and bodily integrity; reasserting our self-determination; restoring our spirituality; dismantling the material and symbolic foundations of the colonial-capitalist state; decentering Western hegemonies of knowledge and cultures regarding race, gender, sexuality, etc." (Tamale 2020, 21). In doing so, some chapters take a decolonial approach to Sexual and Reproductive Justice, by how historical and contemporary (neo)colonial power relations and systems produce and maintain sexual and reproductive oppression.

Others call attention to and critique colonising, and therefore homogenising and exclusionary, approaches to knowledge production and activism on reproductive politics and oppression. These authors demonstrate that, far from being "neutral" or inherently just, systems of knowledge and social justice praxis continue to be important sites of sexual and reproductive injustice when based upon colonising and exclusionary approaches. Their work requires us to recognise that a commitment to achieving Sexual and Reproductive Justice for *all* necessitates that we direct our efforts inwards, towards the movement itself as well as internally through personal reflection, just as much as we direct efforts outwards. Indeed, as the long activist and scholarly traditions of visibilising and speaking to power have shown, there are no spaces that are unshaped by systems of oppression and privilege.

EXPANDING THE LENS: SEXUAL *AND* REPRODUCTIVE JUSTICE

The chapters in the first half of this volume raise issues and amplify the experiences of groups that, while sometimes acknowledged, are often not specifically or substantially addressed from a Reproductive Justice perspective, though sometimes covered in sexual citizenship or sexual health and rights scholarship.

Several authors engage with sexual health, rights, and agency in its own right (Le Grice, chapter 3; Mabenge, chapter 5; Abrahams, chapter 6) showing that Sexual and Reproductive Justice can be used as a framework for exploring injustices that may not have reproductive consequences. These chapters illuminate the conditions that undermine sexual freedom and bodily integrity. Others consider the complex and compounding intersections between sexual and reproductive injustices (Nkala-Dlamini and Thwala, chapter 3; Stevens et al., chapter 1). Along with Parker's (chapter 7), these chapters extend understandings of how reproductive oppression occurs through the denigration and denial of various marginalised groups' reproduction.

Sexual Justice

Calling on scholars to think seriously and more expansively about sexual freedom and bodily integrity, both inside and outside of the Sexual and Reproductive Justice framework and movement, the work in this volume expands understandings of these. It shows that efforts to ensure sexual justice must necessarily include: (i) freedom from sexual violence, including freedom to practice and be supported by Indigenous ways of knowing, responding to, and eradicating sexual violence; and (ii) freedom to engage in and to earn a living from sex and sexual intimacies without state or individual intrusion or violence. These freedoms, and the ability to exercise sexual dignity and self-determination, require equitable access to accurate and full information and education about sex. These freedoms just as importantly require queer and gender affirming primary and psychological care.

Le Grice et al. highlight the ways in which tikanga and mātauranga Māori (Indigenous practices and understandings) are devalued and supplanted by Eurocentric mainstream therapeutic approaches to sexual violence. These individualistic approaches clash with the holistic approaches to healing and restitution practised by Māori. The authors demonstrate how individualising therapeutic approaches to sexual violence overlook important familial, cultural, social, and spiritual consequences of sexual violence for Māori, producing further material and symbolic harm and injustice, including the violation of mana (status) and tino rangatiratanga (self-determination), and preventing healing from sexual violence. This study not only highlights Indigenous people's unique contributions to Sexual and Reproductive Justice but also underscores the need to support Indigenous expertise and practices in *decolonial* ways.

Much of the Sexual and Reproductive Justice scholarship tends to view those who are capable of pregnancy as the singular, default subjects of sexual and reproductive in/justice, focusing largely on endosex (i.e. non-intersex) cisgender heterosexual women's experiences. This focus provides a narrow understanding of reproductive injustices faced by people with the capacity to gestate and excludes the experiences of those without this capacity, both of which include intersex, trans, and non-binary people, as well as cisgender men and women. Both Mabenge's and Abrahams' chapters underscore that accessible gender-affirming primary and mental healthcare is indispensable to gender-inclusive *Sexual* and Reproductive Justice, and that attending to the inter-workings of racist and colonial, cis-normative/anti-trans, and classist/ anti-poor systems is essential.

Mabenge shows how these systems rely on binaried (in terms of class and gender) healthcare provision that denies or produces dehumanising "care" so that gender-affirming care is out of reach for many of the black trans and gender diverse South Africans who seek it. Mabenge's chapter makes a crucial South African contribution to trans/Sexual and Reproductive Justice scholarship. Much of the scholarship is produced by Global North scholars and has tended to focus on forced sterilisation. It predominantly centres the reproductive injustices that trans men are subjected to, to the exclusion of trans women (Cárdenas 2016) and non-binary people.

Psychology's role in maintaining dehumanising and harmful systems is spotlighted in Abrahams's chapter. The chapter traces how South African psychological knowledge production and practice reinforce and legitimate cis-heteronormative and anti-queer understandings of gender, sex, and sexual orientation; pathologise queer identities; and render mental healthcare inaccessible. This culminates in "care" that is dehumanising and psychologically harmful to sexually and gender diverse people, especially working class and poor people of colour.

Abrahams shows how psychology professionals can and should use the Sexual and Reproductive Justice approach to understand and disrupt the workings of systems of power, including role in upholding these systems. If psychological healthcare is to be truly *accessible*, it must be socially just: it should always work to affirm queer peoples' sex, gender, and sexual orientation identities. The development of accessible identity-affirming mental healthcare is one way in which the profession can and should answer Grzanka and Frantell's (2017) call to make psychology in service of Sexual and Reproductive Justice.

Connections between Sexual and Reproductive In/Justice

In their sex worker-informed and co-produced contribution (chapter 1), Stevens et al. highlight the interrelated sexual and reproductive injustices perpetrated by the state (police and healthcare), family and communities, and clients against gender non-conforming and cisgender sex workers who are mothers. They show how the criminalisation of sex work is underpinned by capitalist and patriarchal gender relations. In contrast to hegemonic/colonising feminist approaches, which exclude sex workers, and sexual and reproductive health and justice approaches, which preclude sex workers as *mothers*, Stephens and colleagues show how sex work is vital to caring for children and families. The criminalisation of sex work therefore violates sex workers' sexual and reproductive health and rights, including their right to parent safely and free from violence. Their work underscores the fact that the full decriminalisation of sex work is necessary to achieve sexual and reproductive justice.

Disability-focussed research on sexual and reproductive services, health, and rights tends to overlook young people, while adolescence-focussed research neglects disability. Nkala-Dlamini and Twala's chapter (chapter 3) therefore makes a unique contribution to both these bodies of work. Their study concerns the re/production of sexual and reproductive injustices in a South African residential care facility for disabled youth. The chapter shows the limitations of sexual and reproductive health, rights, and justice, when informed by ableist and ageist ideals of sexual and reproductive citizenship/subjectivity and norms about sex and reproduction inform. Coercive practices undertaken to 'protect' intellectually disabled adolescents from sexual violence and pregnancy preclude their agency and deny them the right to self-determination and dignity, sexual freedom, and pleasure, as well as the right to have children under conditions of their choosing, and to parent them in safe and supportive environments.

Parker's exploration of "maternal obesity" through a Reproductive Justice lens (chapter 7) uses a form of critical discourse analysis, incorporating intersectionality. This analysis illuminates the intersection of fat reproductive oppression with other axes of oppression, including racism and classism, showing the particularly harmful effects on fat pregnant people who are poor and/or of colour. Parker pinpoints the role of the neoliberal discourse of healthism as a technology of social control that places responsibility on individuals for attaining normative prescriptions and restricts fat people's bodily and reproductive agency. Parker's work not only demonstrates the ways that pregnancy fatness is problematised in health-care spaces, but also speaks to using the findings of Reproductive Justice research to construct resistant "counter stories" of reproductive bodies and to stimulate social change. Parker's chapter thus offers an expanded view of reproductive *health* and *justice*, both of which must be re-envisioned and re-shaped around the reproductive dignity and self-determination of fat, poor, queer people of colour.

SEXUAL AND REPRODUCTIVE
JUSTICE FOR YOUNG PEOPLE

Normative socio-cultural discourses infantilise adolescents and prescribe abstinence as the best solution to the "problems" of teenage sexuality and reproduction (Hans and White 2019; Macleod 2001). Although some sexual and reproductive health research recognises young people's agency in sexual decision-making, mainstream researchers tend to assume that youth sexual and reproductive health necessarily excludes parenthood (Mavuso and Macleod 2020). The emphasis is therefore on "safer sex" and preventing "unplanned pregnancy." The risk discourse that dominates discussions of youth sexuality focuses on individual choice and responsibility. It obscures the social, systemic, and structural systems of power delimiting choices and action and also masks the gendered ways in which adolescents are responsibilised for young parenthood (Chiweshe, Fetters and Coast 2021; Morison and Herbert 2018).

In contrast, several contributions in this volume (Nkala-Dlamini and Twala, chapter 3; Nkala-Dlamini and Nkomo, chapter 6; Alexander, chapter 10; and Ngabaza and Shefer, chapter 11) contribute to a critical understandings of young people as rights-bearing sexual and reproductive subjects with the right to parent in supportive conditions. These chapters, as we discuss below, explore the ways in which various systems, including the ageism/adultism supported by developmental psychology, constrain decision-making, agency, and freedoms.

Expanding the analytical focus beyond cisgender women's experiences, Nkala-Dlamini and Nkomo's (chapter 6) critical reading of young cisgender men's desire for fatherhood demonstrates how a Reproductive Justice approach can shift analyses of the negotiation of heterosex and reproduction beyond the inclusion of men simply as (problematic) actors in women's reproductive lives. This allows for a more nuanced approach, in which young men can be viewed as reproductive subjects whose desires, decision-making, and practices are informed by hetero-gendered narratives of sexuality, reproduction, and parenthood.

Furthermore, using the power-focussed lens of Reproductive Justice, it is also possible to illuminate how dominant hetero-patriarchal understandings create power imbalances in the negotiation of heterosex and heterosexual procreation and how these are reinforced by the structural context (Morison and Macleod 2015). The focus for intervention in problematic practices related to sex and reproduction (such as reproductive coercion or gender-based violence) shifts from problematic young men (and young people more generally) to conscientising young people and creating spaces conducive to resisting problematic hetero-patriarchal scripts and generating alternative understandings that promote equity and justice.

Another important way through which young people's sexual and reproductive decision-making, freedoms, and dignity are governed is through gendered, race-, and class-based norms. Thus, Alexander (chapter 10) shows how gender norms that prescribe respectable femininity for coloured women are entwined with classed and racialised ideals of respectability for coloured people. She demonstrates how shaming works to enforce these ideals and to ensure that the "ordentlike" (decent/respectable) coloured woman reserves sexual engagement and childbearing for (married) adulthood. Young women are shamed for "early" sexuality and reproduction, deemed "vrot" (rotten or spoiled), and their mothers are chastised for "failing" to produce "ordentlike" coloured women.

Alexander's work underscores the importance of centring young mothers' own accounts of their sexual and reproductive experiences, decision-making, and desires. Doing so spotlights instances where families normalise and accept young mothering and demonstrates how raced, classed, and gendered identity meaning-making are dynamic, ongoing processes. It also enables us to envision Sexual and Reproductive Justice where young women's sexual agency is supported, and where young mothers are supported in their parenting.

Underscoring the preceding chapters, Ngabaza and Shefer's (chapter 11) critical literature review highlights the fundamental shift that needs to take place in the conceptualisation of "youth" to allow for sexuality education pedagogy that works towards gender, sexual, and reproductive justice. Their critical literature review highlights how, similar to other countries, South African sexuality education problematises youth (hetero)sexuality and reproduction as "irresponsible", positioning young people as simultaneously "at-risk" and "a risk" to themselves, others, and society at large. The authors invite readers to envisage pedagogy that addresses youth as sexual subjects capable of co-constructing knowledge, rather than passive recipients of adult instruction.

THE RIGHT TO SUPPORTIVE CONDITIONS
FOR BIRTHING AND PARENTING

Birth Justice is a component of Reproductive Justice that spotlights the racial, socio-economic, gender, and sexual inequalities that lead to negative birth experiences and outcomes, particularly for queer people, women of colour, low-income women, survivors of violence, immigrant women, and women in the Global South (Diaz-Tello and Paltrow 2020; Oparah & Chinyere 2015). Following the values and principles of the Sexual and Reproductive Justice movement, Birth Justice advocates and scholars argue for "the right to choose whether or not to carry a pregnancy, to choose when, where, how, and with whom to birth, including access to traditional and indigenous birth-workers, such as midwives and doulas, and the right to breastfeeding support" (Black Women Birthing Justice 2020). Birth Justice also underscores the right to access culturally safe, affordable, timely, high-quality, equitable, and dignified care during and after pregnancy.

Obstetric care is recognised as a potential site of reproductive oppression in both research on obstetric violence (Chadwick 2021) and Reproductive Justice scholarship (Luna and Luker 2013). These hitherto separate bodies of work are brought together in Dutton and Knight's (chapter 8) analysis of provider–patient interactions in obstetric care. Focussing on the interacting systems of power that structure obstetric care, and through which midwives are simultaneously privileged and oppressed, they avoid a simplistic perpetrator/victim dichotomy that often arises in mainstream reproductive health and rights research. Instead, they offer a nuanced understanding of midwives and nurses working in under-resourced public obstetric care. They are at once perpetrators (of material and symbolic violence) and victims (of the wider denigration of reproductive labour), and their individual acts of compassion also rupture dominant ways of being in these settings. While demonstrations of compassion in an otherwise fraught space are important, individual acts cannot engender reproductive justice. Rather, reproductive justice requires working to end the injustices faced by both patients and midwives by dismantling the systems and structures supporting oppressive practices.

Turning to the right to parent under safe and supportive conditions, Saunders (chapter 9) focuses on economically marginalised mothers living in a wealthy country (Scotland). She highlights the structural and political barriers to having and raising children faced by these women in her Bourdieusian analysis of everyday accounts of raising children and parenting practices. The analysis attends to the ways motherhood is disciplined through neoliberal and class-based ideals of motherhood that are articulated in policy and subtly and insidiously re/produced in mundane everyday practices. Saunders shows how conceptions of "good" motherhood are predicated upon neoliberal and middle-class norms that uphold classed inequalities. These ideals stipulate an individualised and entrepreneurial parenting approach to be considered a "good" mother, and ultimately absolves the state from its responsibilities to provide supportive and equitable conditions for parenting. This chapter usefully adds to Reproductive Justice scholarship on motherhood and parenting by showing how wider systems of oppression and inequity impinge upon commonplace caregiving practices, reinforcing class-based and racialised hierarchies of "good motherhood."

REPRODUCTIVE DECISION-MAKING AND
THE RIGHT NOT TO HAVE A CHILD

The right to decide whether or not to carry a pregnancy is a long-standing focus of Reproductive Justice activism and scholarship (Macleod et al. 2017). However, restricting or denying abortion access is not the only way that the state intervenes in this decision. Two contributions to this volume expand understanding of reproductive oppression in this area by attending to the reproductive politics of the prosecution of women for infanticide and concealment of birth (Burry et al., chapter 12) and contraceptive agency in healthcare consultations (Morison et al., chapter 13).

Burry et al.'s analysis of judicial cases in the Pacific Islands (Fiji, Papua New Guinea, Solomon Islands, Vanuatu, Samoa, and Tonga) where women were tried for infanticide and concealment of birth illuminates how Pasifika women's right to choose whether or not to carry a pregnancy is restricted by a hetero-patriarchal, colonial construction of motherhood. The authors show how laws on infanticide and concealment of birth invoke a highly circum-scribed ideal of femininity, punishing any deviation, including seeking not to have (more) children. This essentialising and individualised construction of motherhood also obscures the highly unsupportive conditions and the vari-ous injustices the women face, attributing their attempts to end pregnancy or conceal birth to personal "failings" or "deficiency," thereby absolving state and social responsibility for their lack of support.

The authors argue that understandings of motherhood upon which laws and policies are based need to take "proper account of the nuanced nature of women's lives, their capacity for reproductive autonomy, and the contexts in which they are trying to parent." This chapter thus brings home the signifi-cance of physical, emotional, material, social, and economic support in rela-tion to pregnancy decisions (Macleod 2018). Importantly, when considering if a pregnancy is supportable, it ought to be those facing unwanted or unin-tended pregnancy who should ultimately define what supportability means in their unique circumstances on the basis that they are best placed to do so.

Morison et al. (chapter 13) use a post-structuralist theoretical framework to "operationalise" Reproductive Justice theory in their analysis of patients' accounts of contraceptive counselling and decision-making. The analysis shows the value of using this theoretical lens to extend analyses and under-standings of contraceptive coercion, such that agency can be limited even in contexts where voluntary rights-based care is endorsed by contraceptive providers. Using a Reproductive Justice lens to highlight the intersecting relations of power in participants' constructions of interactions with con-traceptive providers, the authors show how contraceptive agency is limited by hierarchical patient–provider interactions, as well as racial and gendered power relations based on classist and racist determinations around who should/should not procreate.

In the last chapter (chapter 14), Mavuso et al. extend thinking on Reproductive Justice and abortion, as well as understandings of abortion safety, by focussing on South African abortion counselling services. Their analysis highlights how anti-abortion discourses and the directive anti-abortion counselling they engender, rely on cis-normative and anti-trans discourses that unproblematically construct of abortion-seekers, and pregnant people more generally, as (cisgender) women. These discourses are harmful and their use in abortion counselling undermines the "safety" of abortion care for pregnant people, including intersex, trans, gender non-conforming people, and cisgender women. Abortion-seekers who are black and working-class/poor are especially marginalised by capitalist and racist systems that create inequitable access to mental healthcare, leaving them to self-manage the harms produced by anti-abortion counselling. Mavuso et al. thus argue that achieving humanising and dignified abortion care and service provision means that abortion counselling must be underpinned by counselling guidelines that recognise the sexual and gender diversity of abortion-seekers, and counteract patriarchal anti-abortion discourses that "awfulise" abortion (Hadley 1997).

CONCLUSION

In many ways, *Sexual and Reproductive Justice: From the Margins to the Centre* challenges what has become normative for understanding sexual and reproductive health and justice: the issues and topics which a Sexual and Reproductive Justice approach is perhaps considered appropriate to explore; what Sexual and Reproductive Justice is and what it can and should look like; who the beneficiaries-actors of Sexual and Reproductive Justice activism are (and should be); who Sexual and Reproductive Justice knowledge producers and consumers are (and should be); and who is acknowledged as a sexual and reproductive citizen and subject.

Simultaneously, however, this volume reflects normative ways of speaking/writing about and imagining sexual and reproductive subjects. Thus, while our volume contributes to scholarship that recognises the sexual and gender diversity of sexual and reproductive subjects and victims of sexual and reproductive oppressions, most of the chapters in this volume speak to the perspectives and experiences of cisgender women with uteri, and none addresses sexual and reproductive injustices faced by intersex people. This pattern reflects much of the English-language literature referenced throughout this book, which similarly casts pregnancy-capable cisgender women as the default and primary subjects of sexual and reproductive health and justice scholarship and activism. In doing so, much sexual and reproductive scholarship excludes and marginalises various people with and without uteri, including intersex, trans, non-binary, and gender non-conforming people, women, and men, *as well as* some cisgender women and cisgender men. Just as importantly, the assumption that sexual and reproductive subjects are non-disabled operates as an unacknowledged presence shaping much sexual and reproductive health and justice research and scholarship. Our book is no exception: only one chapter attends to the intersection of ableism with other oppressions. So, too, there is only a single chapter that addresses weight stigma and fat oppression in reproductive injustice, while none addresses the ways in which the criminalisation of migration shapes sexual and reproductive injustices (Keygnaert, Guieu, Ooms, Vettenburg, Temmerman, and Roelens, 2013).

Thus, while we believe that the value of this collection of chapters offered here is that it makes visible systems of power and the ways that they work in interacting and intersecting ways to constrain and devalue sexual and reproductive decision-making, capacities, and freedoms, we also recognise how our book is just as much a *product* of these systems in the ways they shape knowledge production. In other words, in telling stories of the sexual and/or reproductive oppressions of various groups, identities, and subjects and their resistances to these oppressions, we are keenly aware that our book is predicated on the privileging of certain identities and subjects in/through that telling. We hope, then, that the strengths *and* limitations of this volume encourage further critical and reflexive engagement from a Sexual and Reproductive Justice perspective with the stories told about sex, gender, sexuality, pregnancy, and reproduction, those told about Sexual and Reproductive Justice, and the ways in which these stories are themselves implicated in and shape sexual and reproductive injustices.

We return to the question posed at the start of this final chapter, keeping in mind that most people's sexual and reproductive lives are shaped by occupying identities that are at once privileged/centred and oppressed/peripheried. What can the centre learn from those who "stand at the edges and claim them as central" (OluTimehin Kukoyi 2021)? Many, many books' worth. We offer our own book as *part* of that multitude.

REFERENCES

Cárdenas, Micha. 2016. "Pregnancy: Reproductive Futures in Trans of Color Feminism." *TSQ: Transgender Studies Quarterly* 3(1–2): 48–57.

Chadwick, Rachelle. 2021. "Breaking the Frame: Obstetric Violence and Epistemic Rupture." *Agenda* 1–12. doi: 10.1080/10130950.2021.1958554.

Chiweshe, Malvern Tatenda, Tamara Fetters, and Ernestina Coast. 2021. "Whose Bodies Are They? Conceptualising Reproductive Violence Against Adolescents in Ethiopia, Malawi and Zambia." *Agenda* 1–12. doi: 10.1080/10130950.2021.1964220.

Eaton, Asia A., and Dionne P. Stephens. 2020. "Reproductive Justice: Moving the Margins to the Center in Social Issues Research." *Journal of Social Issues* 2: 208–18. https://doi.org/10.1111/josi.12384.

Hadley, Janet. 1997. "The 'awfulisation' of abortion." *Choices* 26(1): 7–8.

Itriyeva, Khalida. 2018. "Use of Long-Acting Reversible Contraception (LARCs) and the Depro-Provera Shot in Adolescents." *Current Problems in Pediatric and Adolescent Health Care* 48 (12): 321–32.

Keygnaert, Ines, Aurore Guieu, Gorik Ooms, Nicole Vettenburg, Marleen Temmerman, and Kristien Roelens. 2013. Sexual and reproductive health of migrants: Does the EU care? *Health Policy* 114: 215–25.

Kukoyi, OluTimehin. 2021. "Your Power Ends Where Mine Begins: The Redeeming Freedom of Queerness." *The Republic.* https://republic.com.ng/august-september -2021/redeeming-freedom-queerness/.

Luna, Zakiya, and Kristin Luker. 2013. "Reproductive Justice." *Annual Review of Law and Social Science* 9: 327–52. https://doi.org/10.1146/annurev-lawsocsci -102612-134037.

Macleod, Catriona Ida. 2001. "Teenage Motherhood & Regulation of Mothering in the Scientific Literature: The South African Example." *Feminism & Psychology* 11 (4): 493–510.

Macleod, Catriona Ida. 2018. "Expanding Reproductive Justice through a Supportability Reparative Justice Framework: The Case of Abortion in South Africa." *Culture, Health & Sexuality* Online fir: 1–17. https://doi.org/10.1080 /13691058.2018.1447687.

Macleod, Catriona Ida, Siân Beynon-Jones, Merran Toerien, and Merran Gurney Macleod, Catriona Ida; Beynon-Jones, Sian Maeve; Toerien. 2017. "Articulating Reproductive Justice through Reparative Justice: Case Studies of Abortion in Great Britain and South Africa." *Culture, Health & Sexuality* 19 (5): 601–15. https://doi .org/http://dx.doi.org/10.1080/13691058.2016.1257738.

Mavuso, Jabulile M. J., and Catriona Macleod. 2020. "Pregnancy decision-making: Abortion and adoption." In *The Encyclopaedia of Child and Adolescent Development*, edited by S. Hupp and J. D. Jewell. New Jersey: John Wiley & Sons Inc. doi:10.1002/9781119171492.wecad494.

Morison, Tracy, and Catriona Ida Macleod. 2015. *Men's Pathways to Parenthood: Silence and Heterosexual Gendered Norms.* Cape Town, South Africa: HSRC Press.

Morison, Tracy, and Sarah Herbert. 2020. "Muted resistance: The deployment of youth voice in news coverage of young women's sexuality in Aotearoa New Zealand." *Feminism & Psychology* 30 (1): 80–99. doi: 10.1177/0959353519864376.

Ross, Loretta J. 2017. "Conceptualising Reproductive Justice Theory: A Manifesto for Activism." In *Radical Reproductive Justice: Foundation, Theory, Practice, Critique*, edited by Loretta Ross, Erika Derkas, Whitney Peoples, Lynn Roberts, Pamela Bridgewater, and Dorothy Roberts. New York: Feminist Press at CUNY.

Ross, Loretta J., and Rickie Solinger. 2017. *Reproductive Justice: An Introduction.* Oakland: California University Press.

Tamale, Sylvia. 2020. *Decolonization and Afro-Feminism.* Ottawa: Daraja Press.

Index

abandonment, in primary families and communities, 25–27

abortion, 9–10, 34–35, 276–77; awfulisation discourse of, 252–53; case study, 250–51; counselling services, 248; discourses deployed in directive counselling, 251–55; micro-narratives, 255–58; in South Africa, 249–50

abuse: police of sex workers, 29; in primary families and communities, 25–27; sexual, 210, 215, 216, 218

acceptable masculinity, 113–14

adolescents: human rights of, 74; with intellectual disabilities, 69, 72; obstacles, sexual and reproductive health, 62; sexual and reproductive health in, 62–64. *See also* young people

adolescent sexuality, 178

Alteration of Sex Description and Status Act 49 (2003), 80, 81

ambiguous deaths, 214–16

antenatal care clinic (ANC), 146

anti-abortion counselling, 250

"antiwelfare commonsense," 160

Aotearoa New Zealand: contraceptive care in, 230–31; curtailing Māori community agency, to sexual violence, 48–50; kaupapa Māori research methodology, 46, 47; Māori ingenuity disconnected, through cultural appropriation, 52–54; Māori innovators and experts, 50–52; Māori women, 41; pūrakau approach, 47; sexual violence specialists, 44; use of weight-based criteria, 123

Aversion Project, 80

awfulisation discourse, of abortion, 252–53

binaristic gender and sexual normativity, 196

binary health system, 82–85

biogenetic parenthood, 6

Birth Justice, 274

black: abortion seekers, 250–51, 260; teenagers, 110; transgender, 86–88; women, 6–8, 141, 149, 159

Body Mass Index, 123

Bourdieu, Pierre, 161, 162

Bourdieusian theory, 157

breakfast clubs, 165, 166, 171n4

British colonial law, 212

British Infanticide Act 1922, 212

British social policy, problematising of poor parents in, 160–61

Butler, Judith, 229

About the Editors and Contributors

ABOUT THE EDITORS

Jabulile Mary-Jane Jace Mavuso (they/he) is a postdoctoral fellow at the *University of Pretoria* and a 2020 recipient of the *International Centre for Research on Women's* Paula Kantor Award. Dr. Mavuso holds a PhD in Psychology from *Rhodes University*, where they are a research associate for the Critical Studies in Sexualities and Reproduction research programme. His research interests are in gender, race, sexualities, and reproduction, and sexual and reproductive justice, with his current research focussing on cis-gendered men's desires to be pregnant. They have published on abortion, adolescent pregnancy decision-making, sexual violence policy at higher institutions, and African feminisms and decolonial psychology in international and local journals.

Tracy Morison is a senior lecturer in health psychology at Massey University (New Zealand), an Honorary Research Associate of Rhodes University's *Critical Studies in Sexualities and Reproduction* programme (South Africa), and an editor of international journal *Feminism and Psychology*. Her research is located at the intersection of critical psychology, health psychology, and feminism. Her latest research, funded by the *Marsden fund* of *Royal Society of New Zealand*, explores the transnational reproductive politics around Long-Acting Reversible Contraception and aims to develop Reproductive Justice theory. She is the lead editor of *Queer Kinship* (Morison, Lynch, and Reddy, 2019) and co-author of *Men's pathways to parenthood* (Morison and Macleod, 2015).

ABOUT THE CONTRIBUTORS

Aneeqa Abrahams (she/they) is an emerging feminist scholar. She graduated from the *University of the Western Cape (UWC)* in 2017 with a bachelor's degree majoring in Psychology, Gender Studies, and Sociology. She completed her Honours Degree in Psychology in 2018. She is currently completing her master's degree in research with the Gender Studies department at the same university with a focus on critical men's studies and 'coloured' identities among 'coloured' young men in South Africa. She is currently a supportive and trauma counsellor at the *South African Police Service (SAPS)*. In addition to this, she was the Provincial Community Development leader and Western Cape Regional Representative for the *Psychological Society of South Africa*. Their research interest concerns the education and positionality of young people, intergenerational trauma among families of colour, masculinities, and racial identities. They have guest lectured on masculinities at UWC, and provided insight on masculinities, patriarchy and sexual violence for SAPS and the National Shelter Hotline.

Andrea Alexander is a feminist scholar and activist with an Honours in Gender and Transformation and an undergraduate degree in Sociology and Gender Studies from the *University of Cape Town* (South Africa). She is currently completing a master's degree in Gender Studies at the same institution. Her research interests lie at the intersections of race, class, and gender and how they relate to people in the Global South. She aspires towards a career in academia and has lectured in the Gender Studies department on intimate labour and coloured identity. Ms. Alexander has developed a boardgame, *Clue & A*, as an interactive tool that seeks towards social justice and transformation agendas within communities and academia.

Kristen Beek is an academic from the School of Population Health, *University of New South Wales* (Australia). She is a social scientist with research interests in sexual, reproductive, maternal, adolescent, and child health and rights, particularly in humanitarian settings. Kristen has researched and worked throughout the Asia Pacific on engaging and strengthening capacity to respond to sexual and reproductive health needs in complex contexts.

Kate Burry is a PhD candidate at the *Kirby Institute, University of New South Wales*. She has worked as a sex educator in Vanuatu and New Zealand and has worked in the sexual and domestic violence sectors. She has led various research projects including on the sexual and reproductive health and rights of sex workers and barriers to family planning uptake in remote communities in Vanuatu, and on reproductive coercion in New Zealand.

Duduzile (Dudu) Dlamini is a sex worker activist and human rights defender, fighting for the decriminalisation of sex work. An award winner of the Prudence Mabele Prize, she has been a part of the *Sex Workers Education and Advocacy Taskforce (SWEAT)* for eight years as a peer educator. She progressed to Advocacy and program manager and eventually founded an organisation—Mother's for the Future and Sex workers Empowerment. Ms. Dlamini is also a National Organiser/Mobiliser for *Sisonke*—a union for Sex Workers in South Africa.

Ryan du Toit is a registered Research Psychologist and independent lecturer at the *University of Kwa-Zulu Natal* and the *South African College of Applied Psychology*. He is a PhD candidate in the Critical Studies in Sexualities and Reproduction research programme at Rhodes University. Using conversation analysis and discursive psychology, his thesis explores how pre-abortion counselling is conducted within the public sector. He has presented his research at national and international conferences. His research findings have been used to inform a step-by-step counselling guide for providers, a policy brief document, and the development of workshops that explore pre-abortion counselling talk.

Jessica Dutton is a PhD student at the School of Public Health, *University of Western Cape*, and her study focus is on barriers to quality of care within Cape Town MOUs from the perspective of nurses and midwives. Jessica trained as a midwife in Toronto, Canada.

Nicola Gavey (Pākehā) is a professor in the School of Psychology at the *University of Auckland*. Her research has focussed on understanding the connection between sexual violence and everyday taken for granted norms around gender and sexuality. This broad interest has led to several collaborative projects examining, for example, critical conversations about the sexism, racism, and misogyny within mainstream pornography, experiences and responses to image-based sexual abuse, and, most recently, a project examining a model of working with boys and young men around gender, sexism, and online ethics (*Shifting the Line*). The second edition of her book, *Just Sex? The Cultural Scaffolding of Rape*, was published in 2019.

Bridget Haire is a senior research fellow at the Kirby Institute, *University of New South Wales*. She conducts research in the areas of research ethics, public health, and human rights, particularly regarding HIV and other blood-borne infections, sexual health, and emerging infectious diseases. She is also the *University of New South Wale's* LGBTIQ Champion (2019–2020) and a former President of the *Australian Federation of AIDS Organisations* (AFAO). Bridget is currently conducting research into the impacts of quarantine.

Lucia Knight is a social scientist with research interests in sexual and reproductive health, access to health care, and social interventions to support care. She is an associate professor and the Head of Social and Behavioural Sciences at the School of Public Health and Family Medicine at the *University of Cape Town* and an Extraordinary Professor in the School of Public Health at the *University of the Western Cape.*

Jade Le Grice is Indigenous to Aotearoa New Zealand, from Northern tribes Te Rarawa and Ngāpuhi. She works as a senior lecturer at the *University of Auckland.* Her research explores the socio-cultural contexts of Indigenous lives informed by colonial pressures and the vibrancy of Indigenous ways of knowing and being. Current research projects explore sexual violence prevention, youth well-being, reproduction, and sexual health. Jade is inspired by Māori people working collectively and innovatively in community contexts, and their aspirations for future generations. Her work informs academic publications, psychology curriculum, health policy, and she is a member *of Ngā Kaitiaki Mauri,* of *Te Ohaakii a Hine: National Network Ending Sexual Violence Together* & *He Paiaka Totara,* a network of Māori Psychologists.

Lance Louskieter is a health policy and systems researcher with a particular interest in queer and decolonial feminist scholarship and praxis. They are a PhD candidate and senior Atlantic Fellow for Health Equity in South Africa. Their PhD explores health systems responsiveness to queer users in primary health care settings. Lance's activism includes partnering with Sex Workers Education and Advocacy TaskForce (SWEAT) and is a board member of the Sexual and Reproductive Justice Coalition (SRJC) to advocate for the rights and access to health for sex workers, queer folk and other marginalised populations by contributing to policy and implementation processes. Lance uses creative participatory methodologies to facilitate local, national and global advocacy spaces to enable transformative approaches to achieve health equity.

Landa Mabenge is the author of *Becoming Him: A Trans Memoir of Triumph.* He holds a BCom P.P.E degree from the *University of Cape Town* and a BA Hons cum laude from the *University of the Western Cape,* where he also guest lectures in gender studies. He is an MA candidate in Gender Studies at the *University of Sussex,* which is funded by prestigious *Chevening Scholarship Programme.* Landa is a transgender educationalist through his independent consultancy, *Landa Mabenge Consulting.* He is the first known transgender man in South Africa to successfully motivate a medical aid for the payment of his gender alignment surgeries and has extensive experience working in the private and public health care sectors in South Africa. Landa also works with the *Stellenbosch University Equality Unit*, where he is a community partner for their Programme for International Students. He also works with other institutions of higher learning as a guest speaker and facilitator, specifically for their equality and transformation units. He is an alumnus of the *Mandela Washington Fellowship* (MWF), the flagship programme of President Barack Obama's *Young African Leaders Initiative* (YALI) and currently serves as non-executive director on the South African MWF Alumni Council. Landa is passionate about community youth engagement and is serving on the USAID's youth advisory board and is a 2019 Human Rights Campaign Global Fellow. He also serves on various boards within the human rights space and currently serves on the *University of Cape Town* Electoral College and was part of the delegation that appointed the current Chancellor, Dr Precious Moloi-Motsepe.

Catriona Ida Macleod is a distinguished professor of Psychology at the University still known as Rhodes (South Africa), where she chairs the *Critical Studies in Sexualities and Reproduction* programme. She has published extensively on teenage pregnancy, abortion, sexuality education, pregnancy support, reproductive decision-making, and feminist and decolonial theories. She is editor-in-chief of the international journal *Feminism and Psychology*. She has authored, co-authored, or co-edited four books, including the *Palgrave Handbook of Ethics in Critical Research*.

Yanela Ndabula is a PhD candidate in the *Critical Studies in Sexualities and Reproduction* research team based at Rhodes University, South Africa. She completed her master's thesis on Xhosa women's sexual socialisation in 2017. Her presentation of this work received the *Sexuality and Gender Division/Feminism and Psychology* Student Presentation Award at the *1st Pan African Psychology Congress* (2017). Her doctoral research focusses on the constructions of women who use long-acting reversible contraception in the Eastern Cape.

Sisa Ngabaza is an associate professor in the Department of Women and Gender Studies at the University of the Western Cape, South Africa. Her teaching and research interests are in contemporary gender issues; sexuality education, young people and sexualities, gender-based violence, and women with disabilities, as well as gender and development matters. Prof. Ngabaza has published extensively on sexuality education and school-age pregnancy in South Africa. She has also taken interest in feminist pedagogies particularly focussing on photovoice and young people's activism in higher education contexts and issues of gender and social justice.

Linda Waimarie Nikora is Indigenous to Aotearoa New Zealand, from tribes Te Aitanga-a-Hauiti and Tūhoe. She works as a professor of

Indigenous Studies at the *University of Auckland* where she is also co-director of *Nga Pae o te Maramatanga*, New Zealand's Maori Centre of Research Excellence. Her specialty interest is in the development of Indigenous psychologies to serve the interests and aspirations of Indigenous peoples. She has been involved in research about Maori flourishing; Tangi: Māori ways of mourning; traditional body modification; ethnic status as a stressor; Māori identity development; cultural safety and competence; Māori mental health and recovery; social and economic determinants of health; homelessness; relational health; social connectedness; and human flourishing.

Dr. Busisiwe Nkala-Dlamini is a senior lecturer at the University of the Witwatersrand's Department of Social Work. She has been involved in a number of HIV prevention clinical trials; vaccines, microbicides, and community engagements. She is passionate about teenage and adolescence (boys and girls) research and program development; HIV management, sexual and reproductive health services, socio-behavioural research, parental involvement in teenagers' sexual and reproductive health issues, teenage pregnancy prevention and management, and historical and socio-cultural factors' contribution to teenager sexual and reproductive health problems including services and families. She is involved in international collaborative interdisciplinary research projects investigating teenage and adolescent sexual and reproductive health and services.

Dr. Thobeka Nkomo is an esteemed researcher, published author, and academic at the *University of the Witwatersrand*. Her research interests include spirituality and health concerns, forgiveness, gender issues, ethics, and values specifically related to cultural sensitivity, young women leadership, HIV/AIDS and sexual reproductive health, and social work. She is actively involved in collaborative research projects with peers from all over Africa, such as menstrual hygiene in partnership with *AIDS Foundation of South Africa* (AFSA) and *Women Intellectuals Transforming Scholarship in Education*. She supervises many undergraduate and postgraduate students to promote, nurture, and advance education in the South African context.

Dr. George Parker (Pākehā) is a lecturer in Health Service Delivery in the School of Health, *Te Herenga Waka | Victoria University of Wellington*. Prior to this, Dr. Parker taught in the School of Midwifery at *Otago Polytechnic* and in the School of Medicine at the *University of Auckland* and acted as the Strategic Advisor at *Women's Health Action Trust*. A registered midwife, Dr. Parker has spent several years working in women's health policy and research and is passionate about applying critical perspectives in the pursuit of equitable and just care. Their research includes critical perspectives on maternal obesity, rainbow inclusive maternity care, and reproductive justice in sexual and reproductive healthcare.

Dr. Kristina Saunders was awarded a PhD in 2019 from the *University of Glasgow* (Scotland) where she now holds a lectureship in sociology. Her broad research interests are in the areas of gender, class, and inequalities in sexual and reproductive health.

Tamara Shefer is a professor in Women's and Gender Studies, Faculty of Arts, *University of the Western Cape*. Her work primarily addresses youth, gender, and sexualities. Most recent co-edited books are *The Routledge International Handbook of Masculinity Studies* (2019, with L. Gottzén and U. Mellström); *Engaging Youth in Activist Research and Pedagogical Praxis: Transnational and Intersectional Perspectives on Gender, Sex, and Race* (2018, with J. Hearn, K. Ratele, and F. Boonzaier) and *Socially Just Pedagogies in Higher Education: Critical Posthumanist and New Feminist Materialist Perspectives* (2018, with V. Bozalek, R. Braidotti, and M. Zembylas).

Marion Stevens has an academic background as a midwife, in medical anthropology, and in public and development management. She has worked in the area of Sexual and Reproductive Justice for over 30 years. Her work has included conducting participatory research, policy analysis, and development and advocacy. She has worked with a range of stakeholders both locally and internationally. She is the outgoing founding director of the Sexual and Reproductive Justice Coalition in South Africa and PhD candidate/SARChI Chair in Gender Politics, Department of Political Science, Stellenbosch University.

Cheryl Turner is Indigenous to Aotearoa New Zealand, from Northern tribes Ngāpuhi and Ngātiwai. She works as a senior registered nurse at *Hokianga Health Hospital*, in her tribal area. Cheryl has many roles at the hospital, including senior nurse, mentor, educator, acting health services manager, and mental health credentialing. Cheryl also occupies the esteemed role of chairperson of Pakanae marae (Māori kinship group connected to ancestry and place), including roles of cultural and spiritual significance—kaikaranga (ceremonial role of an esteemed woman), and taumata kaumatua (leaders of a collective). She has also held roles of status for her tribe as her hapū kaikorero (Māori kinship network delegated speaker) for te Tiriti o Waitangi (Māori and Crown) negotiations.

Sanele Twala is an emerging scholar; she is a highly motivated and positive individual with excellent organisational and communication skills.

She recently graduated in social work degree from the University of the Witwatersrand. She has extensive exposure to theoretical and practical components of social work, with skills in psychology, social sciences, and research design. In addition, she has good interpersonal, counselling, interviewing, and assessment skills. Her research niche is in sexual and reproductive health rights and service provision.

Heather Worth has recently retired from academia. For the past two decades, she led teams of researchers studying sexual and reproductive health issues, particularly in the Pacific.

www.ingramcontent.com/pod-product-compliance
Lightning Source LLC
Chambersburg PA
CBHW022302280326
41932CB00010B/957